COMPLEX SOCKET DEFORMITIES

ADVANCES IN OPHTHALMIC PLASTIC AND RECONSTRUCTIVE SURGERY
Stephen L. Bosniak, M.D., Editor

Volume One (1982): *Ptosis*
Volume Two (1983): *The Aging Face*
Volume Three (1984): *The Lacrimal System*
Volume Four (1985): *Blepharospasm*
Volume Five (1986): *History and Tradition*
Volume Six (1987): *Orbital Trauma, Part 1*
Volume Seven (1988): *Orbital Trauma, Part 2*
Volume Eight (1990): *The Anophthalmic Socket*
Volume Nine (1991): *Complex Socket Deformities*

COMPLEX SOCKET DEFORMITIES

ADVANCES IN OPHTHALMIC PLASTIC AND RECONSTRUCTIVE SURGERY

STEPHEN L. BOSNIAK
EDITOR

BYRON C. SMITH
FOUNDING EDITOR

McGRAW-HILL, INC.
Health Professions Division

New York St. Louis San Francisco Auckland Bogota Caracas
Lisbon London Madrid Mexico Milan Montreal New Delhi
Paris San Juan Singapore Sydney Tokyo Toronto

NOTICE

Medicine is an ever-changing science. As new research and clinical experience broaden our knowledge, changes in treatment and drug therapy are required. The editors and the publisher of this work have checked with sources believed to be reliable in their efforts to provide information that is complete and generally in accord with the standards accepted at the time of publication. However, in view of the possibility of human error or changes in medical sciences, neither the editors nor the publisher nor any other party who has been involved in the preparation or publication of this work warrants that the information contained herein is in every respect accurate or complete. Readers are encouraged to confirm the information contained herein with other sources. For example and in particular, readers are advised to check the product information sheet included in the package of each drug they plan to administer to be certain that the information contained in this book is accurate and that changes have not been made in the recommended dose or in the contraindications for administration. This recommendation is of particular importance in connection with new or infrequently used drugs.

Complex Socket Deformities

1 2 3 4 5 6 7 8 9 0 MAL MAL 9 8 7 6 5 4 3 2 1 0

ISBN 0-07-105383-2

Malloy Lithographers, Inc., was the printer and binder.

ISSN 0276-3508

Contents

CONTENTS

List of Contributors

Raffaele Bonanni
Institute of Ophthalmology
University of Siena
Siena, Italy

Giulio Bonavolontà
Institute of Ophthalmology
University of Naples School of Medicine
Naples, Italy

Stephen L. Bosniak
Manhattan Eye, Ear, and Throat Hospital
New York Eye and Ear Infirmary
New York, NY

Mark Bowden
University of Louisville
University of Kentucky
Lexington, KY

Randy Burks
Northwest Regional Hospital
Margate, FL, and
Coral Springs Medical Center
Coral Springs, FL

Richard Collin
Moorfields Eye Hospital
London, England

Greg L. Dootz
Kellogg Eye Center
University of Michigan Medical Center
Ann Arbor, MI

Richard Downes
Moorfields Eye Hospital
London, England

Juan Echeverri
School of Dentistry
Louisiana State University
New Orleans, LA

Don S. Ellis
University of California, and
Pacific Presbyterian Medical Center
San Francisco, CA

Israel M. Finger
School of Dentistry
Louisiana State University
New Orleans, LA

Renato Frezzotti
Institute of Ophthalmology
University of Siena
Siena, Italy

Luis R. Guerra
School of Dentistry
Louisiana State University
New Orleans, LA

Bahman Guyuron
Mt. Sinai Medical Center, and
Case Western Reserve University
Cleveland, OH

M. L. Herdan
Fondation Ophtalmologique
Adolphe de Rothschild
Departement de Chirurgie Plastique
    Ophtalmologique
Paris, France

T. Hurbli
Fondation Ophtalmologique
Adolphe de Rothschild
Departement de Chirurgie Plastique
    Ophtalmologique
Paris, France

Ira S. Jones
Harkness Eye Institute
Columbia Presbyterian Hospital
New York, NY

Sara A. Kaltreider
Medical College of Virginia
Richmond, VA

James W. Karesh
University of Maryland
Baltimore, MD

Robert E. Kennedy
University of Rochester
Rochester, NY

Henry LaFuente
Dean A. McGee Eye Institute
University of Oklahoma
Health Sciences Center
Oklahoma City, OK

Michael Lavin
Moorfields Eye Hospital
London, England

Charles R. Leone, Jr.
University of Texas
Health Science Center
San Antonio, TX

Virginia Lubkin
New York, NY

Clinton D. McCord, Jr.
Atlanta, GA

Donald Mitchell
University of Oklahoma
Oklahoma City, OK

Serge Morax
Fondation Ophtalmologique
Adolphe de Rothschild
Departement de Chirurgie Plastique
　Ophtalmologique
Paris, France

Alessandro Nuti
Institute of Ophthalmology
University of Siena
Siena, Italy

Ennio Polito
Institute of Ophthalmology
University of Siena
Siena, Italy

Allen M. Putterman
University of Illinois
Chicago, IL

Algernon B. Reese (deceased)

James M. Richard
Dean A. McGee Eye Institute
University of Oklahoma
Health Sciences Center
Oklahoma City, OK

Barry Shipman
Community Cancer Center
Johnston-Willis Hospital
Richmond, VA

John W. Shore
Harvard Medical School
Massachusetts Eye and Ear Infirmary
Boston, MA

Robert G. Small
Dean A. McGee Eye Institute
University of Oklahoma
Health Sciences Center
Oklahoma City, OK

William B. Stewart
University of California, and
Pacific Presbyterian Medical Center
San Francisco, CA

Bryant A. Toth
University of California, and
Pacific Presbyterian Medical Center
San Francisco, CA

Augustus J. Valauri
New York University School of Medicine
New York, NY

Introduction to Volume 9
Complex Socket Deformities

Shallow, inadequate conjunctival fornices do not provide sufficient stability for an ocular prosthesis. Reduced vertical and horizontal dimensions of the socket soft tissue and bony-orbital apertures do not provide a sufficient cavity for a satisfactory ocular prosthesis. The potential surgical remedies for these problems may be complex and are performed with varying degrees of success. Exenterated sockets provide no lids and no fornices for prosthetic stability. Until a comfortable and convenient means of prosthetic fixation was developed, the black patch was the only aesthetic alternative. And so, contracted and exenterated sockets present the surgeon and prosthetist with difficult circumstances and limited options. Advanced technology and refined surgical techniques have expanded the potential for the rehabilitation of these complex socket deformities.

We thank our contributors and our subscribers for their continued, energetic support. We thank the American Society of Ocularists and the American Anaplastology Association for their cooperation and support.

Stephen L. Bosniak, M.D., F.A.C.S.
Byron Capleese Smith, M.D., F.A.C.S.

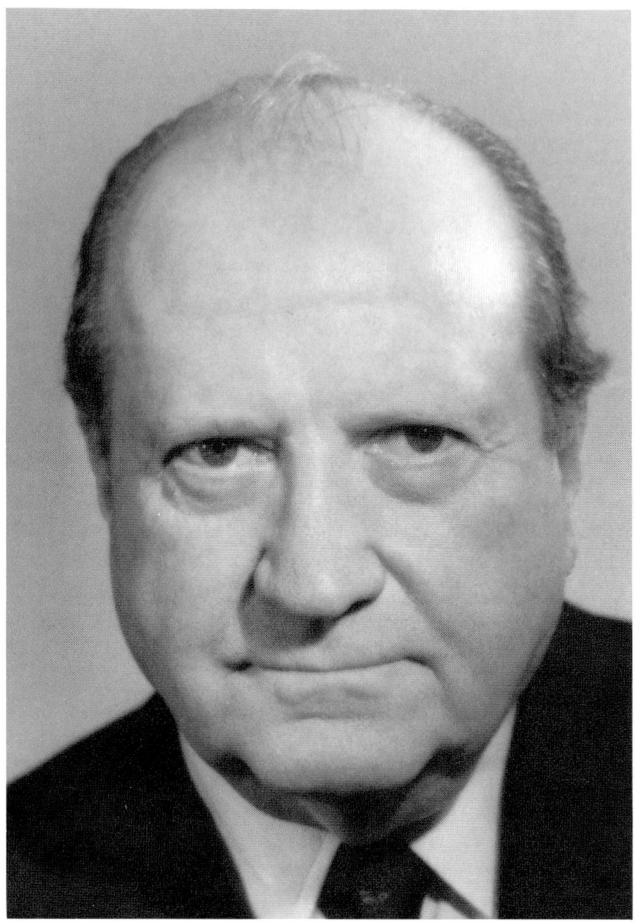

Byron Capleese Smith (1908–1990)

Byron Capleese Smith was a complex individual. Most of us who thought that we knew him well knew him as an inspirational mentor and a surgical guide who defied us to second-guess him. He dazzled us with his prowess and shared with us his cherished possession — his creativity. But I am most moved by the young Byron who knew what he wanted and persevered. He tossed aside his shabby suit, shaved his moustache, and transformed himself from a Kansas farmboy into a Yale man, and finally into the dapper Lord Byron of Broadway. A recent portrait of Byron taken in Spain clearly illustrates why few people could ever guess his age.

Byron, you were a memorable character to the end and you certainly left your indelible mark on me. You will be remembered on the printed pages of your many textbooks, in the minds of every ophthalmic plastic surgeon who ever adjusts an eyelid, and in the hearts of every person who has spent even a moment with you.

Stephen L. Bosniak, M.D., F.A.C.S.

The Effect of Early Enucleation on the Orbit in Animals and Humans

Robert E. Kennedy, M.D.

ABSTRACT

Facial asymmetry and cosmetic deformity can occur following enucleation. The effect of enucleation on the growth of the orbit can be demonstrated in the rabbit and cat by early enucleation, X-ray study and dry skull measurements. In 42 human patients the anophthalmic orbital changes are determined by roentgenograms. The influencing factors of age and the use of implants are discussed as to changes in the rim, orbital walls and volume, and optic foramina measurements. Growth retardation due to roentgen ray therapy and other clinical aspects are considered which would influence the appropriate clinical management.

INTRODUCTION

Significant cosmetic deformity occurs frequently following removal of an eye. This fact does not eliminate the necessity for surgery when the indications are present. Careful surgical technique, the use of an implanted mass in the orbit, and the early use of a prosthesis have done much to reduce the deformity to a minimum. Despite these steps, general dissatisfaction in many cases warrants an attempt at better understanding of the basic changes that occur in the growth of the orbit following enucleation, particularly at an early age. Many clinical impressions are based on a minimum of experimental and clinical reports on this subject. Because of the limited number of these reports, a study was undertaken to determine more accurately the influence of early enucleation on the growth of the orbit in experimental animals, and in infancy and childhood.

REVIEW OF THE LITERATURE

Merkel [1] in 1891 makes the single sentence statement that—since Pétrequin you can find the notation that the orbit gets smaller after enucleation of the eye. This statement is credited to the latter's writings on ophthalmologic subjects around 1840.

In 1898 Byers [2] reported an investigation as to whether there was arrested development in the orbit following enucleation of one eye in childhood. He examined 10 cases as adults, five of whom had lost their eyes before the age of five years and five of whom had lost their

---

This chapter was originally published in *Tr Am Ophthalmol Soc* 1964; 62:459–510. Used with permission.

eyes between age 10 and 13 years. Measurements were made externally through the skin and he reported that no arrest of development had occurred, at least as far as the external orifices of the bony wall of the orbit were concerned.

In 1901 Thomson [3] attempted to determine the influence of the eyeball on the growth of the orbit by experimental enucleation of one eye in young animals. He chose young rabbits approximately three weeks of age, finishing with six survivors, which he sacrificed at seven to nine months of age. Only three of these skulls were macerated and direct readings taken from the dry bone skulls. Readings were also taken from the other wet specimens. With this limited number, his results showed conclusively that, in rabbits, a deficiency of growth occurs in the anophthalmic orbit. Averaging his figures for the anteroposterior (width) measurement with the vertical measurement of the orbit of the three dry skulls, this decrease was found to be in the magnitude of 11.1%. He concluded that in certain animals the growth of the orbit was influenced by the presence of the eye. He assumed by inference that the same would hold true in other animals and in man.

In a series of experiments [4–6] from 1909 to 1921, Wessely demonstrated that the bony orbit will show retardation of growth, with a reduction of the orbital contents, even without enucleation. He decreased the size of the eye by various glaucoma procedures and by doing discissions of the lenses in young rabbits. This was followed by microphthalmos of 1 to 2 mm and a decrease in the diameter of the orbits by a similar amount. Following reduction of the orbital volume by removal of the gland of Harder in very young rabbits, Wessely also demonstrated reduction of growth of the bony orbit. He reported a 16-year-old patient, with microphthalmos (phthisis) after a penetrating injury at age one and a half years, whose roentgenograms revealed a smaller orbit on the affected side.

Sattler [7], in 1922, in recommending fat transplant to the orbit to improve the cosmetic results after enucleation, made the following statement: "In nine one-eyed patients, age three to 18, I always found a clear difference between the sizes of the orbits on x-rays, and this as soon as one year after enucleation in spite of continuously wearing a glass eye." This was not further elucidated.

As recently as 1922, Heckel [8] reported three cases of enucleation in infants in which he stated he did not favor the implantation operations, nor did he believe that it made any difference in the development of the orbit whether or not implantation was performed.

Koch and Brunetti [9], in 1933, reported their roentgenologic technique to determine the volume of the orbit and the measurement of its depth. They applied their method to the measurement of the anteroposterior axis of the orbit in unilateral anophthalmos. They concluded the orbit of the affected side was smaller but retained the same depth as the unaffected side.

A clinical study of the effect of the enucleation of one eye in childhood, and the subsequent development of the face, was made by Taylor [10] in 1939. For this, 51 patients were reviewed in two series. All of the cases were studied by means of external measurements, and 36 had been X-rayed. He confirmed the occurrence of the same arrest in children that Thomson had reported in the experimental rabbits. He found that enucleation before the age of five could lead to a deficiency of the bone growth of the orbital margin, as much as 15% on the enucleated side as compared with the normal side. This change persisted into adult life. He also found that enucleation at nine years and after apparently did not lead to appreciable alteration. He reported that the maxillary antrum of the anophthalmic side underwent overgrowth when the enucleation had been performed before the age of nine. None of Taylor's 51 patients had an orbital implantation [11]. Nine of the 51 patients had worn no prosthesis after enucleation. His findings in these cases, compared with those wearing a prosthesis, revealed no influence of the prosthesis on the development of the bony part of the orbit, but probably some influence on the soft parts around the orbit.

In 1945 Pfeiffer [12] made an excellent report on the effect of enucleation on the orbit. He summarized his observations in a critical analysis of 31 patients who were studied by photographs, external examination, and roentgen study. A group of children were included who had been X-rayed eight or 10 years previously at the time of enucleation for retinoblastoma. He made the observation that removal of the eye arrested development of the orbit and led to a contraction of it, or to a reduction of its capacity. These changes were greater the earlier in life the eye was removed. He also found that the implantation of spheres tended to maintain the intraorbital pressure and counteract the contracting process. Although the orbit still contracted even with a buried implant, it did not do so to the same degree as the orbit in which no implant had been used. The walls were more normal in contour. Diminution of the size of the orbit resulted eventually even with enucleation of the adult eye. He emphasized stereoscopic evaluation and even consideration for laminography. Asymmetry of the face of the child was also noted.

Other short statements or isolated case reports refer to, or show the effect of, this decrease in bone development of the orbit following enucleation [13–21]. A decrease in the size of the optic canal on the enucleated side has been noted [12,19,22].

EXPERIMENTAL PURPOSE

An investigation was made into the influence of early enucleation of one eye and the subsequent development of the orbit in the rabbit, the cat, and in infants and childhood. The purpose was to determine and more firmly establish, both in animals and in humans, what bony changes occur in the orbit, the relation between age of enucleation and the changes in the orbit, the influence of an orbital implant, and the clinical consideration which might be governed by these findings. Furthermore, optic nerve canal and roentgen therapy bone changes were evaluated.

METHOD

A series of studies was carried out in three main parts:

1. The right eyes of a group of young rabbits were enucleated. The rabbits were allowed to mature, were sacrificed, and the skulls macerated for direct measurement study.
2. A similar study on a larger series of cats was performed. Silicone spherical implants were placed in some of the orbits following enucleation to determine their influence on subsequent orbital development.
3. Forty-two humans who had lost one eye in infancy or childhood were studied by skull roentgenograms, and the measurements from these films were correlated. A control group of 20 normal skull roentgenograms from patients without eye pathology was reviewed in a similar manner.

PROCEDURE

RABBITS

This study primarily was to repeat and confirm the previously reported animal work of a similar nature by Thomson [3] on three macerated rabbit skulls. A total of 10 New Zealand

White rabbits comprising two litters was studied. Two rabbits, of a litter of three, had the right eye enucleated under local Xylocaine anesthetic at age seven days, the third rabbit being left as a control. Six rabbits, of a litter of seven, had the right eye enucleated under local Xylocaine anesthetic at age 11 days, with the seventh rabbit being left as a control. These two litters were allowed to grow to maturity and were sacrificed at 228 days and 204 days, respectively. The skulls of the 10 rabbits were macerated and craniometric determinations were made using the measuring rule, spreading calipers, sliding parallel compass, and a hole gauge.

The following craniometric determinations were made on each skull:

1. The anteroposterior or horizontal internal orbital measurement at the rim. This measurement was made anteriorly from the rim of the orbit of the maxilla just below the lacrimal bone, posteriorly to the anterolateral wing of the temporal bone which extends to join with the zygomatic bone.
2. The greatest vertical internal orbital measurement at the rim.
3. The depth of the orbit as measured as close to perpendicular as possible from a vertical plane at the orbital rim to the optic foramen.
4. A measurement from the mid-sagittal suture between the orbits to the cusp of the last molar tooth.

The three orbital measurements 1, 2, and 3 are those described by Davis [23]. The measurements were recorded for the right and left orbits with the percentage difference, or decrease, listed for each comparative measurement. The percentage differences for the two intraorbital rim measurements 1 and 2 were averaged for each rabbit, and these figures averaged for the entire group of operated rabbits and compared with the controls.

CATS

A larger series of cat skulls was studied. This animal was chosen in preference to the rabbit for more extensive study because the skull more nearly simulates the human in that the orbital rim is nearly intact. Also, the visual axis and orbital axis are more nearly similar to that of humans as compared with many other laboratory animals. The cat also matures reasonably quickly and the skulls could be studied without as long a delay for maturation as other animals might require.

A total of six litters was studied, with the size of the litters ranging from three to five cats. Within each litter, one cat was left as a control and the other litter mates had the right eye enucleated under local Xylocaine anesthetic. A total of 25 cats was used initially, four of which died and were disposed of inadvertently during the study. This left a total of 15 cats which had been enucleated, and six control or unoperated animals. They were operated from eight to 23 days after birth and were sacrificed at various stages from 104 to 169 days after birth. Two of the 15 cats died prematurely at age 38 and 87 days and were included in the series.

In three of the six litters an attempt was made to determine the influence of orbital implantation on subsequent development of the orbit. Within each litter a control cat was present, a simple enucleation was performed on a litter mate, and a silicone sphere was placed in the other, or others, of the litters at the time of enucleation. The silicone spheres were of varying sizes, from 5 to 8 mm, and of the type described by Ruedemann [24]. They replaced enucleated eyes which were about 10 mm in diameter. Despite conjunctival suturing and suturing of the lids, all of these implants extruded at various stages, the intervals for which were unknown for some. In two of the cats the implants remained for at least a month. Following sacrifice all 21 cat skulls were macerated and measured in the same manner as the rabbit skulls. The following measurements were taken:

1. Horizontal measurement: posteriorly from the frontal process extending anteriorly to the medial wall near the nasolacrimal canal at the suture junction at the orbital rim of the maxillary and frontal bones.
2. Vertical measurement: the greatest vertical intraorbital measurement at the rim.
3. The depth of the orbit, as measured from the optic foramen to the anterior inferior orbital margin in the region of the infraorbital foramen.

These were recorded for the right and left orbit with the percentage difference, or decrease, listed for each comparative measurement. The two orbital measurements at the rim were averaged for each cat and the average taken for the entire group of operated animals. These averages were compared with the control group.

HUMANS

A series of 42 humans was studied by roentgenograms. All of the cases had one eye removed surgically at varying young ages. They were studied at various intervals after enucleation. One patient with unilateral congenital anophthalmos was included. These patients became available by reviewing the operating room and history room records in five local hospitals to determine the patients who had enucleations performed at a young age. Many of the patients were contacted directly, and with the co-operation of many of my colleagues in supplying additional patients and records, the total of 42 cases was accumulated. Some were referred by opticians who had been fitting them with prostheses.

Their age range at the time of enucleation is shown in Table 1. There were 21 males and

Table 1. Age Distribution at Time of Enucleation

Age	Number
0– 6 months	4
6–12 months	4
$1–1\frac{1}{2}$ years	4
$1\frac{1}{2}$– 2 years	2
2– 3 years	5
3– 4 years	3
4– 5 years	5
5– 6 years	2
6– 7 years	2
7– 8 years	2
8– 9 years	2
9–10 years	2
10–11 years	1
11–12 years	1
12–13 years	1
13–14 years	1
14–15 years	1
Total	42

21 females. The right eye had been removed in 16 and the left eye in 26. The earliest enucleation was on the first day of life, and the oldest enucleation in this series was in the fifteenth year. The age at the time of examination ranged from two and one half years to 42 years of age. The intervals after enucleation ranged from 22 months to 40 years, with the average being $11\frac{1}{4}$ years. The diseases necessitating removal of the eye are shown in Table 2.

The following eight roentgenographic projections were made: (a) The Caldwell view in an exaggerated projection so as to place the petrous pyramids below the rim of the orbit (stereoscopically); (b) A stereoscopic Waters projection; (c) The right lateral skull and the left lateral skull; and (d) The right and left optic foramen. With five of the very young children who were examined, single Caldwell and Waters projections were made, since stereoscopic projections could not be accomplished satisfactorily.

Fifteen cephalometric determinations were made from the roentgenograms of each patient. They are shown in Figure 1 and Table 3. These measurements comparing the right side and the left side were tabulated, together with the percentage difference, or decrease, in that particular measurement. The average for the percentage difference of the four measurements, including the orbital height, width, and two diagonals was also recorded. This is used as the main single measurement to represent the percentage decrease in size of the orbit of the anophthalmic orbit, as compared to its fellow normal orbit.

Roentgenograms for 20 normal adult patients were studied in a similar manner. These had been taken for diagnostic evaluation of some other condition, such as sinusitis or a neurological disorder. These same measurements were made from the roentgenograms in this series. The percentage difference for each measurement, and the average for each measurement, were determined and used as a control group for comparison with the anophthalmic series of patients.

RESULTS

RABBITS

The bony orbital changes presented a characteristic picture. These can be demonstrated in Figures 2 through 7. There was contraction in a purse string effect of all of the bones making up the orbital rim. This was particularly prominent in the region of the supraorbital process of the frontal bone superiorly with its anterior and posterior projections. This showed shrinkage and depression. The zygomatic bone showed elevation and flattening medially. The depth of the orbit was somewhat decreased. The entrance to the orbit and its rim, which is usually nearly circular, had become much more oval with its long axis in a horizontal direction. The optic foramen has an anterior edge which is common to both orbits in the midline and there-

Table 2. Reason for Enucleation

Trauma		25
Tumor		11
Congenital anophthalmos		1
Inflammation		2
Unknown		3
	Total	42

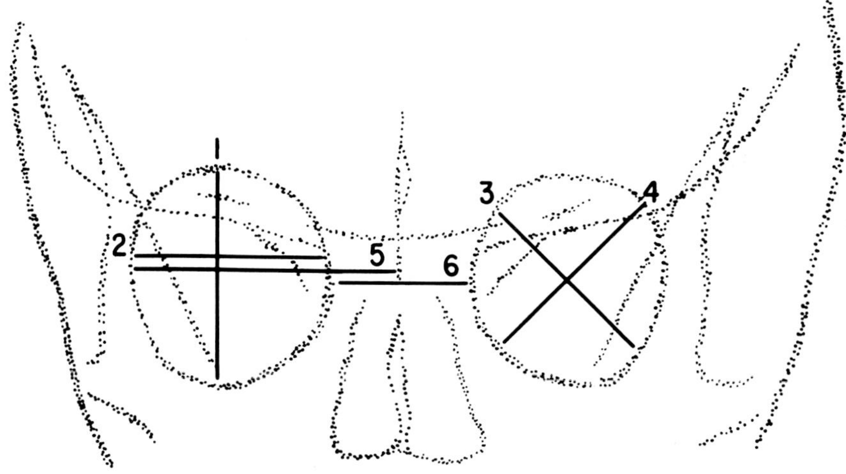

Figure 1. Roentgenographic measurements.

fore could not be compared with the opposite side, but showed little change over the optic foramina of the control rabbits. This is usually about 4 mm in diameter [25].

The craniometric determinations were recorded for each rabbit, an example of which is shown in Table 4. These bony changes resulted in the horizontal and vertical orbital rim measurements being less on the enucleated side for all of the rabbits. The measurements of the depth of the orbit, and the measurements from the mid-sagittal suture between the orbits to the cusp of the last molar tooth, as a suggestion of facial asymmetry, were equal or less on the enucleated side in all cases. The greater orbital rim changes were in the vertical diameter with the average per cent difference for the vertical measurement being 17.4, and for the horizontal distance 8.2. The average of these two was an overall diminution of orbital measurements of 12.8%. This compared with 1.1% variation for the control animals (Table 4).

The age at the time of surgery appeared to be related to the degree of change in the orbit. The 12.8% decrease was the average change for both litters. Litter 2, operated at seven days, showed a 16.2% decrease compared to Litter 1, operated at 11 days, which showed an 11.7%

Table 3. Fifteen Roentgenographic Measurements

1. Greatest vertical orbital dimension, each orbit	2
2. Greatest horizontal orbital dimension, each orbit	2
3. Greatest diagonal (lower temporal-upper nasal) orbital dimension measured at 45° to horizontal, each orbit	2
4. Same measurement, diagonal (lower nasal-upper temporal), each orbit	2
5. Midline to lateral orbital margin, each orbit, approximately nasion to ectoconchion	2
6. Minimum interorbital distance—horizontal line between most medial point of right and left medial orbital margins	1
7. Optic foramen, horizontal diameter, each side	2
8. Optic foramen, vertical diameter, each side	2
	15

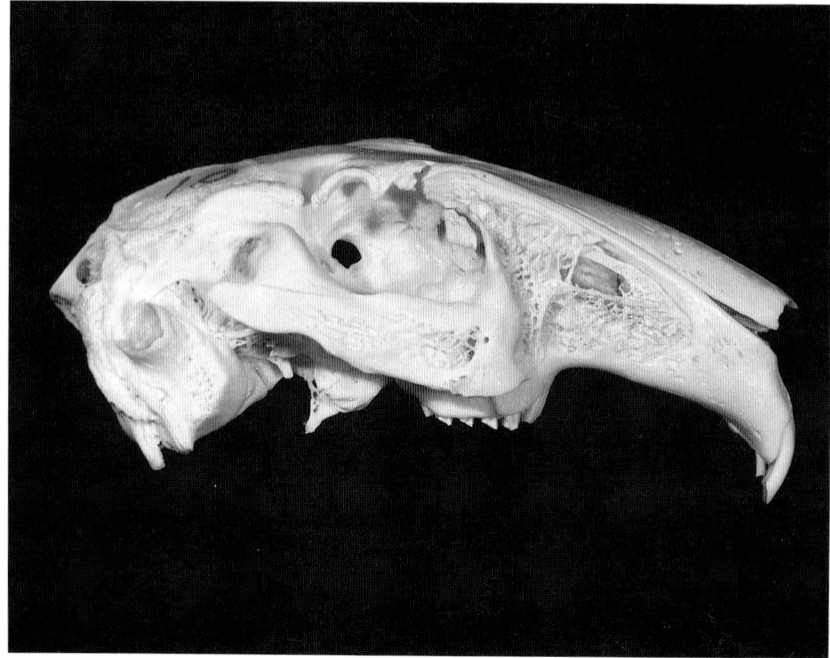

Figure 2. Rabbit 10. Anophthalmic right side, enucleated seven days, sacrificed 228 days. Smaller orbit with drooping and atrophy of supraorbital process of frontal bone and changes in maxilla, zygomatic, and temporal bones causing orbital deformity.

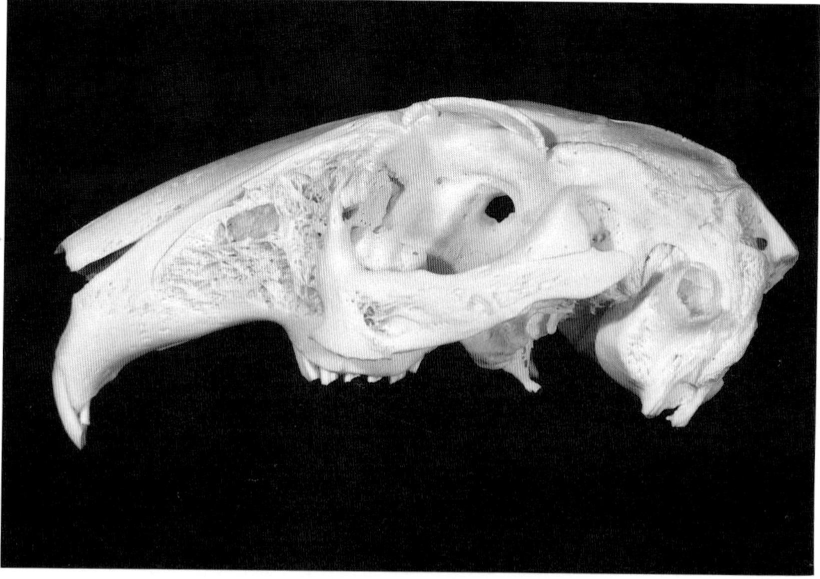

Figure 3. Rabbit 10. Normal left side.

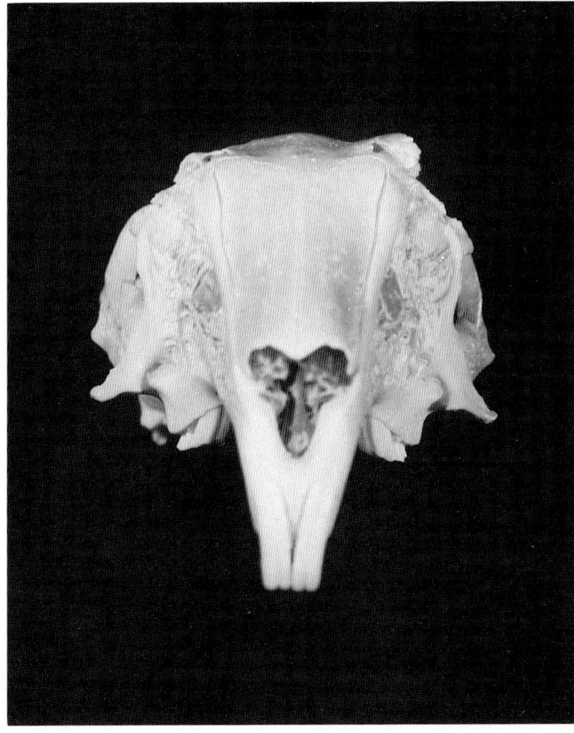

Figure 4. Rabbit 10. Front view. Shows drooping of supraorbital process of frontal bone.

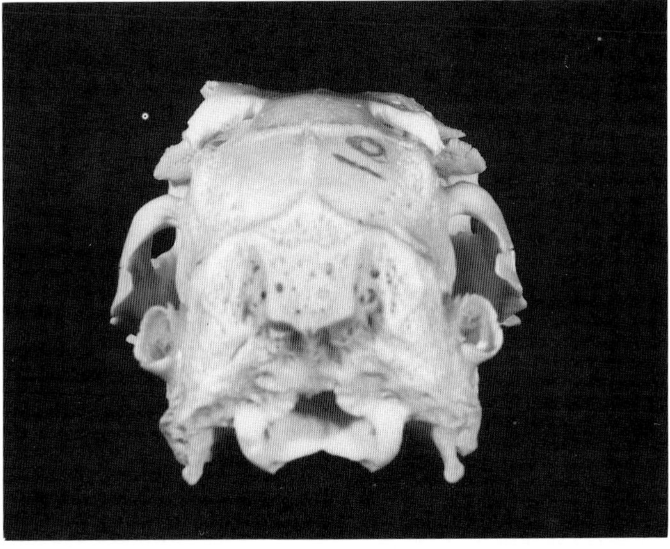

Figure 5. Rabbit 10. Viewed from behind. Showing drooping of supraorbital process of frontal bone.

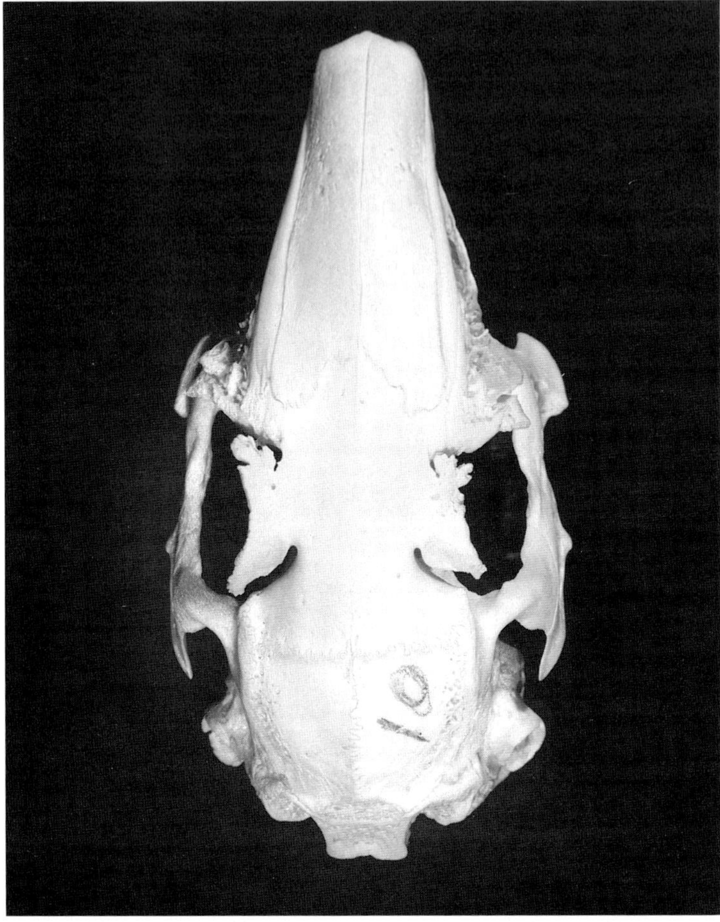

Figure 6. Rabbit 10. Viewed from above. Deformity of right orbit. Atrophy of supraorbital process of frontal bone and zygomatic bone.

decrease. Thomson's series, operated at about 21 days, showed an 11.1% decrease. Thus, the earlier the enucleation, the greater were the changes in the orbit.

In summary, the anophthalmic orbits of the rabbits showed uniform marked contraction of the rim of the orbit, in the magnitude of 12.8%. The changes were more marked the earlier the enucleation was performed.

CATS

The characteristic bony orbital changes can be demonstrated in Figures 8 through 14. The rim of the orbit of the cat skull, which is normally made up of the frontal, maxillary, and zygomatic bones, with a frontal and zygomatic process joined by the orbital ligament, usually shows a 5- to 7-mm gap between these sharp tips. This gap in the enucleated skulls was re-

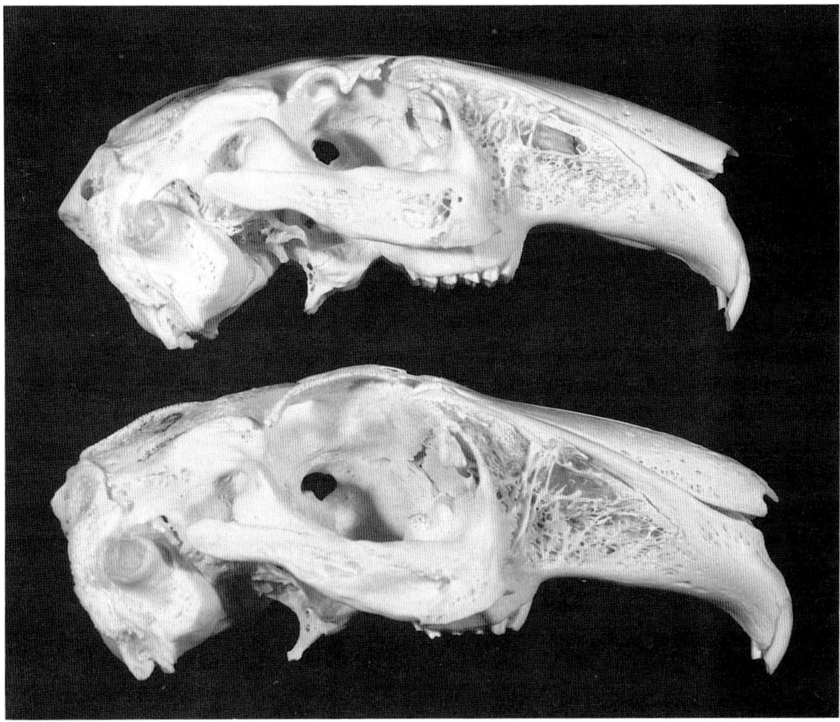

Figure 7. Rabbit 10 (top), compared to litter mate, control rabbit 9 (below), showing marked contracture and deformity of orbital rim.

duced to 2 to 4 mm and the sharp tips of the processes were very blunted. The sharp edges of the rim of the orbit were much more smooth and rounded, and the bone at the rim appeared more porous and less dense. The zygomatic bone was very much flattened and elevated, contributing to a marked reduction in size of the orbital entrance. The oval entrance to the orbit was much more oval, with its long axis in a horizontal direction. The depth of the orbit was decreased. In every case the optic foramen was smaller on the enucleated side than on the opposite side. The orbital fissure at times was smaller. The nasolacrimal fossa was displaced posteriorly 3 to 5 mm and the nasolacrimal canal, which usually measures 1.25 mm, was smaller. The infraorbital canal and foramen in the maxillary bone were always smaller.

The craniometric determinations were recorded for each cat, an example of which is shown in Table 5. These bony changes resulted in the horizontal and vertical orbital rim measurements being less on the enucleated side for all the cats. The greater orbital rim change was in the vertical diameter, with the average per cent difference for the vertical measurement 30.8%, and for the horizontal measurement 22.8%. The average of these two figures was an overall diminution of the orbital measurements of 26.8%. This compared with 0.8% for the control animals. The average decrease in the orbital depth was 11.5%. Whereas roentgenograms of the cat skull demonstrated these bony changes very adequately, as shown in Figure 15, their actual measurement from the dried skull was more practical.

An attempt was made to determine the effect of an orbital implant. In five of the cats from

Table 4. Rabbits: Craniometry and Percentage Differences for Orbital Measurements

	Horizontal (mm)			Vertical (mm)			Avg. % diff. horizontal and vertical	Depth of orbit (mm)			Midline skull to molar tooth, mm		
	R	L	% diff.	R	L	% diff.		R	L	% diff.	R	L	% diff.
Rabbit 10	22	25	12.0	15	21	28.6	20.3	16	17	5.9	29	30	3.3
Range, operated rabbits	22–26	24.5–28	4–12	15–21.6	20–24	10.4–28.6	8.8–20.3	11–18	15–18.5	0–6.7	27–30	28.5–31.5	0–6.9
Control rabbit 9	27	27	0	23	23	0	0	18	18	0	30	30	0
Average % difference operated rabbits (8)			8.2			17.1	12.8			3.4			3.3
Average % difference unoperated controls (2)			1.0			1.2	1.1			0			0

Table 5. Cats: Craniometry and Percentage Differences for Orbital Measurements

	Horizontal (mm)			Vertical (mm)			Avg. % diff. horizontal and vertical	Depth of orbit (mm)		
	R	L	% diff.	R	L	% diff.		R	L	% diff.
Cat 17	17.5	22.5	22.2	11.5	19.5	41.0	31.6	23	26	11.5
Range, operated cats	15–20	18–27	16.7–30.6	11.5–17	16–23	21.9–41.0	19.3–33.6	17–30	19–32.5	6.7–20.8
Control cat 7	32	32	0	24	23.5	2.1	1.1	31	31	0
Average % difference operated cats (15)			22.8			30.8	26.8			11.5
Average % difference unoperated controls (6)			0.4			1.3	0.8			0.8

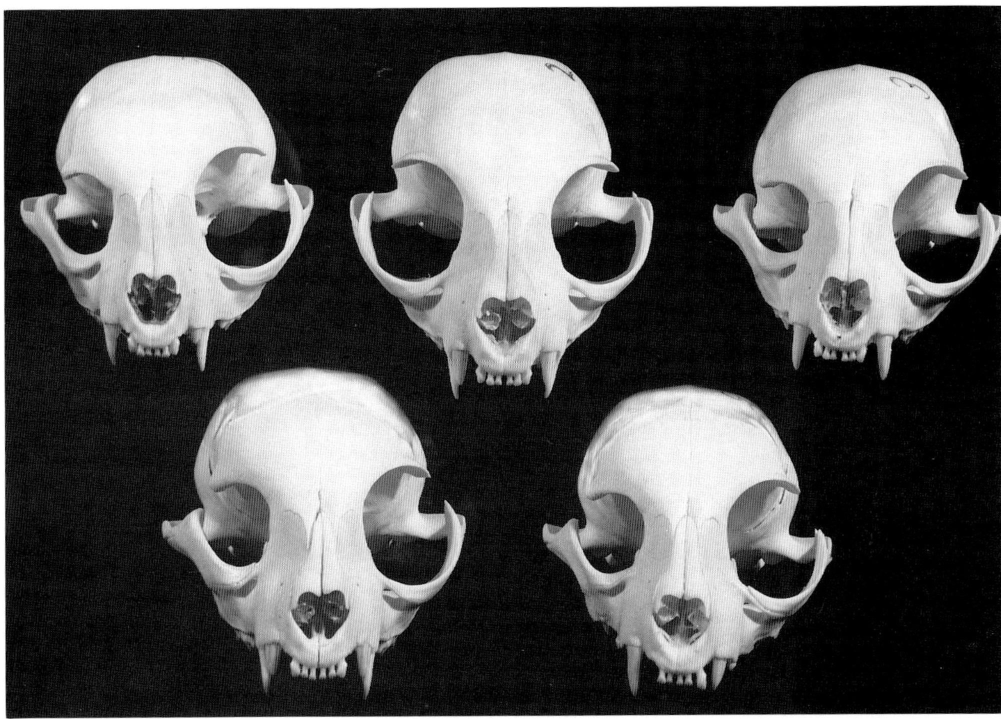

Figure 8. Litter 1, cats 1–5. Four cats have had right eye enucleated showing characteristic changes which can be routinely reproduced. Top center skull is unoperated control. Operated on 15th day, sacrificed 146 days.

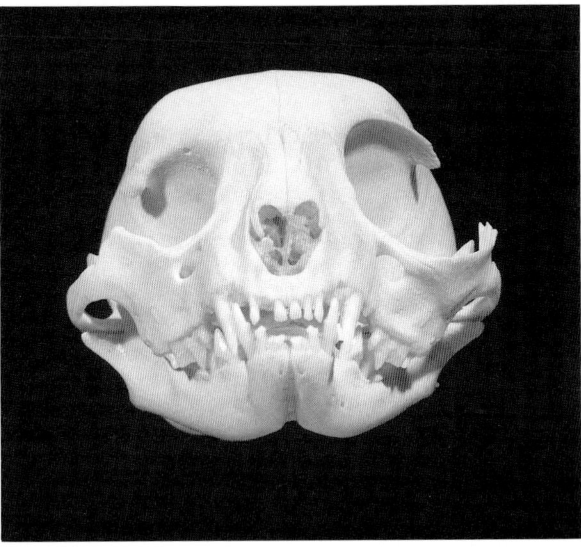

Figure 9. Cat 17. Front view. Smaller right anophthalmic orbit. Irregular orbital rim. Flattened frontal area. Higher zygomatic bone. Smaller infraorbital foramen.

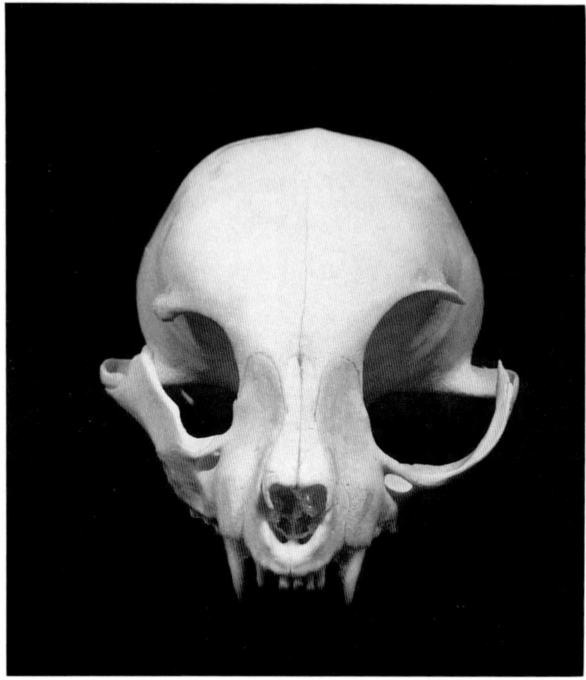

Figure 10. Cat 17. Front view. Anophthalmic right side.

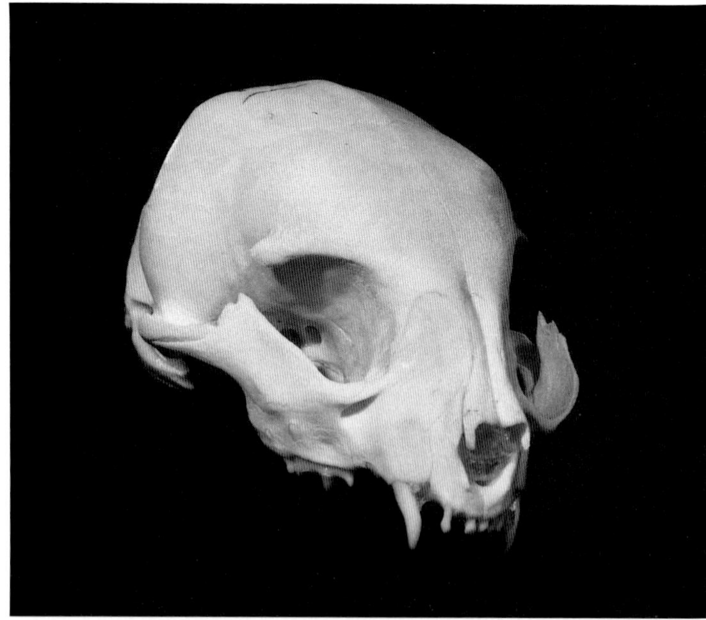

Figure 11. Cat 17. Side view. Anophthalmic right side. Smaller orbit. Thickened orbital processes. Smaller optic foramen.

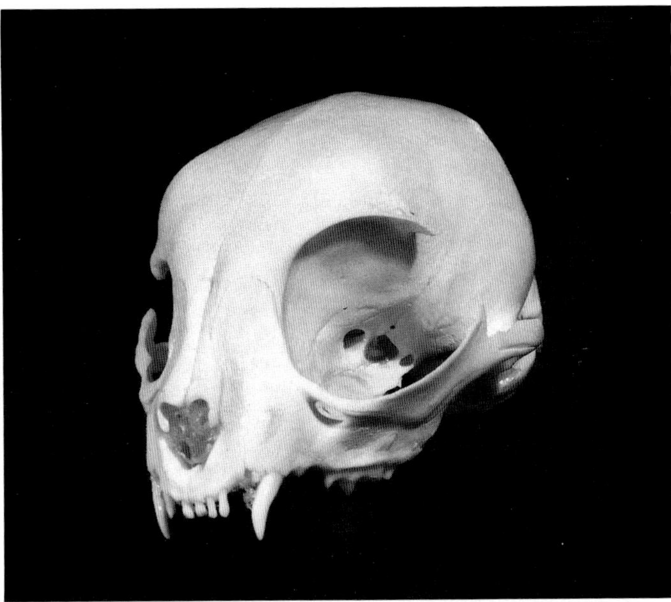

Figure 12. Cat 17. Side view. Normal left side.

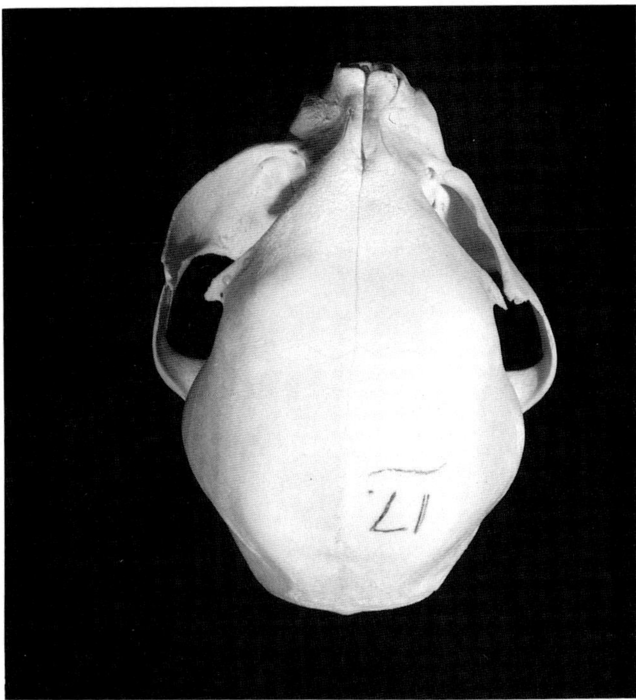

Figure 13. Cat 17. Skull viewed from above. Flattened zygomatic bone on anophthalmic right side.

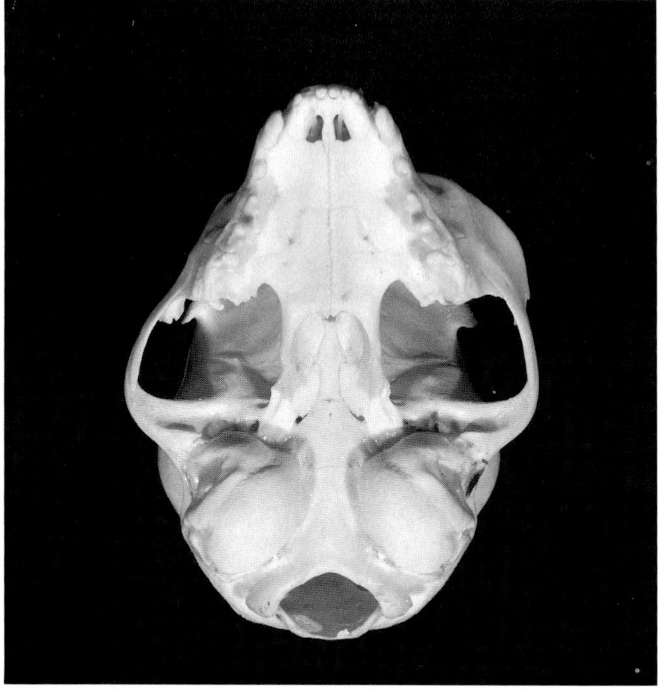

Figure 14. Cat 17. Skull, viewed from below. Flattened zygomatic bone on anophthalmic side.

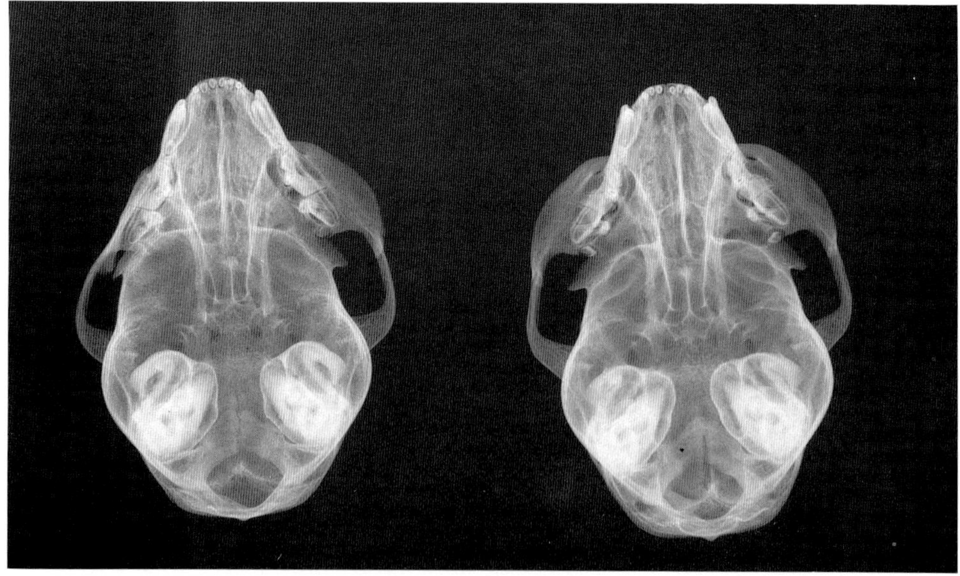

Figure 15. Cat 17 (left) with litter mate, unoperated control cat 18 (right). Roentgenogram shows marked flattening of zygomatic bone of cat 17.

Litters 4, 5, and 6, silicone implants of the type shown in Figure 16 had been placed in the orbits at the time of enucleation. The three implants in the case of Litter 4 all extruded within a few days. However, the one cat in this litter which had an enucleation with no implant showed the greatest percentage of decrease in bone development, suggesting the implants may have had some beneficial effect in the others. In Litters 5 and 6, an 8-mm silicone implant had been placed in the orbit of one kitten in each litter. These remained in position at least a full month before extruding. In both instances the orbit with an implant showed a smaller percentage decrease (22.6%) in the measurements than did litter mates that had a simple enucleation without implant (29.9%). This suggests that an implant results in less change in the bony orbit after enucleation. However, in Litter 1, where none of the kittens had orbital implants, the variation in percentage decrease of the orbital measurements showed a range of difference up to 12.5%.

In summary, the anophthalmic orbits of the cats showed a characteristic, marked decrease in the size, which was in the magnitude of 26.8%. This reduction was not as great in the animals where a silicone implant had been inserted.

HUMANS

The cephalometric determinations were recorded from the roentgenograms of the 42 patients studied; one example is shown in Table 6. Four cases are not included in this section and are discussed separately, because of the marked bone changes and abnormal measurements as the result of roentgen ray therapy for malignancy. The roentgenograms from the other 38 patients showed a smaller orbit on the enucleated side. All measurements of the anophthalmic orbits were equal to or less than the fellow orbits. A greater percentage difference between the height and width of the orbit was about equally divided. The diagonals of the orbits showed a greater percentage decrease in the diagonal from the lower nasal to the upper temporal orbital rim, as compared to the lower temporal to the upper nasal, in the proportion of

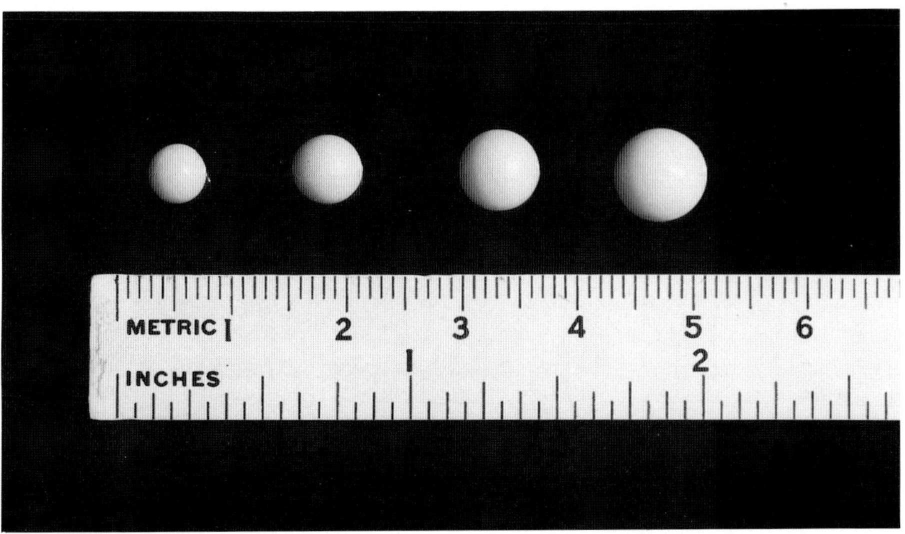

Figure 16. Silicone implants 5 to 8 mm in diameter, for insertion in cat orbit.

Table 6. Humans: Cephalometry and Percentage Differences for Orbital Measurements

Patient	Age surg.	Age exam.	Implant	Orbit height			Orbit width			Diagonal UN−LT			Diagonal LN−UT			Average of measurements 1,2,3,4	Approx. nasion ectoconchion			Inter-orbital distance	Optic canals R		L	
				R	L	% diff.	R	L	% diff.	R	L	% diff.	R	L	% diff.		R	L	% diff.		H	V	H	V
#11, right tumor	$1\frac{1}{2}$	42	0	38	46	17.4	35	40	12.5	43	47	8.5	37	39	5.1	10.9	50	57	12.3	30	2	3	3	4
Variations for measurements from roentgeno-grams of 20 normal patients						1.1 0–4.6			0.9 0–2.7			0.6 0–2.3			0.9 0–3.8	0.86 0–1.8			0.9 0–3.8	28.6 20–34				

three to one. The comparative measurements from the midline to the lateral wall of the orbit showed this to be less on the anophthalmic side in 25, and equal in 13, roentgenograms.

The optic foramina could be compared in the roentgenograms of 33 patients. In some of the others the orbital implants obscured or superimposed the canal. All of these canals on the anophthalmic side were either equal to (6%), or smaller than (94%), the unoperated side by an amount ranging up to 50%, with an average decrease in size of approximately 17%. These measurements were determined by taking the average of a per cent decrease of a vertical and horizontal diagonal of the canal.

The percentage decrease in the size of the orbital entrance can be compared with the age of the patient at the time of enucleation for this group of 38 patients, both with and without orbital implants (Fig. 17). A wide scatter is noted for all age groups. Figure 18 converts this to a line graph showing the percentage decrease in the size of the orbits for enucleations at various ages, for those patients in whom no orbital implantation was made, and for those in whom an implant was inserted. With few exceptions the individual patient with an implant showed less orbital change. The average change for each age group was less for those with implants.

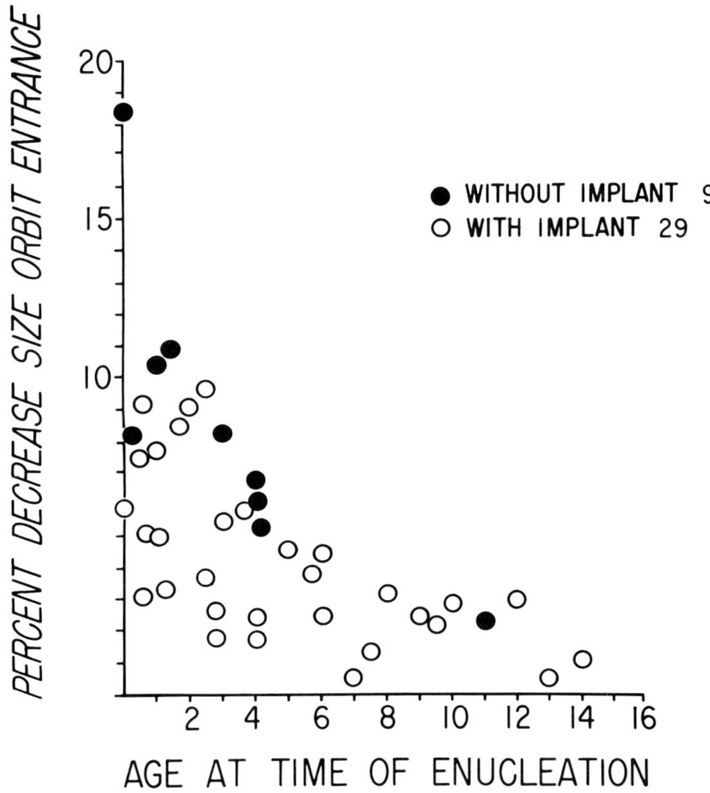

Figure 17. Scatter diagram showing distribution of patients with enucleations at various ages and their percent decrease in size of orbital entrance. Total 38 patients. A wide variation is shown.

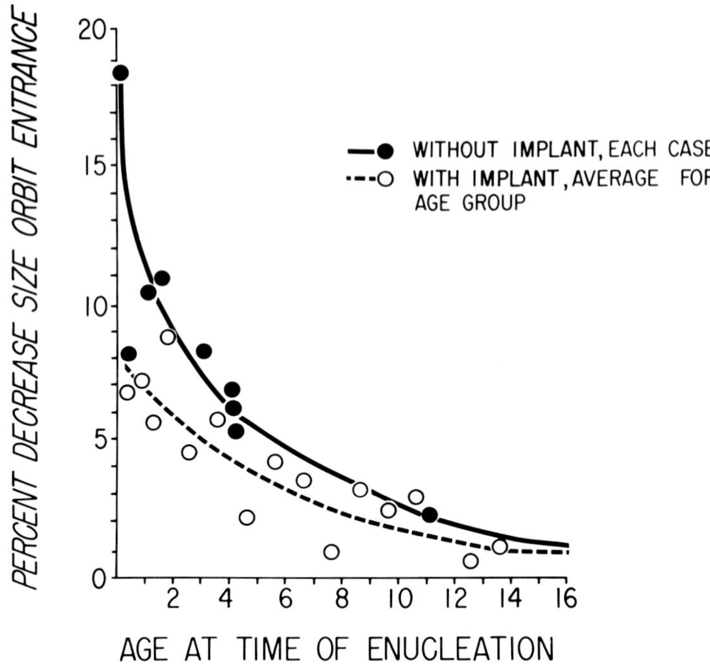

Figure 18. Comparison of percent decrease in size of orbital entrance for patients with and without implants at various ages of enucleation. Total 38 patients.

The length of the postoperative period varies in Figures 17 and 18. In an attempt to eliminate this variable, only those patients who had attained the age of 16 years, or full orbital growth, were plotted in a similar manner (Fig. 19). The curve for percentage of change in size of the orbital dimensions compared to the age at the time of enucleation is shown for the patients without an implant. The coordinates for each patient with an implant are scattered, with all but two falling below the line. Regardless of the age of enucleation, the changes in the orbit at full growth seem to be less for those patients who have had an implant. This variability in the amount of orbital change in patients with implants probably can be accounted for by several factors. The individual growth patterns would differ. Implants of different sizes, variations in surgical technique, hemorrhage at the time of surgery with absorption of orbital fat, all could contribute to this wide variation in the changes in the orbits.

ROENTGENOGRAM FINDINGS

The striking changes found by roentgenographic examination were characteristic but extremely variable. All of the anophthalmic orbits showed arrest in the development of the orbit with reduction in the orbital measurements. These changes tended to be more marked the earlier in life the enucleation had been performed and with a greater interval following enucleation. The orbital walls tended to show contraction and irregularity. The walls of the anophthalmic orbit showed the influence of compensatory changes of the surrounding structures which encroached upon it. This changed the normally concave walls so that they become flat-

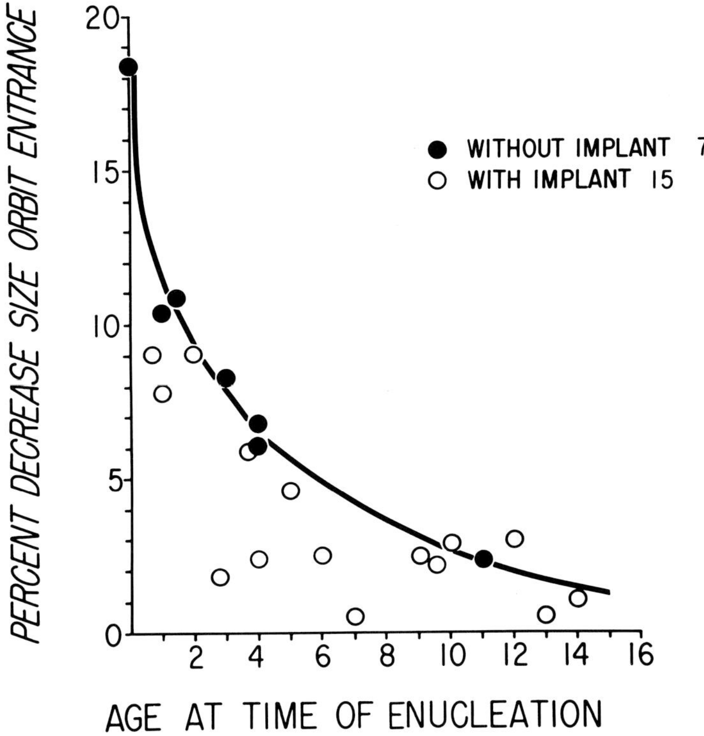

Figure 19. Percent decrease in size of orbital entrance for all patients with full orbital growth, age 16 years or older. Total 22 patients.

tened, or even convex. These changes were the greatest in the roentgenogram (Fig. 20) of a 17-year-old girl who was born with a unilateral anophthalmos. No implant had been placed in the orbit. Figures 21 and 22 show similar changes and have no orbital implants. Figures 23, 24, and 25 have orbital implants and show these changes to a lesser degree. Figure 25 bears out the findings of Pfeiffer that an implant influences the shape of the anophthalmic orbit. Such orbits tend to be larger than the orbits without an implant, though smaller than their fellow orbits, and the walls are more normal in contour.

When the orbit gives up its volume after an enucleation the surrounding structures encroach upon it. Whitnall [13] states that "the orbit conforms to the law of adaptation of the organ to the function it is called upon to fulfill, and if the globe be removed before the orbit is fully formed, growth of the latter is checked." The pull of the extraocular muscles is thought to have a contributing influence in maintaining the normal size of the orbit. Figures 22, 23, and 24 particularly show the enlargement of the maxillary antrum, and ethmoid air cells to cause distortion of the orbit. Figure 21 shows an enlarged air cell in the region of the frontal sinuses, but this was not a consistent finding, and frequently the frontal air cells on the contralateral side were much larger. Figure 23 indicates the flattening of the roof of the orbit, presumably as a manifestation of the influence of the frontal lobe of the brain being willing to encroach upon the orbit. This resulted in the roof and superior rim of the orbit frequently superimpos-

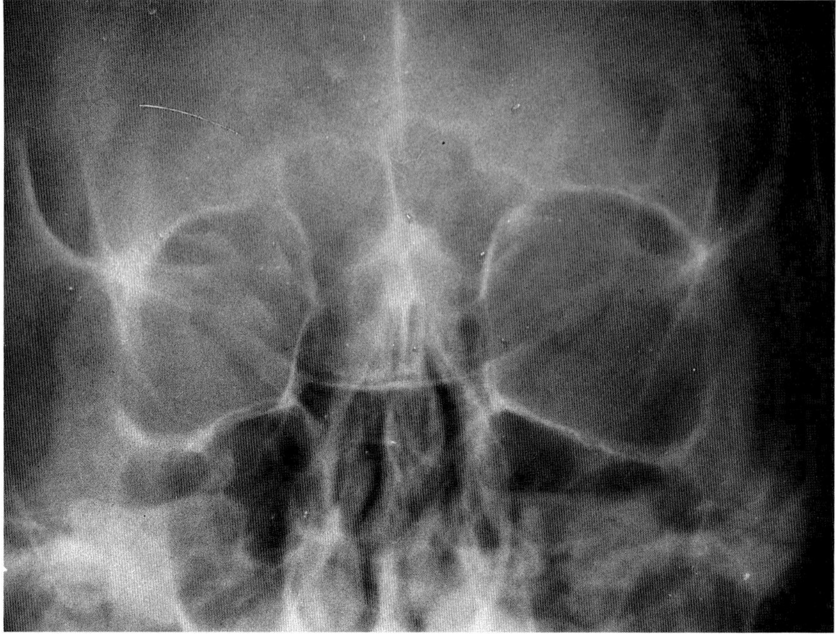

Figure 20. Patient 1. Seventeen-year-old girl, congenital right anophthalmos. Marked contraction of orbit. No implant. 18.4% decrease in orbital dimensions.

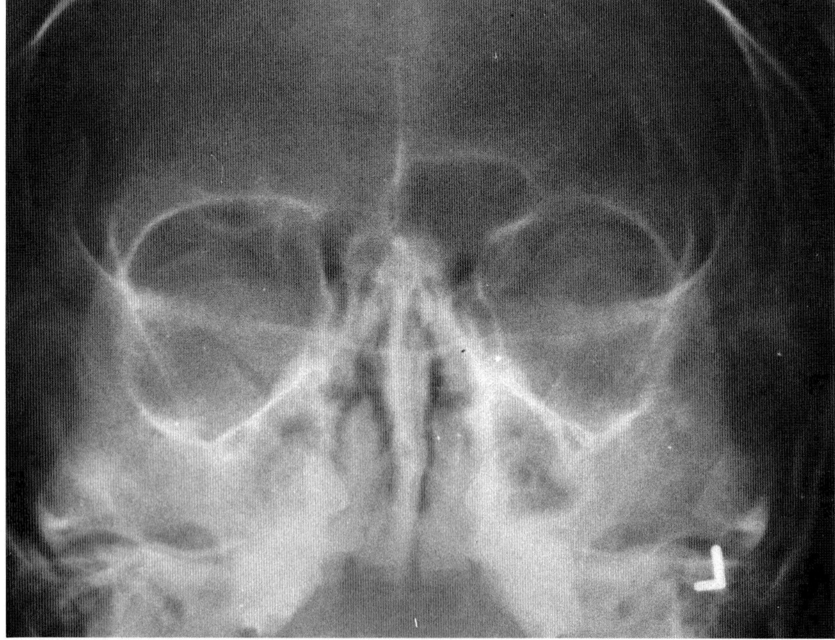

Figure 21. Patient 3. Boy, $9\frac{1}{2}$ years old, enucleated left eye age 4 months. No implant. Irregular contraction left orbital rim; 8.2% decrease of orbital dimensions.

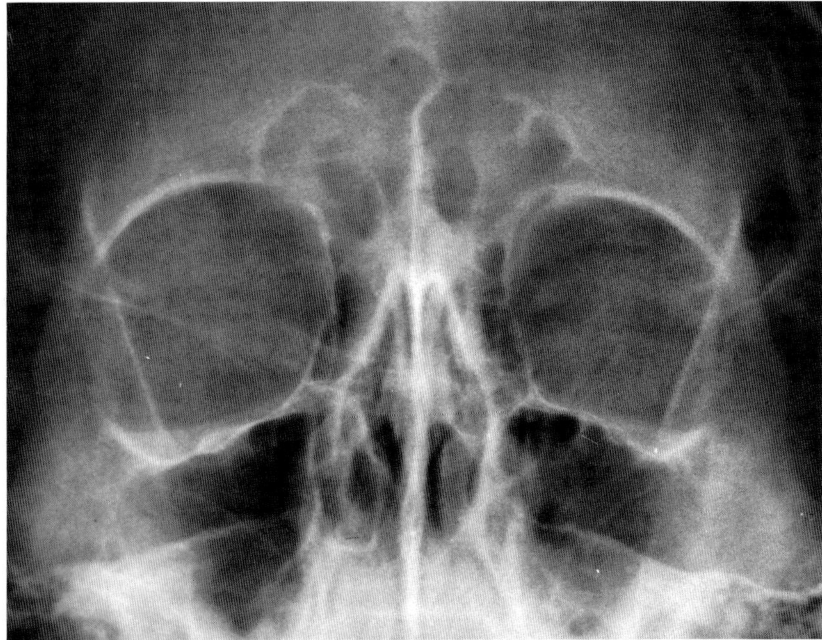

Figure 22. Patient 11. Thirty-three-year-old man, enucleated left eye age 1 year, no implant. Contracted left orbit; 10.4% decrease of orbital dimensions.

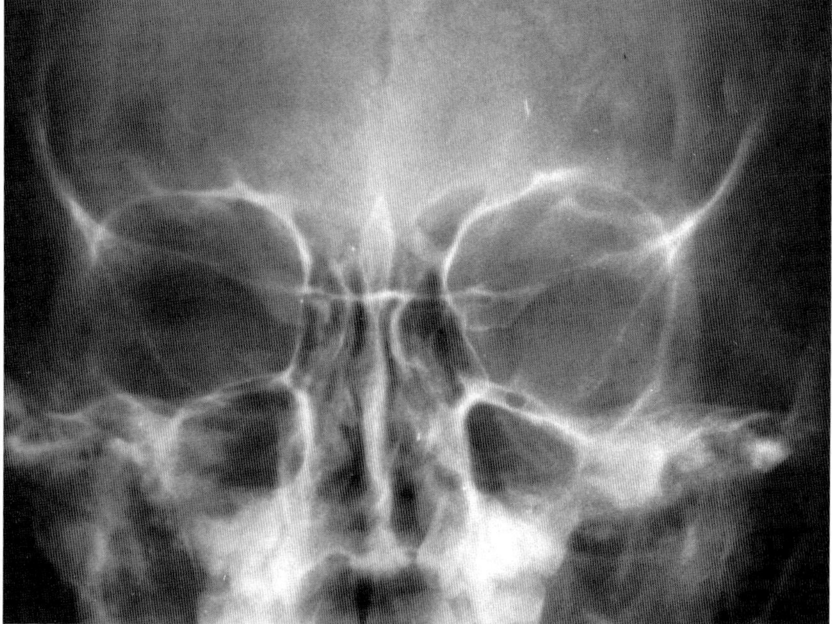

Figure 23. Patient 9. Girl $9\frac{1}{2}$ years old, enucleated right eye age 1 year with plastic sphere orbital implant. More normal contour of anophthalmic orbit. Enlarged antrum on right. Roof of orbit somewhat flattened; 5% decrease of orbital dimensions.

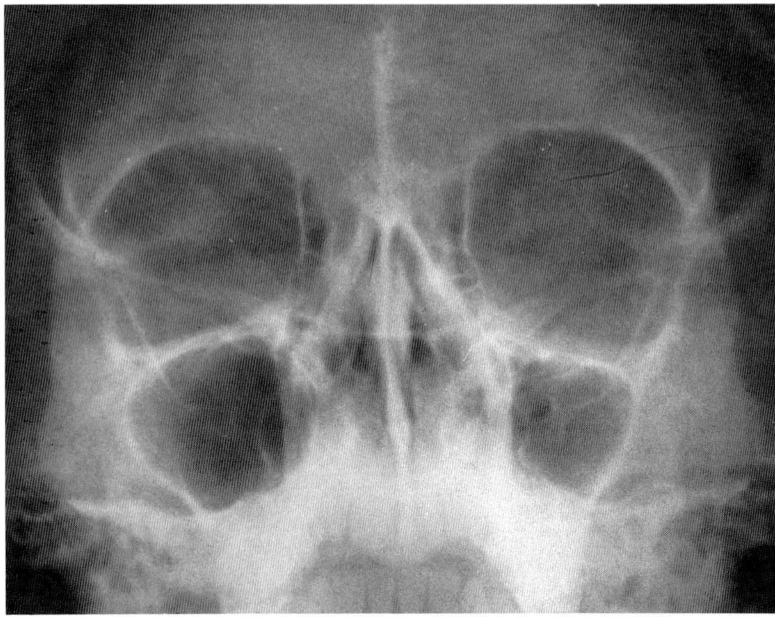

Figure 24. Twenty-year-old patient, enucleated right eye at age 1 year, bone sphere implant. Marked enlargement of antrum on anophthalmic side; 7.8% decrease of orbital dimensions. Bone implant appears to have absorbed.

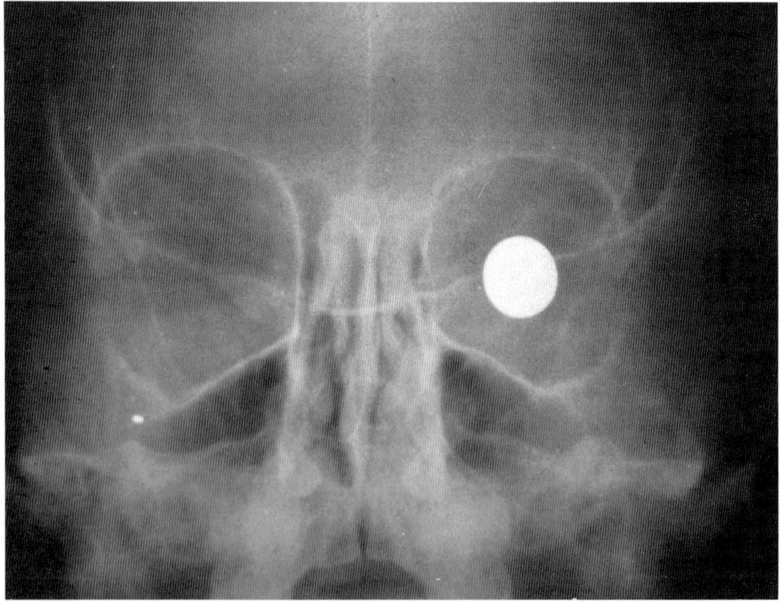

Figure 25. Patient 2. Eight-and-one-half-year-old girl, enucleated left eye age 1 day with gold ball orbital implant. Left orbit is smaller than right but has more normal contour due to implant as compared to orbit without implant; 5.9 % decrease of orbital dimensions.

ing upon each other to appear as a single line, as compared to the two separate lines seen in some of the roentgenographic projections.

Facial asymmetry may be manifested by a decrease in the distance between the midline and the outer wall of the orbit as shown particularly in Figures 20 and 22. Additional changes are evident. The temporal line viewed in the orbit may show either an inconsistent greater or lesser tilt and sometimes appears less pronounced. The temporal margin of the orbit tends to be less distinct and is probably associated with some atrophy of the bone. The decreased density of the anophthalmic orbit associated with loss of tissue volume is quite minimal. Figures 26, 27, and 28 show contraction of the optic canal in patients who lost their left eyes at age four months, four years, and 14 years.

The variations for the measurements from the roentgenograms of 20 normal adults are shown in Table 6. The average of comparable measurements between the two orbits varied between 0.6 and 1.1%. The four orbital rim measurements averaged to just under 1% as the normal variation in the size of the orbit one might expect in the normal skull, with a range up to 1.8%.

DISCUSSION

From these studies it is evident that there can be marked bone changes in the anophthalmic orbit, particularly when the enucleation has been performed at an early age. The changes which were shown in the rabbit by Thomson are here repeated and substantiated. The percentage decrease in the orbital measurement for the rabbit is in the magnitude of 12.8%. Similar findings in the cat skull are in the magnitude of 26.8%. In the human, at birth the percentage decrease in the orbital measurements without an implant would tend to be as high

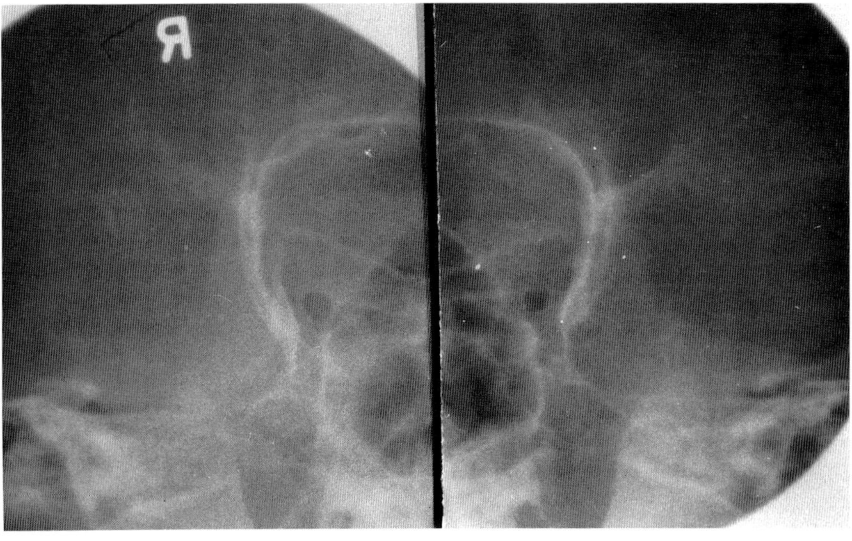

Figure 26. Patient 3. Age $9\frac{1}{2}$ years, enucleated left eye at 4 months, showing smaller left canal for optic nerve.

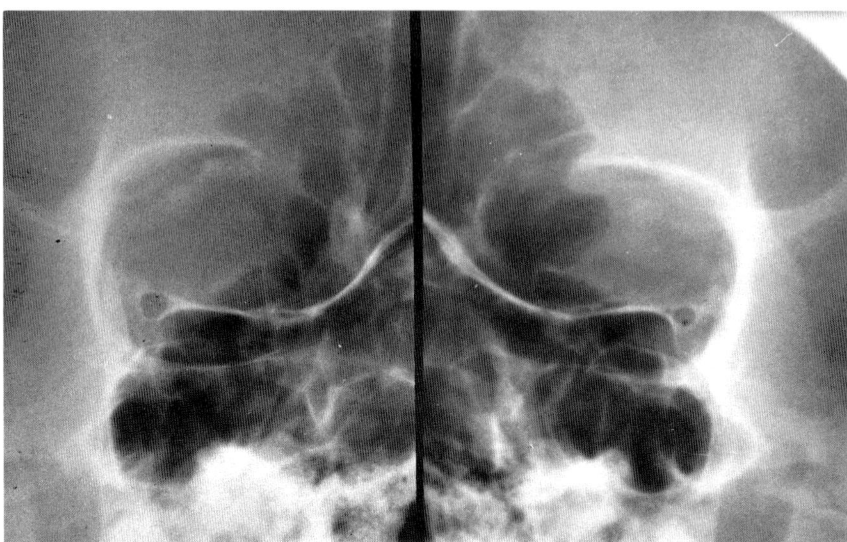

Figure 27. Patient 27. Age 16, enucleated left eye at age 4 years showing smaller left canal for optic nerve.

as 15%, and with an implant about 8%. These figures would be less the later the enucleation was performed. The differential for these figures between the animal and the human might be accounted for because the rabbit and the cat orbits have an incomplete orbital rim, as compared to the solid complete rim of the human. With the incomplete orbital rim of the animals, contraction changes might be expected to occur with more ease, and thus a greater magnitude

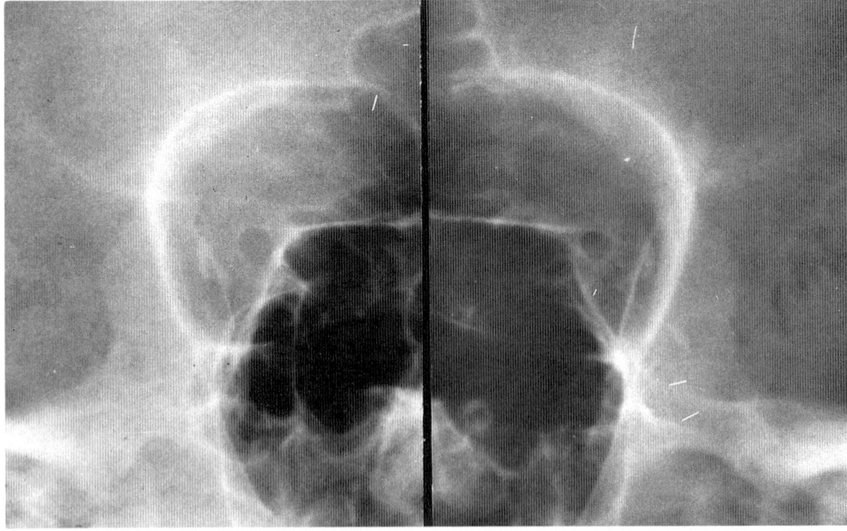

Figure 28. Patient 42. Age 25, enucleated left eye at 14 years, showing smaller left canal for optic nerve.

of change. With measurements taken from Figure 18 the approximate anticipated percentage decrease in the orbital measurements after enucleation is noted in Table 7.

The study of changes in the anophthalmic orbit in the human are dependent upon roentgenographic findings. An attempt was made to locate a dry skull in which it was known that one eye had been enucleated. Several medical centers and the Armed Forces Institute of Pathology were contacted with the hopes that such a skull might be available for examination and direct bone measurements. Unfortunately, none could be located.

A set of roentgenograms captures the moment of growth and change in such an anophthalmic orbit at a particular period of time after enucleation, which could be compared on occasion with preoperative films at an earlier age. It was hoped that films made by the serial roentgenographic cephalometric method might be located to show the progressive changes after enucleation. Two large series of children studied by this technique for their orthodontic problems to show their individual growth progress were evaluated, but, unfortunately, neither of them included a child who had an anophthalmic orbit.

Pfeiffer points out that it is not enough to study the orbital margins, but that the orbit must be considered as a cavity and studied as such. He points out that changes in the walls of the orbit may best be evaluated by stereoscopy and laminography. A much better appreciation of the anophthalmic changes in the walls is offered from the stereoscopic projections. These demonstrate the marked reduction in the volume, or the capacity, of the orbit. The normal concave orbital walls can be seen to flatten, and at times even to become convex as they encroach upon the orbital volume. Because of the irregular walls, no true determination could be made as to the volume changes in this type of orbit. Neither the rabbit skull nor the cat skull, because of the lack of a floor of the orbit, lends itself to volumetric determination of the orbit by any of the usual methods. As was previously mentioned, Koch and Brunetti, in their report of the roentgenologic technique to determine the volume of the orbit and measure its depth, concluded that the orbit of the affected side, in the case of a unilateral anophthalmos, was smaller but retained the same depth as the unaffected side. Alexander et al. [26] studied the orbital volume of 65 skulls by using a sand technique, and by taking roentgenograms of the skulls. Calculations involving three formulas were made from the roentgenograms and compared with those obtained by the sand technique in determining the orbital volume. They could make no relative or absolute correlations between real and X-ray orbital volumes. Therefore, it would be even more difficult to try to make some roentgenologic determination of the volume of these irregular anophthalmic orbits.

Table 7. Percentage Decrease in Orbital Dimensions after Enucleation

Age (years)	Without implant	With implant
Birth	15%	8%
1	11	7
2	9	6
4	6	4.4
6	4.5	3
8	3.5	2.3
12	2	1.3
16	1.1	1

Because a decreased orbital volume must occur after enucleation, some approximate estimate of this decrease seems worthwhile. We might first assume a normal average orbit [13] with the following dimensions: height, 35 mm; width, 40 mm; depth, 40 mm; volume, 30 cc. Empirically, if we assume the shape of the orbit to be a cone with an elliptical base corresponding to the entrance of the orbit, the volume of this form can be determined. For the normal average orbital measurements in the formula for a cone with an elliptical base, the volume would be $14\frac{2}{3}$ cc which actually is about one-half its true volume. If the normal average figures for the orbital entrance are reduced by 10%, as was common with some of the cases presented in this series, the calculated decrease in volume for this cone with the reduced elliptical base would be 19%. Applying this formula to the measurements of patients in this series, the decrease in the orbital volume ranged up to 19.5% in patients with orbital implants, to 27.7% in patients with no orbital implants, and to 36.2% in the one patient with unilateral congenital anophthalmos. The normal orbital diameter is wider by 4 or 5 mm with a depth of 10 mm in back of the rim as compared to its diameter at the rim. Although the changes in enucleation are greater behind the rim, because of encroachment on the volume by surrounding structures, it can be assumed that the volume would be even further decreased, possibly in the magnitude of 35 to 50%.

The study of Hare [27] concerning congenital bilateral anophthalmos is of interest in reference to the per cent decrease in the orbital measurements. He reported two cases, together with their roentgenograms. From these he made four measurements that included the vertical and horizontal, and the two oblique meridians. Comparing these roentgenograms with those of normal children in the same age group, he found approximately 35% decrease in these orbital measurements. Applying the formula for the volume of a cone with an elliptical base to his figures, the volume decrease would be as high as 58%. Mann [28] states that in congenital anophthalmos the orbit is well-formed, though it may be slightly smaller than normal. The fact that the orbit will be present is self-determined, and is in no way dependent on the presence or size of an optic outgrowth. The greater magnitude of change in congenital anophthalmos, however, shows the prenatal influence of the eye.

The orbital entrance at birth is nearly circular, with measurements given for the entrance at birth varying from 18 to 21 mm [13,29,30]. As in both the rabbit and the cat [25] the human eyeball fills the orbit more completely at birth than at maturity. The orbit almost doubles in vertical diameter throughout the growth years [30]. The growth of the anophthalmic orbit increases following early enucleation and only lags behind in measurements up to 15%, or less, by full adult growth. This certainly points to the many other factors that influence the development of the orbit in addition to the globe, which is responsible only for this small amount.

Although the value of an orbital implant has been questioned [8], the findings of Pfeiffer [12], together with the findings in this study, certainly point to the beneficial effect of an implant. The implantation in the cat orbits is also suggestive of a beneficial effect. Pfeiffer [12] demonstrated the roentgenograms of two patients, including one whose eye was enucleated at age seven months in whom no orbital implant was placed. The roentgenogram was taken 11 years later. The second patient had an eye removed at age three years, an implant inserted, and the roentgenogram taken 10 years later. Although these changes are characteristic in each case, there is a marked difference between the two roentgenograms that he demonstrated. The roentgenogram of the patient without an implant showed more irregular contraction of the orbit. However, by taking the average figures from Figure 18, the seven-month-old child might be expected to have a decrease in the size of the orbit of approximately 12%, whereas the three-year-old might have a decrease of approximately 5%. Therefore, more than half of this difference, or about 7%, might be accounted for by the growth interval between the difference of the ages when these children had enucleations.

No report of animal experimentation was found concerning the influence of a buried orbital implant upon the development of the orbit after enucleation. In Litters 4, 5, and 6, the cats that had orbital implants inserted at the time of enucleation, showed less percentage change in the orbital dimensions. The changes in Litter 4 were not as marked because of the early extrusion of the implants. Figures 29 and 30 show the variations within Litter 5 that could be demonstrated. The first skull indicates the decrease in the orbit after simple enucleation, which is a greater change than the second skull in which a silicone implant had been inserted. The third skull is the control. Figure 31 identifies this difference by varying the illumination of the skulls of two enucleated litter mates, one without an implant and one with an implant.

An orbital implant has been used more commonly in recent years. Note that in the series of 51 patients reported by Taylor [10] in 1939 none had a buried implant [11]. More recently, in 1945, DeVoe [31] in reporting his experiences with surgery of the anophthalmic orbit, states that in more than 50% of the patients no implant was in position. In the series now being reported an orbital implant was inserted in 78% of the patients. Since shortly after World War II, with the wide variety of implants of all types, it seems they have found a more common use. Of the nine patients without an orbital implant in this series, four were enucleated as of 1946. Of these, one extruded an implant one week after enucleation because of extensive or-

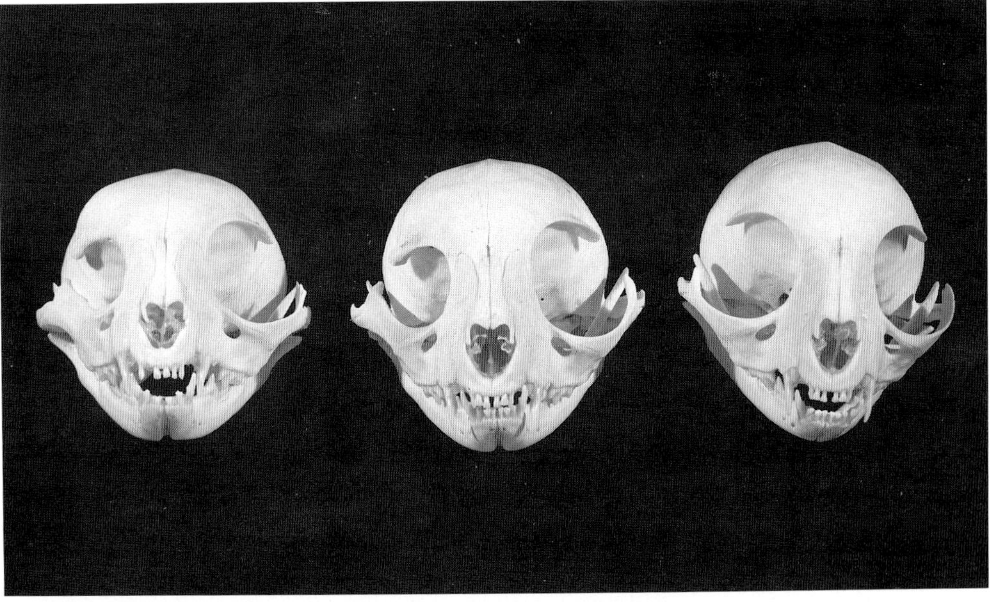

Figure 29. Litter 5, Cats 17, 16, 18, front view. On left, cat 17 with simple enucleation (31.6% decrease orbital dimensions). Compare with cat 16 in center with 8-mm silicone implant inserted at time of enucleation which was retained at least a month (23.9% decrease in orbital dimensions). Implant appears to have reduced the amount of change. Cat 18 on right is the control. Operated on 12th day, sacrificed 116 days.

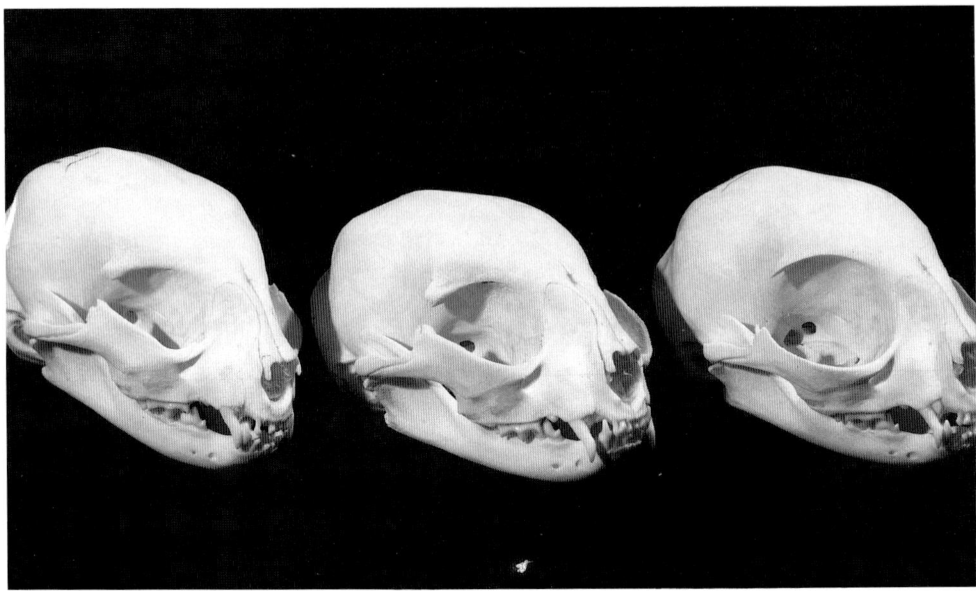

Figure 30. Litter 5, Cats 17, 16, 18. Same as Figure 29. Side view.

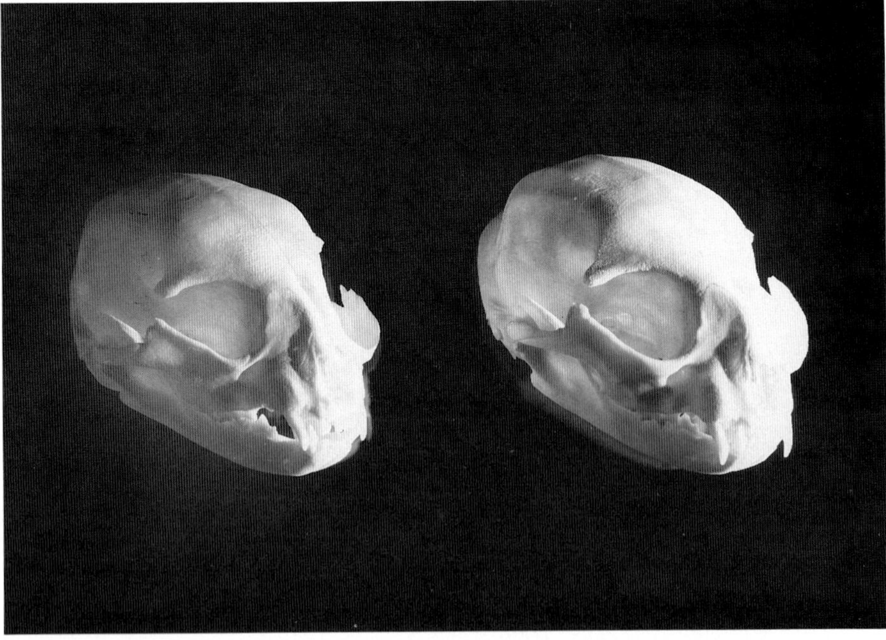

Figure 31. Cats 17 (left), and 16 (right). Showing the larger orbit on the right skull where an implant had been retained at least one month, compared to simple enucleation and smaller orbit in skull on left. Illumination differs from that of Figure 30.

bital hemorrhage, and the other three patients had migrated from the South and no history was available as to whether an implant was considered.

The decreased size of the orbit begins, no doubt, immediately after enucleation. Whitnall [13] refers to Merkel who states that in early childhood the changes occur as soon as 10 weeks after operation. The method of determining this is not described. This appeared in a textbook published in 1901. Unless it was based on a direct anatomical specimen, it, no doubt, did not represent a roentgenologic finding, but must have been based on very astute clinical observations. Sattler [7] found a clear difference between the sizes of the orbit on X-ray as soon as one year after enucleation. The shortest interval after enucleation at which roentgenograms were made in this reported series was 22 months, when a decrease of 5.1% in the dimensions was already evident. A cat (number 8), enucleated on the eighth day, died 30 days after surgery and showed marked changes, in the magnitude of 19% (Fig. 32).

Taylor [10] and Pfeiffer [12] describe the facial asymmetry seen in the human. This can be emphasized in the cat skull (Fig. 33) where the sagittal suture of the skull, as it extends forward to join the midline suture of the nasal bones, can be seen to deviate markedly toward the enucleated side. The external changes evident in the cat are shown in Figure 34.

The interorbital region has been thoroughly studied recently [21]. The authors followed the growth of this region using serial cephalometrograms. They concluded that 50% of growth of the interorbital region occurs by three years of age, and that only slight growth occurs after

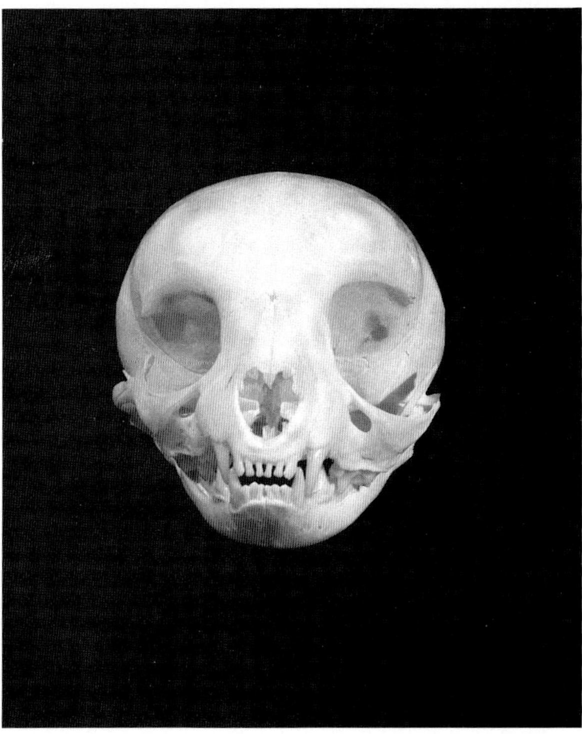

Figure 32. Cat 8. Enucleated right eye eighth day, showing advanced changes at early stage after inadvertent death at 30 days following enucleation.

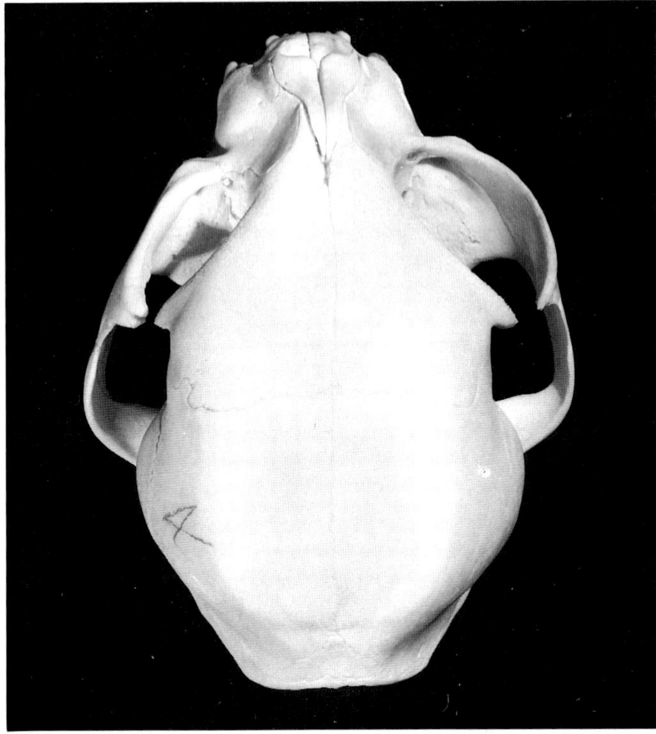

Figure 33. Cat 4. Showing marked deviation toward enucleated side of sagittal suture of skull, with its extension forward to join midline suture of nasal bones.

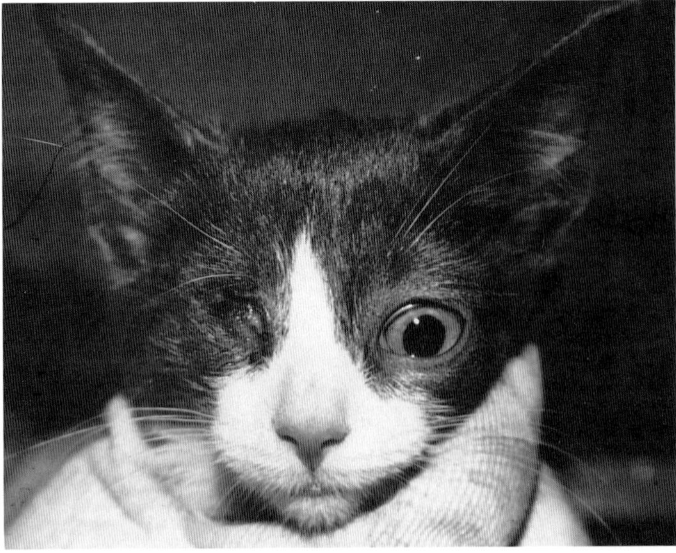

Figure 34. Cat 20. Showing less fullness of face on anophthalmic side with flattening of frontal region of skull. Ear of involved side tended to be turned laterally.

12 years of age. These authors list the growth of the intraorbital structures as one of several forces involved in growth of the interorbital region, the other forces being growth of surrounding structures, growth of sutures, appositional growth, and pneumatization of bone. They mention that a contracted orbit may develop if the eye is removed before growth is completed. No specific mention is made of its effect on the development of the interorbital region. It is assumed the measurement would increase. They give as an adult mean measurement 24.62 mm for the interorbital width after age 20 years. From the series of 40 anophthalmic patients reported in this study, 15 were age 20 years, or older, with an average measurement of 28 mm. This is less, however, than the 28.6-mm average for this measurement taken from the 20 normal adult films studied as a control. It would seem, therefore, that the interorbital measurement is not significantly affected by enucleation of one eye at an early age.

Luzsa [22] has shown the influence of enucleation on the development of the canal of the optic nerve. He examined 37 patients who had one eye enucleated. There was no difference in the size of the canals in 18, four of whom had lost their eye before age 18 years. The remaining 14 were enucleated after age 20 years. Smaller measurements were found on the enucleated side for 15 patients who had one eye enucleated at ages ranging from three to 20. One patient showed an enlargement of the canal of the optic nerve on the enucleated side. Three of the 37 patients were not accounted for. Luzsa believed the development of the canal ceases in the 18th year. The shrinkage of the canal of the optic nerve also has been reported by Pfeiffer [12,15], Pendergrass [19], and Burki [32]. These authors and Goalwin [33] feel the optic nerve canal reaches full adult size at an earlier age ranging from the third to fifth year. Differences between the optic canals of the two sides may exist physiologically according to Goalwin [34]. His findings reveal an absolute symmetry in 45%, a difference of 10%, or less, in 40%, and a difference of 10 to 40% in 14%. As previously noted, in this present series where the optic foramina could be compared in 33 patients, they were equal in two (6%) and smaller in 31 patients (93%) in an amount ranging up to 50%, with an average decrease in size of 17%. Although none of the rabbits in this series showed a change in the canal as compared to the control, a comparison within the rabbit orbits cannot be made since the anterior edge of the optic canal is common to both orbits as a midline foramen. All of the 15 enucleated cat orbits showed a smaller optic nerve canal.

Growth retardation due to roentgen ray therapy of the bones of the orbit has been recognized. Tiburtius and Krokowski [35] have shown its experimental effect on the skulls and orbits of rabbits. Taking seven measurements on 17 rabbit skulls, 114 of the 119 measurements (96%) were smaller on the roentgen-ray-treated side as compared to the normal side. Figure 35 is the roentgenogram of a 14-year-old boy who had roentgen ray therapy for an orbital malignancy at age five with subsequent loss of the globe. The marked bone atrophy of the rim of the orbit, particularly the superior and lateral walls, is evident with a percentage decrease in orbital dimensions in excess of 15%. Normally at his age this would be expected to be about 3% (Fig. 18). In two patients (numbers 7 and 9), in whom an eye had been removed for retinoblastoma, roentgen ray therapy had been given to a retinoblastoma in the contralateral orbit. At the time of their evaluation they showed less decrease in the orbital dimensions of the anophthalmic orbit than the changes that might have been expected for the age of enucleation. This suggests that the roentgen ray therapy retarded development in the unoperated orbit so that the difference between this and the anophthalmic orbit was not as great. Figure 36 is the roentgenogram of a 13-year-old girl who had the left eye removed for a retinoblastoma at age seven months. Roentgen ray therapy was given to the right eye for retinoblastoma at the age of seven months following enucleation of the left eye. Despite therapy to the retinoblastoma in the remaining eye, it progressed and required enucleation. This was performed at age three

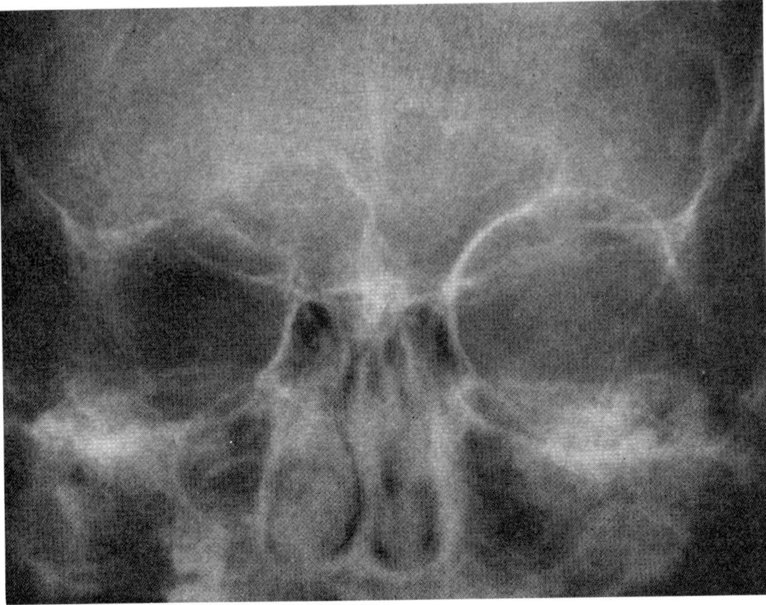

Figure 35. Patient 35. Fourteen-year-old boy who had roentgen ray therapy to right orbit for malignancy age 5 years, with subsequent loss of right eye at age 9 years. Orbit shows 15.2% decrease in size. This marked decrease is associated with irradiation.

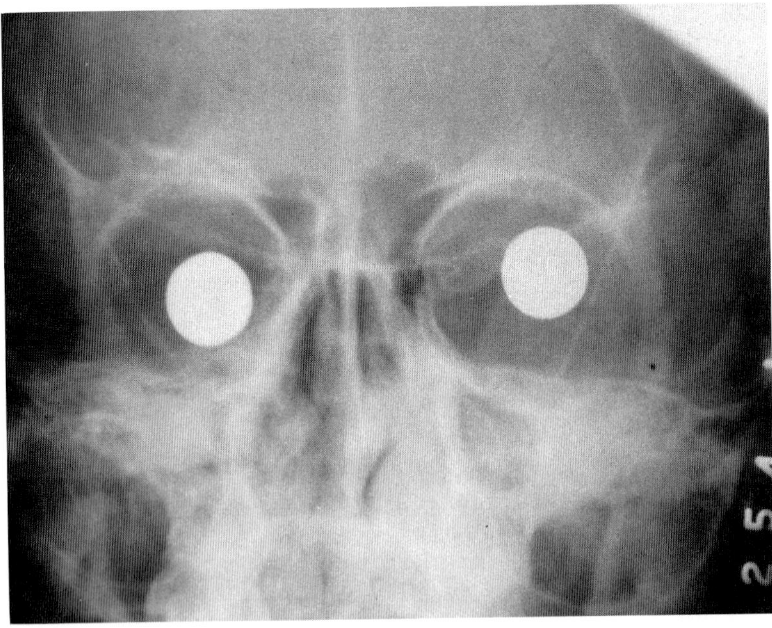

Figure 36. Patient 5. Thirteen-year-old girl. At age 7 months left eye enucleated and right orbit irradiated for retinoblastoma. Right eye enucleated at age 3 years. Implants each orbit. Right orbit is smaller by 11.3% despite enucleation at later age, showing effect of irradiation.

years. This right orbit which had been irradiated, despite being enucleated two and one-half years later, is smaller by about 11.5% than the first orbit that was enucleated. Such changes as the result of therapy will cause additional changes far in excess of those resulting from simple enucleation. The extent of decreased orbital growth on this basis might well be studied further.

CLINICAL CONSIDERATIONS

Because early enucleation may result in lack of development of the orbit, facial asymmetry, and possible interference with the proper fitting of a prosthesis, elective enucleation in infancy is contraindicated. This, of course, cannot apply where there is a malignancy, a recent severe injury, infection, or pain. Because the orbit will decrease in size with a small phthisical eye, there is little reason to defer its removal.

This study further supports the importance of using an orbital implant at the time of surgery, which appears to be in more common clinical use in recent years. Because an orbit may show a decreased size even when a shrunken phthisical eye is present, probably a larger size implant in the range of 18 to 20 mm diameter, as advocated by Sherman [36], would be advisable. This might reduce the amount of diminution of the anophthalmic orbit.

When an orbital implant is being inserted as a secondary procedure, careful roentgenologic study is important if there has been a significant interval since enucleation so that bony changes may have occurred. Alterations in the size and contour of the orbit may call for consideration or modification in the size and shape of the implant. This would hold true for congenital defects such as anophthalmia and microphthalmia. Such an evaluation can be accomplished most satisfactorily by using stereoscopic projections with consideration for laminography.

SUMMARY

The striking and characteristic bone changes that occur in the orbit following enucleation of one eye at an early age are described for the rabbit, cat, and human. The previous experimental work on three rabbits reported by Thomson is repeated and substantiated. These changes are represented by a decrease in the orbital measurements in the magnitude of 12.6% for the rabbit and 26.8% for the cat as determined from the dry skulls.

In the human these bone changes in the anophthalmic orbit were determined from the roentgenograms of a series of 42 patients in whom the enucleation had occurred between the first day and the 15th year. Cephalometric roentgenographic determinations showed a decrease in the orbital measurements up to 15% when no orbital implant had been used, and up to 8% when an implant had been inserted. The magnitude of change decreased the later the enucleation was performed. Tables 8, 9, and 10 supply the complete set of measurements and percentage change determinations for the rabbit and cat skulls, and most of the measurements from the roentgenograms of the patients. (Single examples of each of these have been given in Tables 4, 5, and 6.)

The insertion of an orbital implant results in less contraction of the developing anophthalmic orbit. This is suggested in the cat experimentally, and is evident in the human, with its benefit being greater the earlier in life the enucleation occurs. This supports the findings of Pfeiffer.

Table 8. Rabbits

Litter	Rabbit number	Horizontal (mm)			Vertical (mm)			Avg. % diff. horizontal and vertical	Depth of orbit (mm)			Midline skull to molar tooth (mm)		
		R	L	% diff.	R	L	% diff.		R	L	% diff.	R	L	% diff.
1	1	24	25	4	16	20	20	12	27	29	6.9	14	15	6.7
	2	25.5	27	5.6	17	22	22.7	14.2	29	30	3.3	17.5	18	2.8
	3	24	26	7.7	18	20.5	12.2	10.0	30	30.5	1.6	16	16.5	3.0.
	4	23	26	11.5	19	22	13.6	12.6	29.5	30.5	3.3	16	17	5.9
	5	22.5	24.5	8.2	17	20.5	17.1	12.7	28.5	28.5	0	16	16	0
	6	26	28	7.1	21.5	24	10.4	8.8	30	31.5	4.8	18	18	0
	7 (control)	26	25.5	1.9	20.5	21	2.4	2.2	27	27	0	17	17	0
2	8	23.5	26	9.6	20.5	24	14.6	12.1	30	31	3.2	18	18.5	27
	9 (control)	27	27	0	23	23	0	0	30	30	0	18	18	0
	10	22	25	12	15	21	28.6	20.3	29	30	3.3	16	17	5.9
Average % difference operated rabbits				8.2			17.4	12.8			3.3			3.4
Average % difference unoperated controls				1.0			1.2	1.1			0			0

Litter 1: operated 11 days, sacrificed 204 days; litter 2; operated 7 days, sacrificed 228 days.

The altered orbital volume cannot be determined satisfactorily from either the dried animal skull or from the roentgenograms in the humans. Empirically, however, the decreased orbital volume in the human might be 20 to 30%, and even as high as 50%. An orbital implant appeared to reduce the loss in volume.

Facial asymmetry, as evidenced by increase in the midline to lateral orbital margin measurement, can occur in two-thirds of the patients. The interorbital region measurements show little variation.

The canal of the optic nerve is smaller on the enucleated side as reported by Luzsa and others. This was evident in all of the cats and in 93% of the humans. The average decrease in humans was approximately 17%, but may be as high as 50%.

Roentgen ray therapy to the orbital region may cause additional decreased orbital measurements far greater than those resulting from simple enucleation. Elective enucleation in infancy is contraindicated.

Acknowledgment — I am indebted to many colleagues for their kind permission to include their patients in this series and for supplying additional information concerning these patients. They include Doctors W. C. Caccamise, B. F. Donovan, E. Emerson, K. T. Fairfax, J. R. Fitzgerald, J. F. Gipner, S. J. Ianacone, E. W. Kennedy, P. H. Landers, H. A. Lerner, O. Pearson, G. A. Platt, M. H. Presberg, C. T. Sullivan, E. R. Vernou.

I am most grateful to Dr. Albert C. Snell for his interest, encouragement, and advice. He kindly read an early draft of the manuscript and offered suggestions on revision.

Mrs. Anne Smith devoted much effort in locating the patients and accomplishing their roentgenograms. Her perseverance was tested with the typing of several revisions of the manuscript. I am most grateful both for this and for her help in many other ways during the preparation of this material.

Table 9. Cats

Litter	Cat number	Implant (mm)	Horizontal (mm)			Vertical (mm)			Avg. % diff. horizontal and vertical	Depth of orbit (mm)			Age at surgery (days)	Sacrificed
			R	L	% diff.	R	L	% diff.		R	L	% diff.		
1	1	0	18	25	28.0	13	21	30.1	29.1	27	30	10.0		
	2	C*	25	25	0	21	21	0	0	32	31	3.1		
	3	0	17	24.5	30.6	13	20.5	36.6	33.6	27	31	12.9	15	146
	4	0	19	25	24.0	15	21.5	30.2	21.1	28	30	6.7		
	5	0	20	24	16.7	14.5	21	31.0	23.9	28	31	9.7		
2	6	0	20	27	25.9	17	23	26.1	26.0	30	32.5	7.8	23	169
	7	C*	32	32	0	24	23.5	2.1	1.1	31	31	0		
3	8†	0	15	18	16.7	12.5	16	21.9	19.3	17	19	10.5		
	9	0	18.5	25	25.0	15.5	22	29.5	27.3	28.5	31	8.1	8	158
	10	C*	25.5	25.5	0	21	21.5	2.3	1.2	30	30	0		
4	11	5	15	19.5	23.1	12.5	18	30.5	28.3	19	24	20.8		
	12	8	18.5	23.5	21.3	14	20.5	31.2	26.3	23	28	17.9		
	13‡	0	16.5	23.5	29.8	14.5	21	31.0	30.4	22	27	18.5	12	116
	14	7	18	23	21.7	13.5	21	34.1	28.1	23	27	14.8		
	15	C*	23	23	0	20	20.5	2.4	1.2	27	27	0		
5	16	8	20	24	16.7	14.5	21	31.0	23.9	24.5	26.5	7.6		
	17	0	17.5	22.5	22.2	11.5	19.5	41.0	31.6	23	26	11.5	12	116
	18	C*	22.5	22.5	0	19	19	0	0	26.5	26	1.8		
6	19	0	19	23	17.4	13.5	20.5	31.1	28.2	25.5	28	8.9		
	20	8	18	22	18.2	12.5	18.5	32.4	21.3	25	27	7.4	9	104
	21	C*	21.5	22	2.3	19	19	0	1.2	27	27	0		
Average % difference operated cats					22.8			30.8	26.8			11.5		
Average % difference unoperated controls					0.4			1.3	0.8			0.8		

*Control.
†Cat 8 died 38 days.
‡Cat 13 died 87 days.

Table 10. Humans

Patient number	Eye	Age surgery	Age exam.	Implant	Orbit height			Orbit width			Diagonal UN–LT			Diagonal LN–UT			Avg. % diff.
					R	L	% diff.	R	L	% diff.	R	L	% diff.	R	L	% diff.	
1	R	—	17	0	35	40	12.5	28	38	26.3	40	44	9.1	29	39	25.6	18.4
2	L	1 d.	$8\frac{1}{4}$	+	45	40	11.1	35	34	2.9	41	41	0	42	38	9.5	5.9
3	L	4 mo.	$9\frac{1}{2}$	0	41	40	2.4	34	32	5.9	43	37	14.0	35	32	8.6	8.2
4	L	6 mo.	$4\frac{1}{2}$	+	46	43	6.5	34	33	2.9	46	40	12.9	40	37	7.5	7.5
5*	R	7 mo.	$14\frac{1}{2}$	+	38	41	7.3	33	38	13.2	36	45	20.0	36	38	5.2	11.4
	L	3 yr.	$14\frac{1}{2}$	+													
6	L	7 mo.	35	+	46	43	6.5	36	33	8.3	47	42	10.6	37	33	10.8	9.1
7*	L	7 mo.	$12\frac{1}{3}$	+	46	44	4.3	34	34	0	43	42	2.3	36	34	5.6	3.1
8	R	8 mo.	$2\frac{1}{2}$	+	38	40	5	28	30	6.7	34	35	2.9	34	36	5.6	5.1
9*	R	1	$9\frac{1}{2}$	+	38	42	9.5	35	37	5.4	39	40	2.5	38	39	2.6	5
10	R	1	20	+	36	42	14.3	36	38	5.2	43	46	6.5	36	38	5.2	7.8
11	L	1	33	0	46	41	10.9	40	35	12.5	48	43	11.4	39	36	7.7	10.4
12	R	$1\frac{1}{4}$	$3\frac{3}{4}$	+	43	44	2.3	30	31	3.2	39	41	4.9	36	37	2.7	3.3
13	R	$1\frac{1}{2}$	42	0	38	46	17.4	35	40	12.5	43	47	8.5	37	39	5.1	10.9
14	L	$1\frac{3}{4}$	$5\frac{3}{4}$	+	40	37	7.5	35	33	5.7	42	38	9.5	36	32	11.1	8.5
15	R	2	22	+	40	47	14.9	35	37	5.4	43	46	6.5	38	42	9.5	9.1
16	L	$2\frac{1}{2}$	14	+	44	39	11.4	37	34	8.1	45	41	8.9	39	35	10.5	9.7
17	L	$2\frac{1}{2}$	$7\frac{1}{2}$	+	46	46	0	35	33	5.7	45	43	4.4	42	40	4.7	3.7
18	L	$2\frac{2}{3}$	9	+	48	48	0	36	34	5.6	45	44	2.2	41	40	2.4	2.6
19	L	$2\frac{3}{4}$	26	+	47	46	2.1	37	37	0	46	46	0	40	38	5	1.8
20	L	3	20	0	45	42	6.7	38	34	10.5	46	42	8.7	42	39	7.1	8.3
21	L	3	9	+	45	43	4.4	35	31	11.4	43	43	0	41	38	7.3	5.5
22	L	$3\frac{2}{3}$	25	+	46	48	4.2	35	39	10.3	46	46	0	40	44	9.1	5.9
23	L	4	11	0	39	37	5.1	34	32	5.9	41	40	2.4	39	36	7.7	5.3
24	R	4	40	0	47	51	7.8	34	38	10.5	44	46	4.3	43	45	4.4	6.8
25	L	4	16	0	50	47	6	39	37	5.1	50	47	6.0	41	38	7.3	6.1
26	L	4	$7\frac{1}{2}$	+	45	43	4.4	35	35	0	43	43	0	42	41	2.4	1.7
27	L	4	16	+	40	38	5	37	37	0	35	35	0	42	40	4.7	2.4
28	R	5	22	+	42	43	2.3	36	37	2.7	42	45	6.7	41	44	6.8	4.6
29	R	$5\frac{2}{3}$	$12\frac{1}{3}$	+	42	41	2.4	35	34	2.9	42	41	2.4	40	37	7.5	3.8
30	R	6	31	+	40	41	2.4	37	37	0	42	43	2.3	37	39	5.1	2.5
31	L	6	$9\frac{1}{2}$	+	42	40	4.7	36	34	5.6	41	40	2.4	38	36	5.2	4.5
32	L	7	28	+	45	45	0	39	39	0	48	47	2.1	46	46	0	0.5
33	R	$7\frac{1}{2}$	13	+	47	47	0	36	37	2.7	49	49	0	42	43	2.3	1.3
34	R	8	11	+	45	46	2.2	32	33	3.0	43	44	2.3	36	38	5.2	3.2
35*	R	$8\frac{5}{6}$	$13\frac{5}{6}$	0	43	47	8.5	33	40	17.5	37	44	15.9	34	42	19.0	15.2
36	L	9	$17\frac{1}{2}$	+	44	43	2.3	35	34	2.9	43	41	2.3	41	40	2.4	2.5
37	L	$9\frac{1}{2}$	23	+	44	42	4.5	39	39	0	45	43	4.4	38	38	0	2.2
38	L	10	16	+	44	42	4.5	36	35	2.7	44	42	4.5	38	38	0	2.9
39	R	11	16	0	41	42	2.4	41	42	2.4	50	51	2	39	40	2.5	2.3
40	R	12	17	+	44	45	2.2	37	37	0	41	43	4.6	38	40	5	3.0
41	R	13	20	+	46	47	2.1	39	39	0	46	46	0	40	40	0	0.5
42	L	14	25	+	45	45	0	40	39	2.5	50	49	2.0	42	42	0	1.1

*Cases 5, 7, 9, and 35 received X-ray therapy.

REFERENCES

1. Merkel F: *Handbuch der topographischen Anatomie, vol. I.* Braunschweig, 1891.
2. Byers WGM: Report of committee of the Ophthalmological Society on excision. *Tr Ophth Soc U Kingdom* 1898; 18:256, 301.
3. Thomson WE: The determination of the influence of the eyeball on the growth of the orbit, by experimental enucleation of one eye in young animals. *Tr Ophth Soc U Kingdom* 1901; 21:258.
4. Wessely K: Ueber Versuche am wachsenden Auge. *München Med Wchnschr* 1909; 56:2249.
5. Wessely K: Ueber Korrelationen des Wachstums (nach Versuchen am Auge). *Ztschr Augenh* 1920; 43:654.
6. Wessely, K: Beiträge zu den Wachstumsbeziehungen zwischen dem Augapfel und seinen Nachbarorganen. *Graefes Arch Ophthalmol* 1921; 105:491.
7. Sattler CH: Operationen zur Verbesserung der Kosmetik nach Enucleation. *Graefes Arch Ophthalmol* 1922; 108:229.
8. Heckel EB: Enucleation in infants. *Am J Ophthalmol* 1922; 5:227.
9. Koch C and Brunetti L: Etude des corrélations morphologiques entre l'orbite et le globe oculaire, déterminées sur le vivant, grâce à un nouveau système d'orbitométrie radiographique (surtout dans les amétropies et les anophtalmies unilatérales). *Arch Ophthalmol* 1934; 51:809. Abstract of a paper appearing in *Ann Ottal Clin Ocul* 1933; 61:342.
10. Taylor WOG: The effect of enucleation of one eye in childhood upon the subsequent development of the face. *Tr Ophthalmol Soc UK* 1939; 59 (Part I):361.
11. Taylor WOG: Oral communication, December, 1963.
12. Pfeiffer RL: The effect of enucleation on the orbit. *Tr Am Acad Ophthalmol* 1945; 49:236.
13. Whitnall SE: *The Anatomy of the Human Orbit and Accessory Organs of Vision.* London, Oxford, 1921.
14. Vorisek EA: Maldevelopment of an orbit. *Am J Ophthalmol* 1933; 16:434.
15. Pfeiffer RL: Roentgenography of exophthalmos with notes on the roentgen ray in ophthalmology. *Tr Am Ophthalmol Soc* 1941; 39:492, *Am J Ophthalmol* 1943; 26:724, 816, 928.
16. Berens C: *The Eye and Its Diseases.* Philadelphia, PA, W.B. Saunders Co., 1949:12.
17. Guyton JS: Enucleation and allied procedures. *Tr Am Ophthalmol Soc.* 1948; 46:472, *Am J Ophthalmol* 1949; 32:1517, 1725, 1950; 33:283.
18. Hartmann E: La Radiographie en ophtalmologie. Atlas clinique. Paris, Masson, 1936 (cited by Duke-Elder S: *Text-book of Ophthalmology, vol. 5.* St. Louis, MO, Mosby, 1952:5522).
19. Pendergrass EP, Schaeffer JP, and Hodes PJ: *The Head and Neck in Roentgen Diagnosis* vol. 1. Springfield, IL, Charles C Thomas, 1956.
20. Hartmann E and Gilles E: *Roentgenologic Diagnosis in Ophthalmology.* Philadelphia, PA, Lippincott, 1959.
21. Morin JD, Hill JC, Anderson JE, and Grainger RM: A study of growth in the interorbital region. *Am J Ophthalmol* 1963; 56:895.
22. Luzsa E: Der Einfluss der Enukleation auf die Entwicklung des Sehnervenkanals. *Klin Monatsbl Augenh* 1938; 101:413.
23. Davis FA: The anatomy and histology of the eye and orbit of the rabbit. *Tr Am Ophthalmol Soc* 1929; 27:401.
24. Ruedemann AD Jr: Use of a silicone implant: For evisceration and enucleation. *Am J Ophthalmol* 1962; 54:868.
25. Prince JH, Diesem CD, Eglitis I, and Ruskell, GL: *Anatomy and Histology of the Eye and Orbit in Domestic Animals,* Springfield, IL, Charles C Thomas, 1960.
26. Alexander JCC, Anderson JE, Hill JC, and Wortzman G: The determination of orbital volume. *Tr Canad Ophthalmol Soc* 1961; 24:105.
27. Hare R: Congenital bilateral anophthalmos. *AMA Arch Ophthalmol* 1943; 30:320.
28. Mann I: *Developmental Abnormalities of the Eye.* London, Cambridge University Press, 1937.
29. Keeney AH: *Chronology of Ophthalmic Development.* Springfield, IL, Charles C Thomas, 1951.
30. Peyton WT: A topographic study of the orbit and bulbus oculi during a part of the growth period. *Anat Rec* 1940; 76:343.
31. DeVoe AG: Experiences with surgery of the anophthalmic orbit. *Am J Ophthalmol* 1945; 28:1346.
32. Burki E: Ueber die Röntgenaufnahme des Canalis opticus und ihre klinische Bewertung. *Schweiz Med. Wchnschr* 1952; 82:354.
33. Goalwin HA: The clinical value of optic canal roentgenograms. *AMA Arch Ophthalmol* 1926; 55:1.
34. Goalwin HA: One thousand optic canals. A clinical, anatomic and roentgenologic study. *JAMA* 1927; 89:1745.
35. Tiburtius H and Krokowski E: Ueber Versuche, die Entstehung der Röntgenkatarakte des Kaninchens auf cellulartherapeutischem Wege zu beeinflussen. *Graefes Arch Ophthalmol* 1961; 163:527.
36. Sherman AE: The retracted eye socket. *Tr Am Ophthalmol Soc.* 1950; 48:615, *Am J Ophthalmol* 1952; 35:89.

The Ocularists' Management of Congenital Microphthalmos and Anophthalmos

Greg L. Dootz, A.A.S.

ABSTRACT

Early socket stimulation is crucial for management of congenital anophthalmos and microphthalmos among infants. Progressive sized hard conformers and lid expansion devices can expand the small socket in these patients. The ocularists' management of these two conditions is discussed and techniques are introduced.

MICROPHTHALMOS

The incidence of microphthalmos seen by the ocularist has appeared to increase over the past decade (Fig. 1). It is difficult to conclude whether this is from additional referrals, or an increased awareness that socket therapy is available. No exact cause for this type of condition is noted [1]. It is suspected that early fetal involvement is related to environmental agents causing poor ocular development (Fig. 2). The microphthalmic eye at birth can be from one-third to three-fourths the size of a normal infant eye at birth. The normal eye size of an infant is two-thirds that of an adult. This condition affects males and females with equal frequency.

The present form of treatment for the microphthalmic patient is the use of progressive sized hard conformers to help stimulate the bony orbit and expand socket tissue [2]. The degree of success with socket expansion depends directly upon the time treatment is started. The length of treatment can vary dramatically depending upon the age of the patient. Two years may be needed for this treatment to be completed even under ideal conditions.

At the initial examination, it is important for the ocularist to evaluate vision potential in the microphthalmic eye. It is not uncommon for a patient to have light perception, and sometimes even useful vision out of this small eye. If vision is possible, then the ocularist needs to re-evaluate the form of treatment with the referring ophthalmologist. Following a complete workup of the patient's ocular history, the ocularist needs to measure the palpebral fissure opening horizontally and vertically in both eyes. This will give the ocularist the measurements needed to determine the amount of expansion necessary to equal the lid opening of the other eye. The ocularist also needs to study the position, size, motility, and corneal diameter of the microphthalmic eye. The fear of corneal irritation, abrasions, subconjunctival hemorrhages, and even corneal ulcerations, is of the utmost concern. The ocularist must understand the friction created by the eye movement on the back of the conformer or prosthesis. Patients with nystagmus of the microphthalmic eye may have an extra difficult time adjusting. If corneal

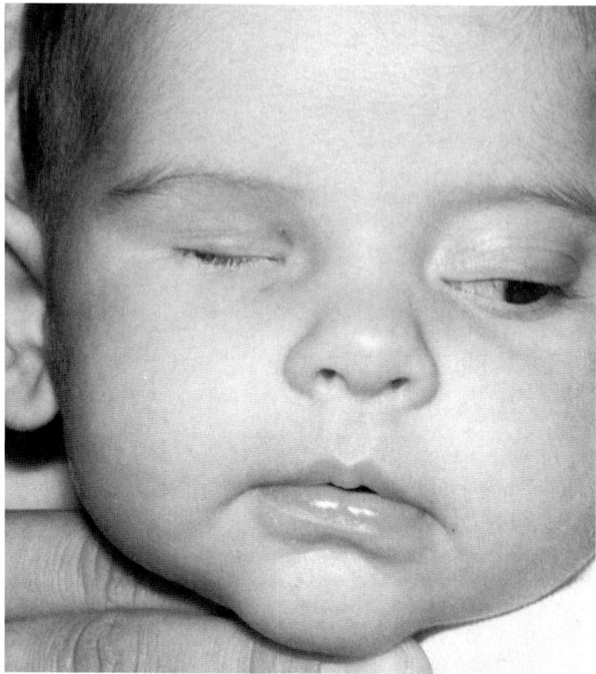

Figure 1. The appearance of a two-month-old female with congenital microphthalmos, showing total ptosis and narrow horizontal palpebral fissure (OD).

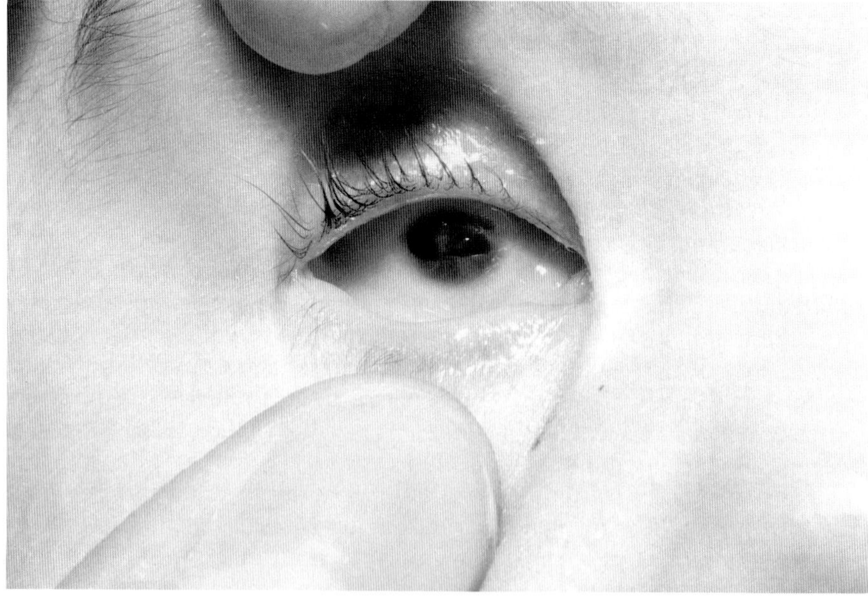

Figure 2. Close-up of a two-month-old microphthalmic eye (OD).

irritation is a constant problem, then it is appropriate for a corneal flap to be placed over the nonseeing microphthalmic eye to reduce its sensitivity. Enucleation of the microphthalmic eye is an unnecessary procedure in the majority of cases [3,4]. The loss of further orbital volume, socket scarring, and the psychological trauma of enucleation is not justifiable with the microphthalmic patient. The literature indicates that the microphthalmic eye does help with socket and orbital development, even if the eye is small [5].

During the management of the microphthalmic patient, the ocularist must be constantly aware of any subconjunctival cysts or subconjunctival hemorrhages that may occur [6]. If any of these situations are noted, then the ocularist must contact the referring ophthalmologist for consultation. Adjusting the conformer or prosthesis can help control these problems in the majority of cases.

In making the first hard conformer, it is mandatory for the ocularist to take a socket impression of the microphthalmic eye. This is often done under general anesthesia with an ophthalmologist present (Fig. 3). An alginate impression material is injected into the small socket to determine the exact shape, size, and configuration of the microphthalmic eye (Fig. 4). The

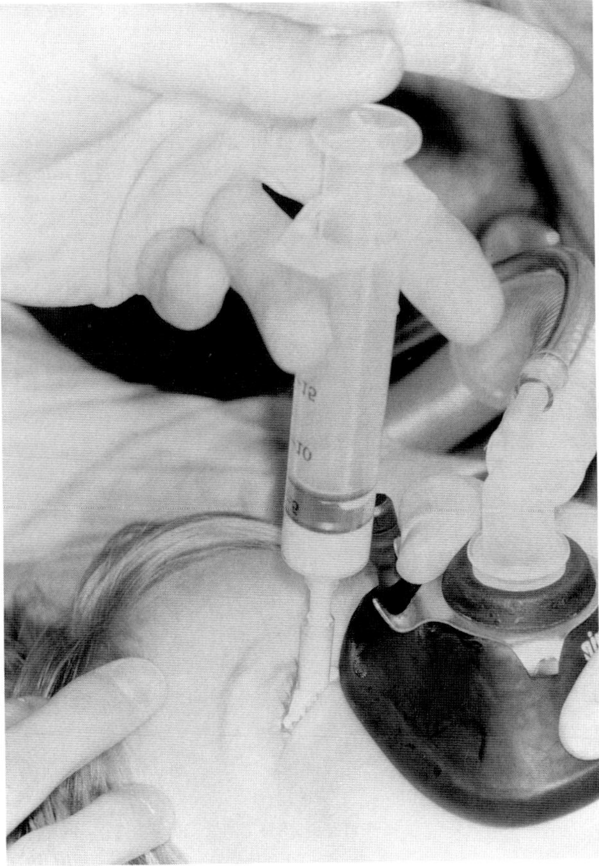

Figure 3. Injecting impression material over a microphthalmic eye (OD).

cornea is protected from the alginate material by inserting a soft contact lens or ophthalmic ointment. Following this procedure, a stone casting is then made of the alginate impression. A clear acrylic conformer (Fig. 5) is then manufactured by using the stone cast as a pattern. The conformer is highly polished to aid comfort and clarity. This allows the ocularist to evaluate the fit and tear flow over the microphthalmic eye. A fluorescein dye and cobalt blue ultraviolet examining light are useful. It is critical that the ocularist be aware of the central corneal clearance and tear pattern of the conformer. If this is not adequate, corneal irritation will exist from added friction or trapped air bubbles in front of the cornea. Following the fitting of the first conformer, the ocularist may place small holes in the conformer to aid in tear circulation. This is important because the patient wears the conformer continuously for weeks. During the insertion of the clear conformer (Fig. 6), an ophthalmic ointment is placed on the back of the conformer to reduce the chance of trapping air bubbles in front of the cornea. Artificial tear drops are also used to help reduce surface friction and dryness. After fitting the first conformer, it is normal for the patient to outgrow it within the first one to two weeks. A larger conformer will be needed to continue socket expansion. This can often be done by adding to the existing conformer, thus avoiding a new impression. Return visits are then scheduled every three to four weeks. It is very common for the socket to expand rapidly at an early age. Once the child becomes one year of age or older, the degree of expansion progresses more slowly. Following one year of age, the patient is seen every two months instead of every three to four weeks. During the return checkup examinations the ocularist will notice a deepening of the lateral and superior fornices (Fig. 7). Once this occurs, and further enlargement of the conformer is difficult, a new socket impression and conformer is needed to help replace this volume change. It is important to observe the changing location of the microphthalmic eye. Often the eye will have moved nasally to its final position. In the majority of cases, the microphthalmic globe rarely increases in size as the socket enlarges, or as the patient becomes older.

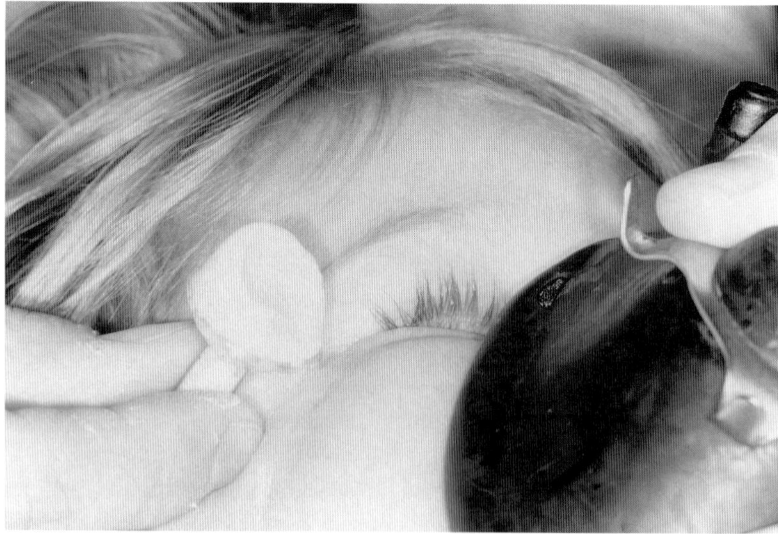

Figure 4. Socket impression of a microphthalmic eye (OD).

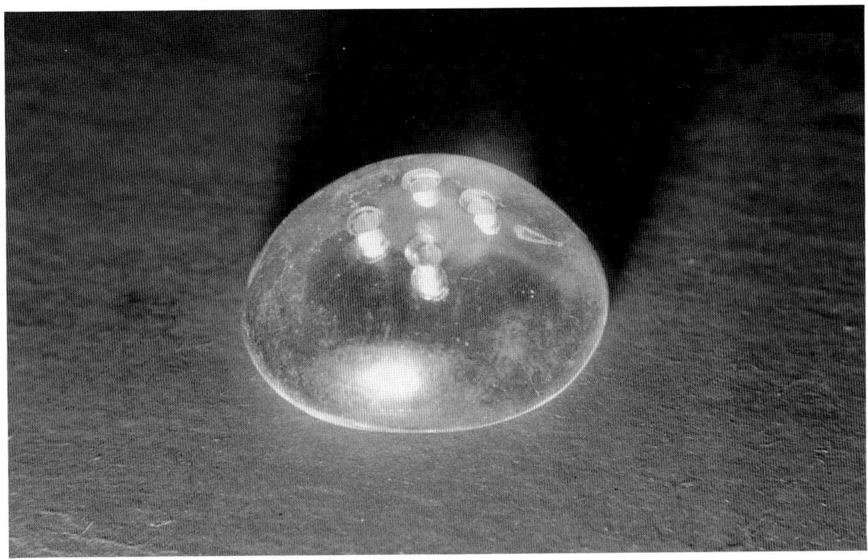

Figure 5. Close-up of a small conformer.

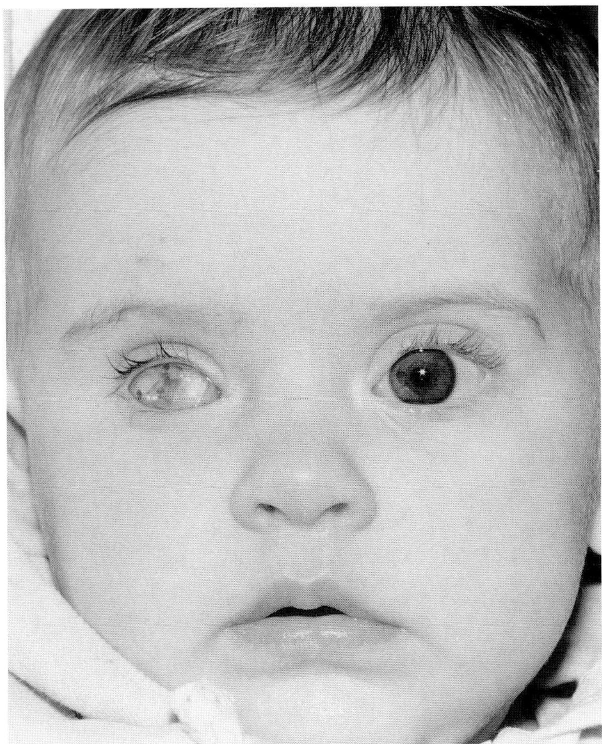

Figure 6. A small conformer in place over a microphthalmic eye (OD) showing expansion of lids.

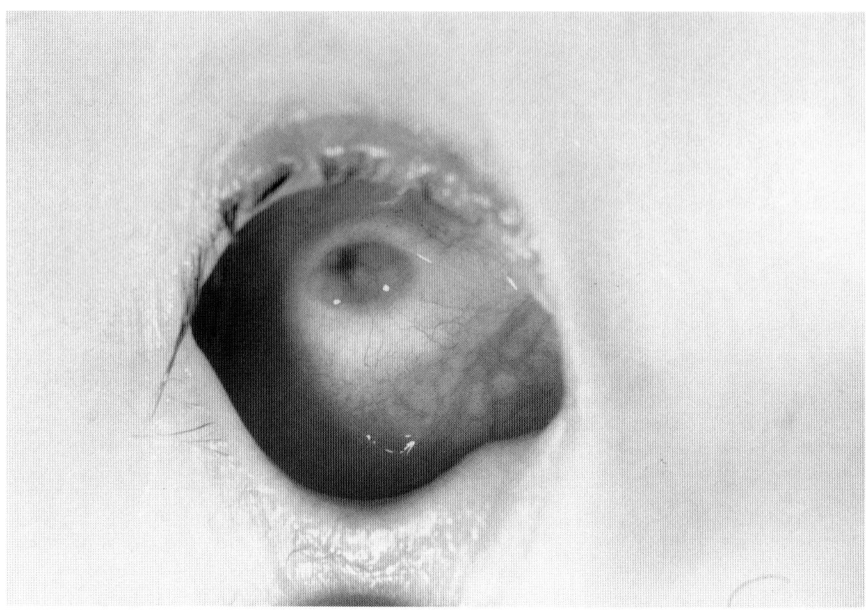

Figure 7. The appearance of a microphthalmic eye and socket (OD) after two years of expansion therapy.

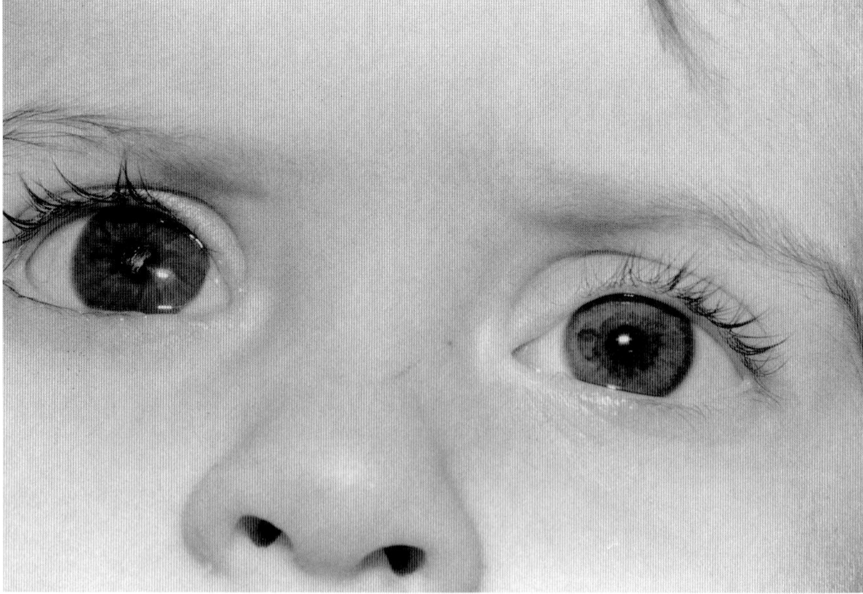

Figure 8. The cosmetic appearance of a painted prosthesis over a microphthalmic eye (OD), after two years of therapy.

During the early expansion of the microphthalmic socket, the palpebral fissure opening enlarges at a slower rate. This in turn makes it difficult to fit larger sized conformers. But, with time the palpebral fissure opening will expand to some degree. During the initial examination, if it is noted that the horizontal palpebral fissure opening of the microphthalmic eye differs from the other eye by more than 5 mm, it is likely that the palpebral fissure opening will always be somewhat different in length. If this difference in length is less than 4 mm, there is a good chance that the palpebral fissure opening can be equalled. For the bilateral microphthalmic patient it is important to have symmetrical lid openings, even if they are small. For those patients whose palpebral fissure openings are not equal, it is possible to do a lateral canthotomy to help increase the opening appearance. This is not always recommended because lateral canthal scarring may occur from this procedure, drawing additional attention to the eye area. It is also possible for an entropion [7] of the microphthalmic lids to occur during therapy. This is often caused by stretching of the lids and cul-de-sac from the conformers. This does not occur nearly as often with the microphthalmic patient as it does with the congenital anophthalmic patient. The length of therapy and amount of the defect may cause this to develop more with the anophthalmic patient. Ptosis may occur with either type of patient. This may be corrected by adjusting the ocular prosthesis, or intervention with surgery. Lid surgery should be held off as long as possible in the hope of correcting the ptosis when the patient is older. It is common during treatment with the progressive sized conformers and even with the final painted ocular prosthesis, for there to be good levator function. It is important to strive to stimulate a normal appearance when blinking.

Note that a *painted* ocular prosthesis needs to be fitted as soon as possible. This in many cases occurs following the completion of socket therapy. This exists in most cases between one and two years of age. If the patient was started with socket expansion therapy at a much older age (two years or older), then it may be necessary for the progressive sized conformers to be painted like a regular prosthesis giving the appearance of a normal, but small, eye. Psychologically this is important for the patient and parents, to achieve signs of cosmetic improve-

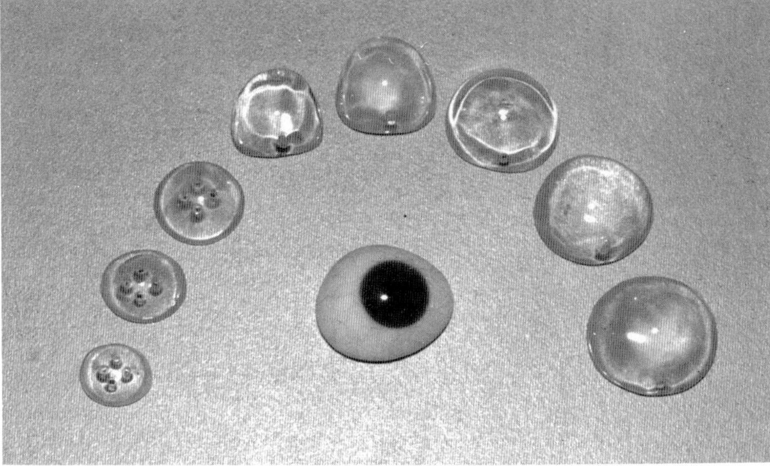

Figure 9. A series of progressive sized conformers along with the first painted prosthesis for a microphthalmic child.

ment and balance. Following the completion of socket expansion therapy (Fig. 8), a new socket impression is taken for preparation of the final prosthesis. After dispensing the new painted prosthesis (Fig. 9), the patient is evaluated two months later. If the patient is doing well, appointments are scheduled every four to six months thereafter until the age of 5. After that, the patient will then be seen every six to nine months until the age of 10 (Fig. 10). Following the age of 10 the patient is seen on a yearly basis for routine checkup examinations. The average microphthalmic patient will need three to four new painted prostheses before the age of 10. Additional prosthesis or build ups will also be needed during the patient's lifetime to ensure a good cosmetic appearance. Once the patient reaches adulthood, the prosthesis will need to be replaced on an average of every 8 to 10 years.

Care and handling of the ocular prosthesis for the microphthalmic patient is very similar to the adult prosthesis. In the majority of cases, the microphthalmic patient wears the prosthesis full-time and removes and cleans it every four to eight weeks, using soap and water. There are some cases where the microphthalmic eye will not tolerate the prosthesis full-time, but does very well during daytime use. In these cases the prosthesis is removed at night and replaced in the morning.

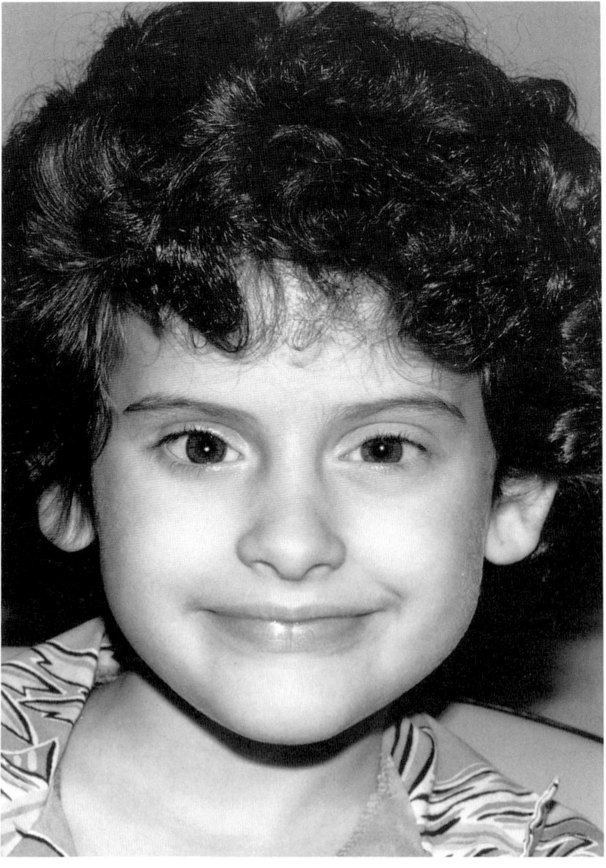

Figure 10. The appearance of the same child as previously shown, now 7 years old.

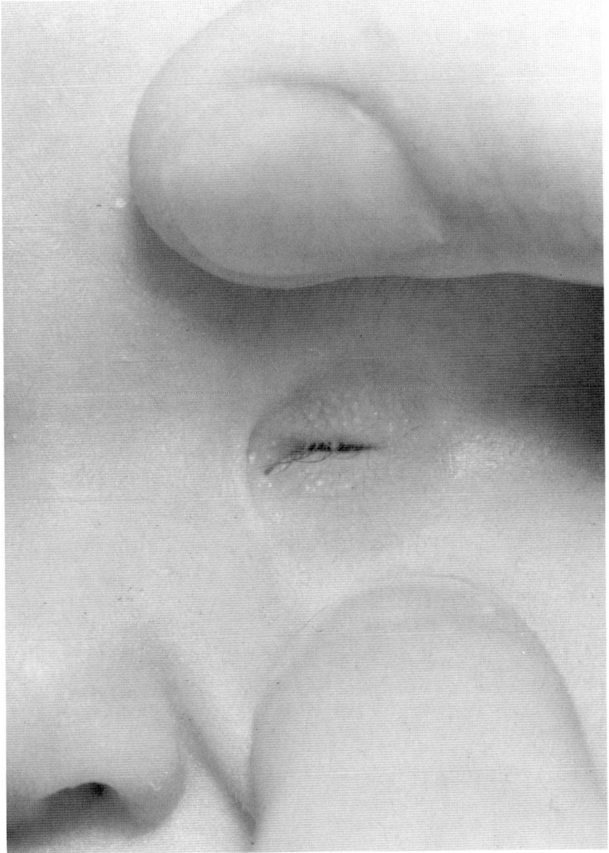

Figure 11. A close-up view of a one-month-old male with a clinical congenital anophthalmic socket (OS).

SUMMARY

The majority of microphthalmic patients can be treated successfully with the use of the progressive size conformer. The degree of success is directly related to the age at which the patient was started with the therapy, and the extent of the defect. The older the patient the more difficult and longer the expansion therapy will be, with often a less than desirable cosmetic result. It is vital that all one-eyed patients wear polycarbonate safety glasses for constant protection. The fear of injury, or the slightest loss of vision to the good eye, is the greatest concern of all.

ANOPHTHALMOS

Clinical congenital anophthalmos [8] is a very rare ocular abnormality [9]. Unilateral anophthalmos is more commonly seen than bilateral anophthalmos. For the ocularist [10] clinical anophthalmos, whether unilateral or bilateral, gives the greatest challenge. Its etiology remains obscure. Environmental agents may be the cause of this abnormality [1]. These may include: (a) irradiation by X-ray treatment, (b) mechanical agitation of the egg, (c) maternal viral infection, such as, rubella, (d) chemical agents, such as, lithium, selenium, or Trypan Blue, or possibly (e) deficiency or excess of Vitamin A. Animal studies [5] have indicated that the degree of deformity is directly related to the development of the fetus during the early stages. The more severe the anophthalmic condition is, the earlier this abnormality must have occurred. This condition can affect males as well as females without preference. The treatment for the anophthalmic patient is similar to that of the microphthalmic patient. However, use of the progressive sized hard conformers is included in series with spring expanders to help further expand the socket. With congenital anophthalmic patients (Fig. 11), more attention is given to developing the inferior and superior cul-de-sacs, and horizontal palpebral fissure length. The ocularist should note that expansion of the anophthalmic socket is directly related to the bony orbital structure, therefore, it is helpful to have an X ray (Fig. 12) of the skull available to guide in the amount of expansion possible.

The congenital anophthalmic patient should be treated with the progressive sized conformers as early as possible [11]. Realistically this occurs within the first two to six weeks of life. Many of these patients often have other severe medical problems causing their treatment to be delayed.

On examination of the congenital anophthalmic socket, the ocularist must measure the difference in the palpebral fissure openings from one eye to the other. It is also important to measure the bony orbital structure. The first form of treatment is to take an alginate impression of the socket to determine the size and shape of the conformer. This is done under general anesthesia in the majority of cases. While the patient is under anesthesia, the ocularist is given the opportunity to evaluate the socket further for orbital cysts, tissue consistency, and cul-de-sac formation. After making the first conformer (Fig. 13), the patient is seen in the office for the insertion of the appliance (Fig. 4). This can often be a very traumatic experience for

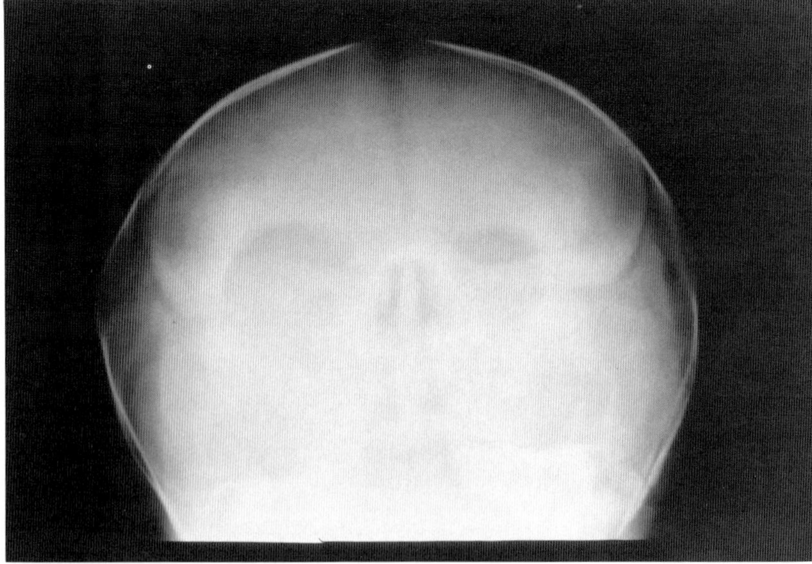

Figure 12. A frontal skull X ray of a one-month-old male showing a small left orbit.

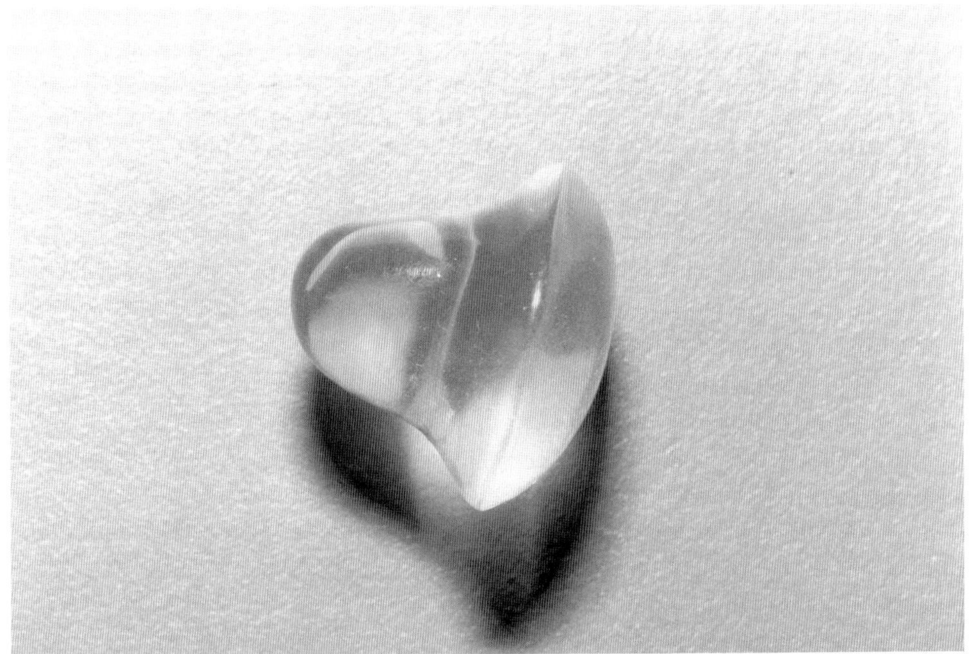

Figure 13. The side view of a conformer used for socket expansion.

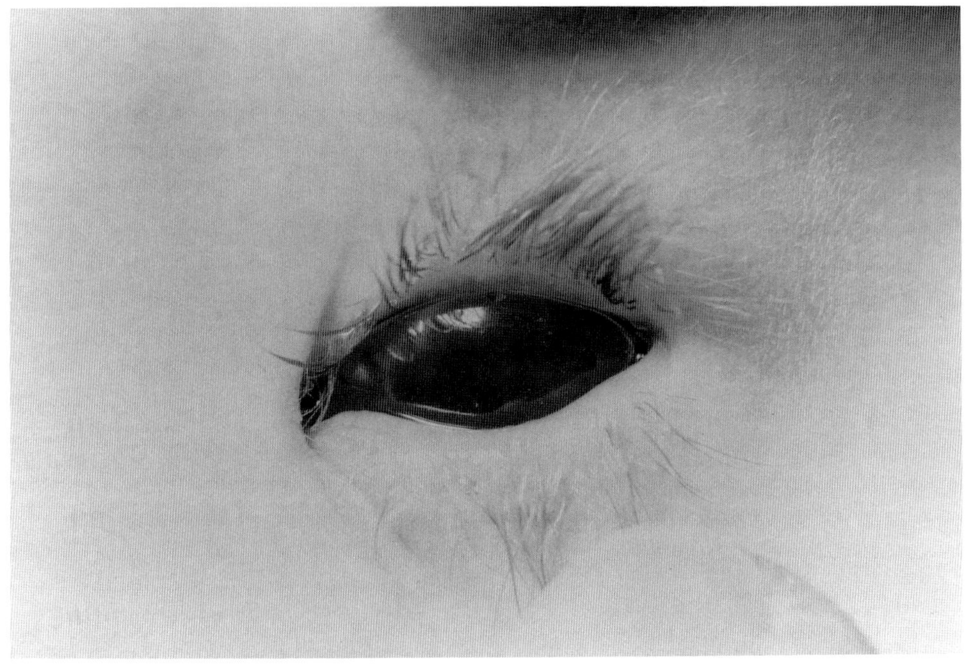

Figure 14. A close-up view of a conformer in place (OS).

both the patient and parents, as well as the ocularist. It is not uncommon to have to redesign the conformer to allow for insertion. The patient wears the first conformer (Fig. 14) for approximately two weeks, and is then re-evaluated for a larger one. If the first conformer appears to be loose and is easily removed, then a larger one is needed. This can be achieved by adding on to the existing conformer to increase its size without taking a new impression. The patient is seen every four to six weeks for evaluation of the conformer. Whenever possible, a larger conformer is made to help with expansion. During the first 12 months of therapy the greatest expansion will be noted.

During the 6th to 24th month of therapy, the ocularist may notice that the socket has expanded at a rate greater than the horizontal palpebral fissure opening. This creates a problem in further expansion of the socket because of the limitation of the lid opening and size of conformer that will pass through. There are presently three forms of treatment to help increase the horizontal palpebral fissure opening. They are: (a) surgical intervention with the use of a lateral canthotomy, (b) the use of a progressive spring expander to put constant pressure on a medial and lateral canthus to encourage expansion, and (c) bony orbital reconstruction, along with a lateral canthotomy. All of these procedures have advantages and disadvantages. The advantage of the lateral canthotomy is its ease of execution, and the instant expansion of the palpebral fissure. The disadvantage is the unpredictable scarring of the lateral canthal area, along with an uncontrollable lid margin configuration. The progressive spring expander (Figs. 15 and 16) [10] is a single spring device designed to place constant pressure on the medial and lateral canthus (Figs. 17 and 18) to increase the horizontal palpebral fissure opening (Figs. 19 and 20). The spring expander offers the advantage of a nonsurgical form of treatment. It expands the palpebral fissures slowly, in turn eliminating the scarring problem. The disadvantage is its slow process. The expander is worn full-time for two to three weeks or longer, then removed and replaced with a larger conformer. The spring expander is

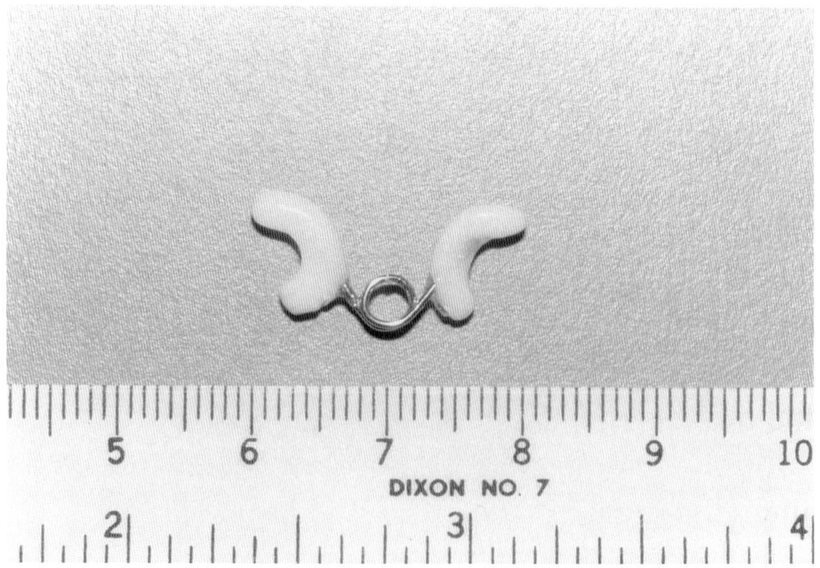

Figure 15. A very small spring expander.

used alternatively with the conformer during the 6th to 24th month of therapy. Note that orbital bone reconstruction has been mentioned in the literature [12] as a form of treatment to help expand the congenital anophthalmic socket. This procedure is risky, and should only be considered as a last alternative when the patient is older.

Following the first year, the degree of expansion takes much longer. The patient is seen every one to two months for the next year. During the start of the second year a painted prosthesis should be considered, even if the openings are not equal. After the age of 3, the patient needs to be seen every six months until the age of 10. Following 10 years of age, yearly appointments are then scheduled. As a child the painted prosthesis is replaced three to four times before the age of 10. Once an adult, the prosthesis is replaced every 8 to 10 years.

It is helpful during the first one to two years of therapy for clear progressive sized conformers to be used. This helps the ocularist in the fitting and ease of manufacturing. However, it is important that a child be fitted with a painted ocular prosthesis by the age of two. A childs' psychological development after the age of two can be permanently scarred without the presence of a painted ocular prosthesis. This is important even if the palpebral fissure openings are not equal, or even close to one another. The use of cosmetic optics is very helpful in giving the appearance of a much larger or longer eye. The image created by prescription lenses worn in glasses can be the difference between satisfaction or disappointment for the congenital anophthalmic patient, and the parents.

The majority of these patients [13] have normal lacrimal excretory systems function, although the eye is absent. This is demonstrated with the normal crying of a child. This will cause mucous and oil coating across the conformer or prosthesis, which is normal for most prosthetic patients. It is important for the surface of the conformer or prosthesis to be kept clean along with the lashes. Removal and cleaning of the device is recommended for every four to eight weeks. Lid scrubs are also helpful in keeping the lashes clean. The use of soap and

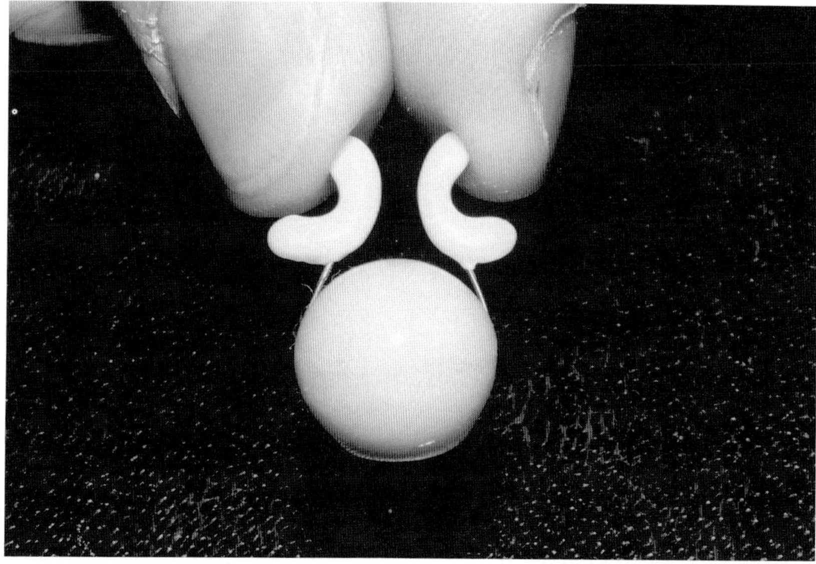

Figure 16. A large spring expander.

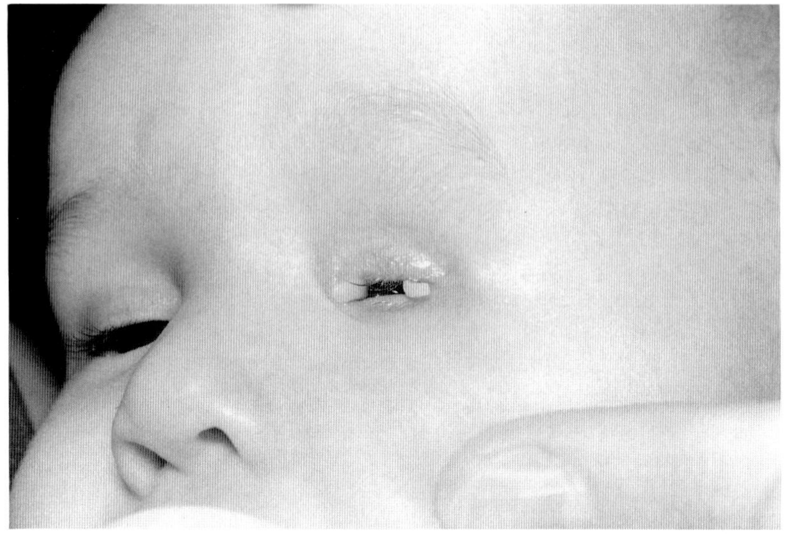

Figure 17. A close-up view of a small spring expander in place, showing horizontal expansion (OS).

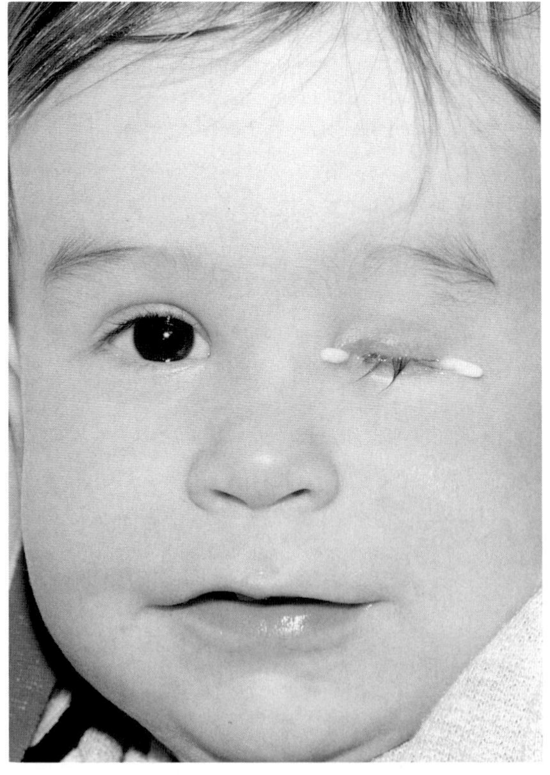

Figure 18. The appearance of a large spring expander in place, showing additional horizontal expansion (OS).

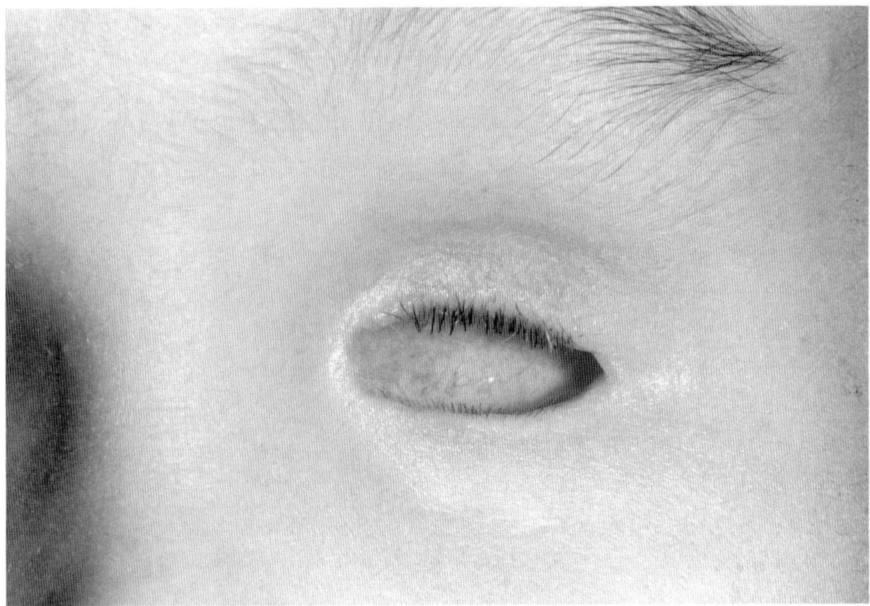

Figure 19. The appearance of an expanded left clinical congenital anophthalmic socket following six years of therapy.

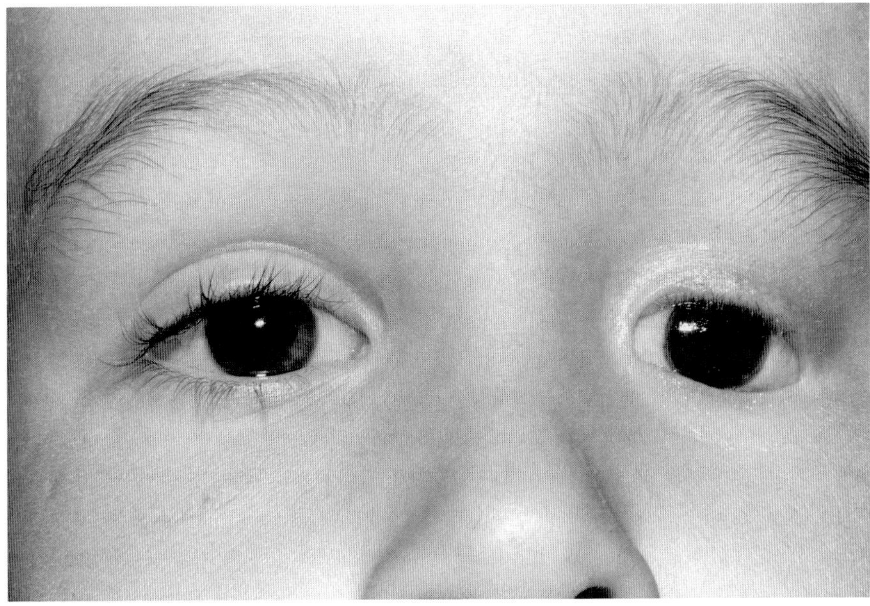

Figure 20. The cosmetic appearance of a custom prosthesis (OS) following six years of socket therapy.

water is the main solution for cleaning. If an infection is suspected, the patient is referred back to the ophthalmologist for evaluation and treatment. If infected, it is advisable *not* to remove the conformer or prosthesis, unless for cleaning. Topical medication can be used over the conformer or prosthesis without removal. The possibility of socket contraction is most likely at this stage.

SUMMARY

Whether the congenital anophthalmic is unilateral or bilateral, the earlier the expansion treatment is started the greater the cosmetic result will be. The current form of treatment as previously discussed, allows for dramatic increases in the underdeveloped socket. Note that the total cosmetic result may not be determined for many years (Fig. 10), therefore, clear communication with the patient, parents, and the referring ophthalmologist is of the utmost importance in achieving the best results possible.

REFERENCES

1. Trannick WR: Congenital anophthalmia & microophthalmia; an overview for the ocularist. *J Am Soc Ocul* 1984; 14:10–13.
2. Price E, Simon JW, Calhoun JH: Prosthetic treatment of severe microphthalmos in infancy. *J Pediatr Ophthalmol Strabismus* 1986; 23:22–24.
3. Small RG, Dalton E: Influence of the ocularist and ophthalmologist in microorbit and microphthalmos. *J Pediatr Ophthalmol Strabismus* 1986; 23:107–112.
4. Van Limborgh J, Tonneyk-Muller I: Orbital growth pattern in experimental microphthalmia. *Mod Probl Ophthalmol* 1975; 14:1–4.
5. Van Limborgh J, Tonneyk-Muller I: Experimental studies on the relationships between eye growth and skull growth. *Ophthalmologica* 1976; 173:317–325.
6. Kok-Van Alphen CC, Manschot WA, Frederiks E, Van Beusekom GT: Microphthalmus and orbital cyst. *Ophthalmologica* 1973; 167:389–392.
7. Lamb VR: Congenital deformities: Maturation in microorbit and microphthalmos. *J Pediatr Ophthalmol Strabismus* 1986; 23:97–106.
8. Skydsgaard H, Hildestad P: Prosthetic treatment of congenital anophthalmia. *Arch Ophthalmol* 1968; 46:513–520.
9. Pritikin RI: The rarity of true congenital bilateral anophthalmos. *Metab Pediatr Ophthalmol* 1980; 4:165–167.
10. Dootz GL: Lid expander for the treatment of anophthalmic patients. *J Am Soc Ocularists* 1984; 14:7–9.
11. Steahly LP: Congenital anophthalmos: Problems in management. *Trans—Ophthalmol Soc U.K.* 1978; 98:28–29.
12. Marchac D, Cophignon J, Achard E, Dufourmentel C: Orbital expansion for anophthalmic and micro-orbitism. *Plast Reconstr Surg* 1977; 59:486–491.
13. Roy FH: Cosmetic treatment of bilateral anophthalmos. *Am J Ophthalmol* 1969; 67:580–583.

Hydrophilic Expanders for the Congenital Anophthalmic Socket

Richard Downes, F.R.C.S., Michael Lavin, F.R.C.S., and Richard Collin, F.R.C.S.

ABSTRACT

The congenitally contracted socket often poses a challenging management problem; early surgery may be necessary in spite of the attendant difficulties.

A series of patients is presented, with particular emphasis upon the use of a new hydrophilic expander in the severely contracted socket, to illustrate our current management protocol. Factors pertinent to orbital development and growth are discussed. Two types of contracted sockets are identified that appear to correlate with the presence or absence of an eye or ocular remnant. Use of a hydrophilic expander in the severely contracted anophthalmic socket with marked lid phimosis has enabled subsequent fitting and retention of a hard conformer in many of these cases, thus obviating early interventional surgery.

INTRODUCTION

Congenitally contracted sockets are unusual but often devastating conditions in which the problems of poor vision or blindness in an infant can be compounded by major facial cosmetic deformity. This combination of handicaps is distressing to the family, and on occasion parents may have difficulty accepting the child. There is clearly great pressure to achieve good cosmesis. Although this is the major goal of treatment in the child with socket contraction, it must be balanced against the adverse effects frequent hospitalization may have on a young child.

Management of the congenitally contracted socket can be one of the most challenging problems encountered by the ophthalmologist. Currently available treatments may be broadly divided into two groups: conservative and surgical. Both aim at expanding the socket with the final common goal of a comfortable prosthesis with good cosmesis.

METHODS

A series of congenitally contracted sockets is described to illustrate our approach to the management of this difficult condition. All patients had been seen by the senior author at Moorfields Eye Hospital, and the hospital notes were reviewed retrospectively.

Those patients requiring fitting of a hydrophilic expander were analyzed separately, and form the bulk of this report. The socket expander used in this study was fashioned from a blank of hydrophilic soft contact lens material (poly-L-hydroxyethylmethacrylate, or HEMA) into a diabaloid shape. A central shaft is drilled in an anteroposterior direction and the shape is attached to a mandrel (a type of prosthetic handle) for ease of manipulation; HEMA has a water uptake of 38.6 units per 100 units of material, thus giving an expansion ratio of 1.19. In principle when this hydrophilic expander (HE) is inserted into a socket, the material hydrates by uptake of adjacent tears or topical lubricants. Young infants have poor aqueous tear production [1] and we have found that adequate hydration of the expander in these patients is often only achieved after use of frequent topical lubricants. Hydration is further facilitated by the central channel in the HE. The effect is one of soft tissue expansion within the socket such that subsequent fitting with a conventional conformer is facilitated.

Some patients required a larger HE following initial socket expansion prior to insertion of a conventional prosthesis. The HE was easily fitted in all cases by an experienced ocular prosthetist without general anesthesia; socket fit and ocular tolerance were assessed at least twice daily during HE wear.

The term ocular remnant is used to refer to a disorganized, vestigial structure, rounded and often cystic, which may be found at any location in the orbital soft tissues. These structures can vary widely in size and position.

RESULTS

Thirty-eight patients were identified with 57 congenitally contracted sockets; the sex ratio was almost even with 20 females and 18 males. Although most patients presented in infancy or early childhood, a small number presented in late childhood or adulthood. The presenting ages ranged from 6 weeks to 15 years, with a mean of 44.1 months. The average follow-up time was 22 months.

Sixteen sockets of 11 patients required HEs to achieve later artificial eye wear. In four sockets a previous hard shape fitting had failed, whereas the remaining patients were deemed to have sockets impossible to fit by any other means from the outset. These patients averaged 8.7 months of age at the time of fitting, with a range of 6 weeks to 3 years. All of these patients had HE fitting for at least 24 hrs (Figs. 1 and 2), with an average of 72 hrs (range 1–9 days). In all cases subsequent fitting with a conventional artificial eye was possible (Fig. 3).

Of the sockets requiring HEs, 14 were anophthalmic and two microphthalmic. The number of anophthalmic sockets in which ocular remnants were present was noted. Only one of the 14 anophthalmic sockets requiring HE fitting had an ocular remnant. This was compared to the 18 remaining anophthalmic sockets (i.e., those not requiring HEs), 12 of which had ocular remnants. This difference is significant (chi square = 11.5, Yates correction = 9.23 $p < 0.01$).

Lid phimosis was common in the group of patients requiring HE, being seen in 11 of the 14 anophthalmic sockets. By contrast, lid phimosis was uncommon in the group of patients not requiring HEs, and was seen in only one of the 20 anophthalmic eyes in this group. This difference was significant (chi square = 19.5, Yates correction 16.4, $p < 0.01$).

Finally, the age at presentation differed between the two groups. Patients requiring HEs presented at a mean age of 8.7 months, whereas the remaining patients presented at a mean of 115 months. This difference in ages was significant (paired t test, $p < 0.05$).

Detailed objective analysis of our patients is difficult because socket measurements, namely palpebral apertures and socket dimensions were both approximate and not always documented. In all patients a moderate or good initial socket expansion was achieved and documented, such that, successful conventional conformers were fitted in all patients. The longer term results (>6 months) after HE show that three of the 17 sockets have not been able to satisfactorily tolerate a conformer. No significant complications have occurred in this series.

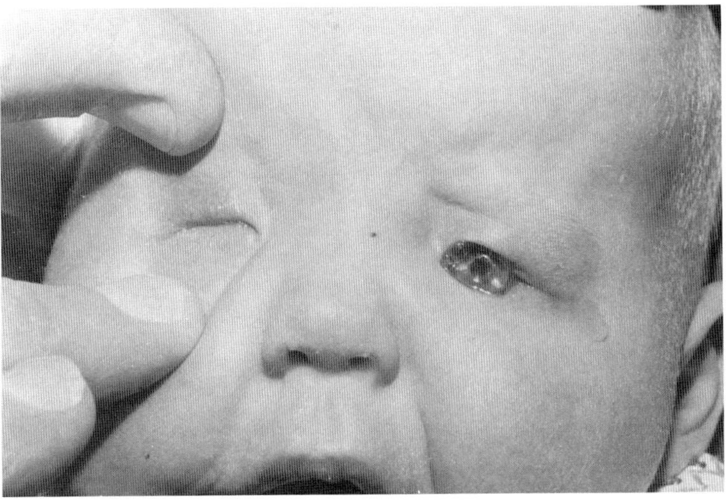

Figure 1. A 3-month-old infant with bilateral anophthalmia demonstrates marked socket contraction on the right. The left socket has been fitted with a hydrophilic expander.

DISCUSSION

The management of the congenitally contracted socket has not been well-addressed in the literature, although the difficulties of management have been noted [2–4].

Note that patients requiring HE fitting presented at a significantly younger age, and had significantly more lid phimosis and fewer ocular remnants than other patients with congenitally contracted sockets.

The factors controlling growth and development of the orbit and its soft tissues are not

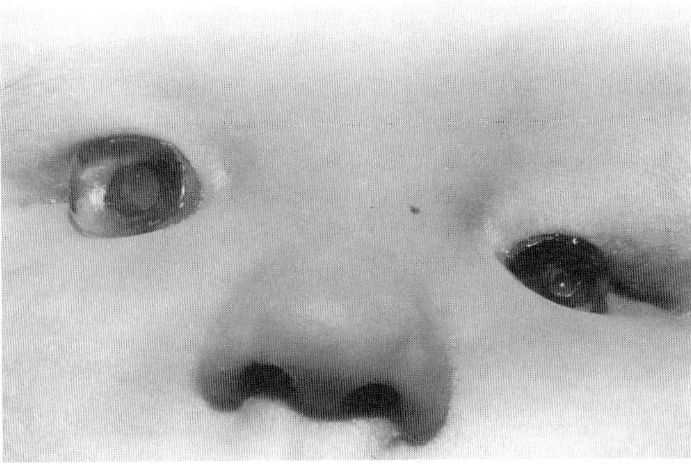

Figure 2. The same infant 24 hrs later with hydrophilic expanders in position. (Note hydration of HE material.)

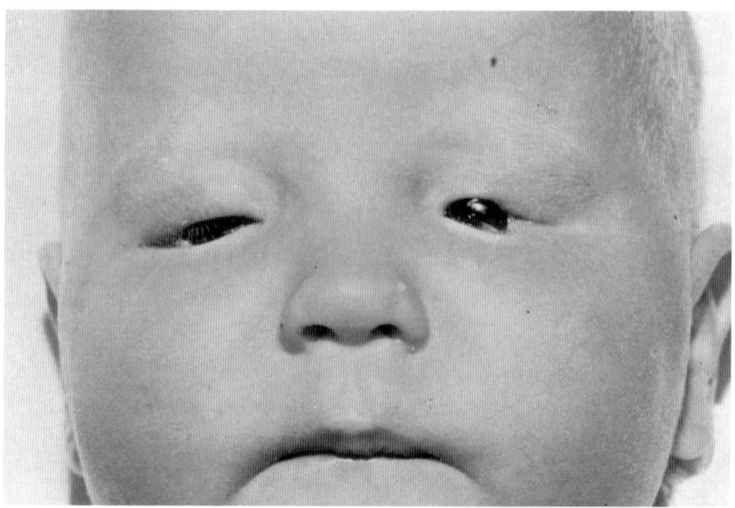

Figure 3. The same child several months later following successful artificial eye fitting, using standard hard materials.

well-understood. The dimensions of the orbital margins, palpebral fissures, and conjunctival fornices at birth are significantly correlated with birth weight [5].

The major determinant of orbital growth appears to be the presence or absence of an eye, and if present its size. Enucleation in infancy results in impaired orbital growth [6,7].

Clinical experience would suggest that microphthalmic eyes have larger sockets than anophthalmic sockets. These observations explain our finding that anophthalmic sockets requiring HEs (i.e., the smallest sockets) had significantly fewer ocular remnants than those not requiring HE fitting (i.e., the larger sockets).

Our clinical impression is that orbital growth can be stimulated by fitting a suitable sized prosthesis to the socket, and that the prosthesis size must be progressively increased to stimulate progressive growth [2–8]. This is supported by the data on orbital growth, and by experimental studies [8–10].

The management of the congenitally contracted socket falls naturally into three phases:

1. In infancy, when significant bony and soft tissue growth is occurring, the aim is to stimulate bony growth from as early an age as possible.
2. In childhood, when bony growth is much less, the aim is to achieve maximal possible bony growth, with soft tissue expansion; enlargement of the mucosal lining frequently requires surgery.
3. In adulthood, when both bony and soft tissue growth have ceased, socket reconstruction is the major tool.

Congenitally contracted sockets generally fall into one of two groups. The first is that of minimal or moderate socket contraction associated with either microphthalmos or significant ocular remnant occurring in a clinically anophthalmic socket. Generally, management of this group is straightforward, with the use of conformer or cosmetic shells of gradually increasing size, which are felt to enhance the orbital development associated with microphthalmos or ocular remnants.

The second category presents a much more difficult management problem; these are the severely contracted sockets occurring with anophthalmos in the absence of significant ocular, albeit disorganized, structures. This group has a very poor prognosis with regard to conservative management. In addition, even multiple surgical procedures may prove singularly disappointing. These patients often have sockets so small as to preclude the fitting of conventional conformers, with marked palpebral phimosis as a regular feature. Procedures designed to allow conformer fitting are often required, although early interventional surgery in these patients causes significant postoperative scarring which limits the eventual success of any surgery performed at a later stage. A new type of socket expander has been used in this group of patients in an attempt to achieve early socket expansion and thus delay or obviate some of the surgical procedures that would otherwise have been indicated.

Use of the HE provided sufficient initial socket expansion to enable fitting with conventional conformers in all cases. This technique therefore reduced the numbers of general anesthetics required in these children. In three sockets this initial improvement was not sustained. One of these cases was fitted at a relatively late age (3 yrs) with simultaneous fornix deepening sutures at the start of the trial. This patient has subsequently required a lateral periosteal flap with mucous membrane grafting, achieving a significant improvement in the dimensions of the palpebral aperture. The other two cases had poor tolerance of any conformer with marked palpebral fibrosis. One patient has had a successful lateral periosteal flap with mucous membrane grafting; the other is awaiting lid surgery. Of the remaining cases satisfactorily tolerating a socket conformer, three are on the waiting list for surgery; two require lengthening of the horizontal palpebral aperture, and one requires a medial lower lid entropion correction.

Note that although the HE has enabled successful fitting of conformers in the majority of cases, it has had little effect on severe palpebral fibrosis which is often seen in the severely contracted socket. Surgery aimed at enlarging the palpebral aperture and deepening the fornices will probably be required eventually in many cases.

In conclusion, the HE represents a significant advance in the early management of the infant with a severely contracted socket. The soft tissue expansion obtained enables successful fitting of a hard conformer in the majority of cases. Although this expander is unlikely to significantly affect palpebral fibrosis it would appear to minimize the requirement for otherwise early surgery and as such represents a significant advance in the management of the severely contracted socket associated with microphthalmos or anophthalmos. Note that, in the management of congenital socket contraction, the earlier treatment with HE is introduced, the more likely is avoidance of early surgery.

REFERENCES

1. Murube-del-Castilla J: Development of the lacrimal apparatus. In Miller B, Weil BA (eds): *The Lacrimal System*, Connecticut, Appleton-Century-Crofts, 1983:12.
2. Steahly LP: Congenital anophthalmos: Problems in management. *Trans Ophthalmol Soc U.K.* 1978; 98:28–29.
3. Pritikin RI: The rarity of true congenital bilateral anophthalmos. *Metab Ped Ophthalmol* 1980; 4:165–167.
4. Collin JRO, Moriarty PAJ: Management of the contracted socket. *Trans Ophthalmol Soc U.K.* 1982; 102:93–97.
5. Isenberg SJ, McCarthy JW, Rich R: Growth of the conjunctival fornix and orbital margin in the term and preterm infant. *Ophthalmology* 1987; 94:1276–1280.
6. Apt L, Isenberg S: Changes in orbital dimensions following enucleation. *Arch Ophthalmol* 1973; 90:393–395.
7. Kennedy RE: The effect of early enucleation on the orbit in animals and humans. *Am J Ophthalmol* 1965; 60:277–305.
8. Sarnat BG: Eye and orbital size in the young and adult. *Ophthalmologica* 1983; 185:74–89.
9. Schultz AH: The size of the orbit and of the eye in primates. *Am J Phys Anthrop* 1940; 26:389–408.
10. Duke-Elder WS: *System of Ophthalmology, Vol XIII, Part II* 1974:1012–1014.

An Expansion Prosthesis for the Microphthalmic Socket

Robert G. Small, M.D., Henry LaFuente, Ocularist, and James M. Richard, M.D.

ABSTRACT

An expansion prosthesis has been developed for the anophthalmic or microphthalmic socket. Orthodontic wire covered with silicone tubing is fused onto a conventional methyl-methacrylate ocular prosthesis. The use of this device is illustrated in a case report.

INTRODUCTION

Infants with microphthalmos or anophthalmos present a challenging problem to the ophthalmologist and ocularist. The goal of treatment is to enlarge the microphthalmic socket so that a prosthesis the size of a normal eye can be worn. Stretching of the anophthalmic socket with acrylic conformers of increasing size as the infant grows into childhood was described in 1949 by Kiskadden et al. They cite the work of Prijibylskaya, from Russian literature in 1931, which may be the earliest report of this method [1]. This technique continues to be recommended in current textbooks of oculoplastic surgery [2,3]. Most authorities recommend nonoperative socket stretching rather than eyelid or socket surgery [2].

One of the authors (HLF) developed an expansion prosthesis for anophthalmos or microphthalmos that uses the principle of progressive socket stretching with two advantages over conventional acrylic socket expanders. The first is the immediate use of an expansion prosthesis that looks like an eye. The achievement of a more normal appearance early in infancy reduces the anxiety of parents distraught by the occurrence of microphthalmos in their child. Secondly, silicone-covered metal posts project anteriorly from the medial and lateral margin of the prosthesis. These posts are bent outward at intervals by the ocularist or parents to progressively stretch the medial and lateral canthi. The use of the device is illustrated in a case report.

MATERIALS AND METHODS

A standard methyl-methacrylate prosthesis is fabricated by sculpting dental wax to fit the microphthalmic socket. A small prosthetic expander is made from the sculpted wax in the same way as a conventional ocular prosthesis. A hole is drilled in the back of the prosthesis to accommodate a piece of orthodontic wire (Tru-chrome orthodontic wire, Rocky Mountain Co., Denver, Colorado, Size .045″ = 1.14 mm). The wire is bent 90° where it exits medially and laterally from the prosthesis so that two metal posts extend anteriorly approximately

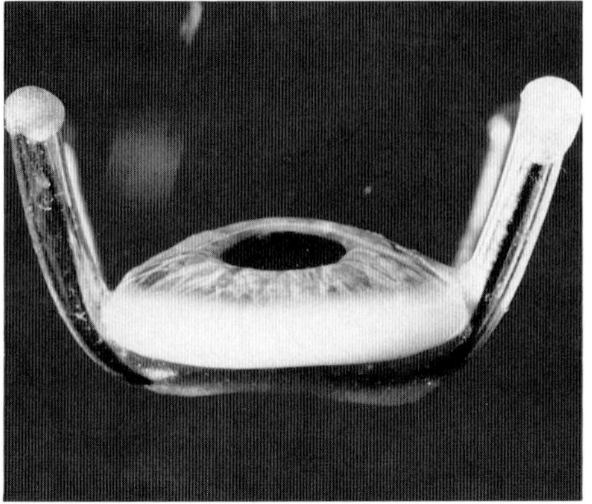 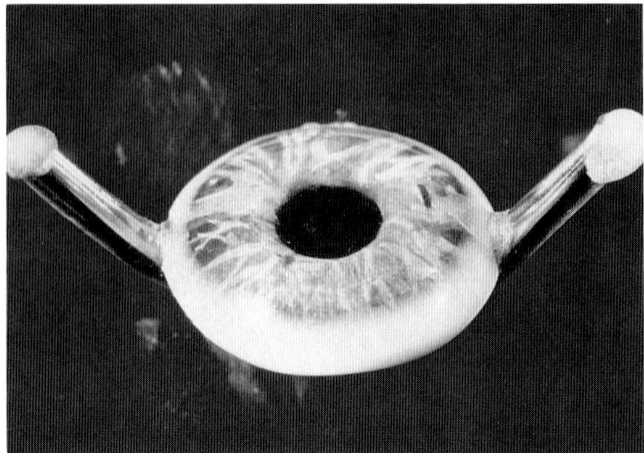

Figure 1. Expansion prosthesis—arms upright.   **Figure 2.** Expansion prosthesis—arms bent outward.

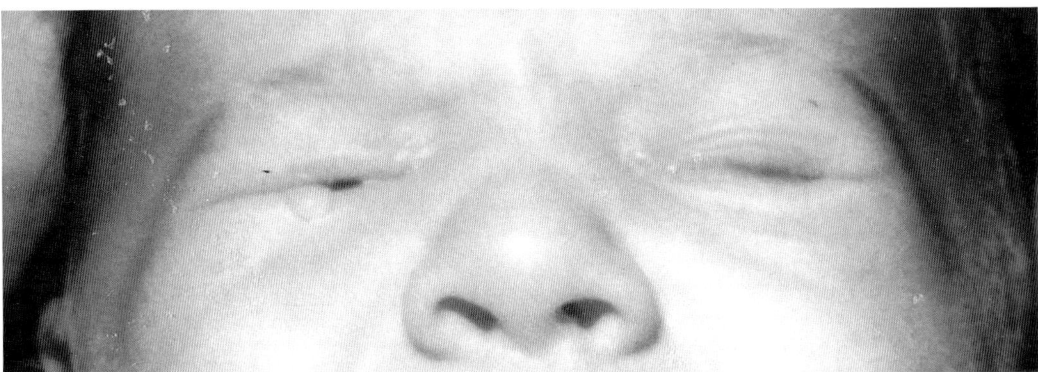

Figure 3. Patient age three months before fitting of prosthesis.

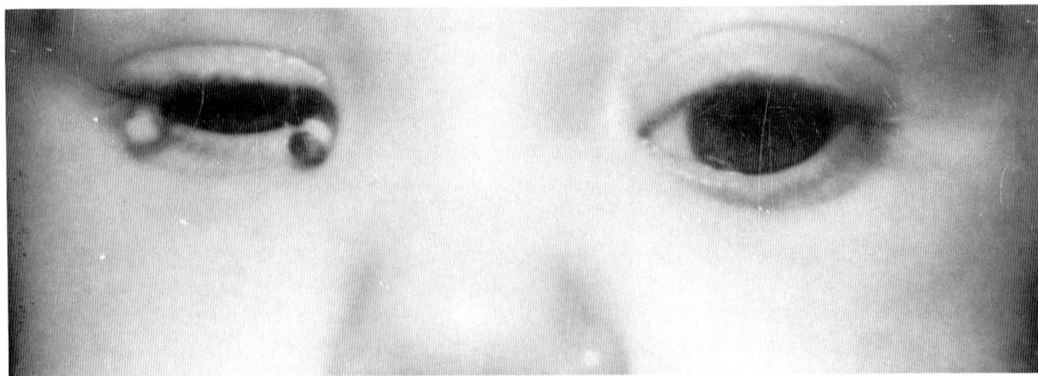

Figure 4. Patient age nine months; expansion prosthesis in place.

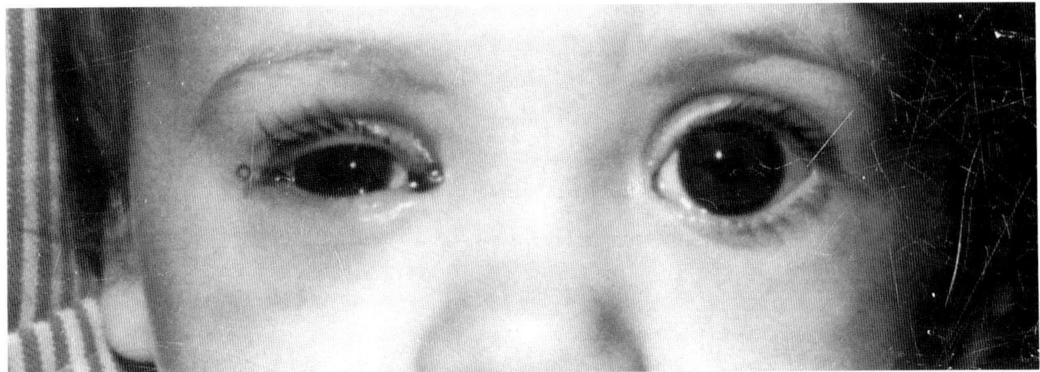

Figure 5. Patient age 15 months; expansion prosthesis in place.

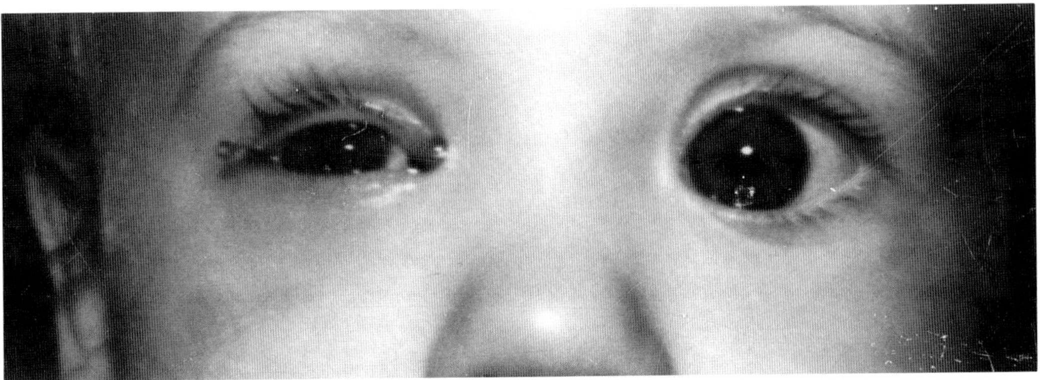

Figure 6. Patient age 18 months; expansion prosthesis in place.

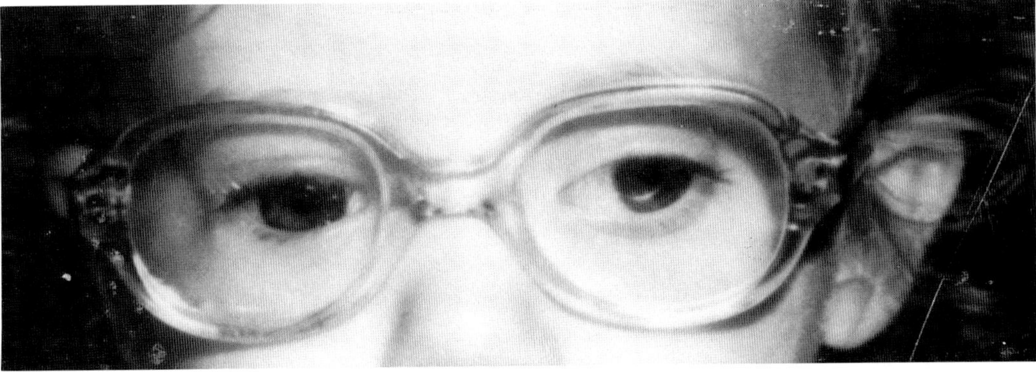

Figure 7. Patient age 24 months with conventional ocular prosthesis.

8 mm. When the prosthesis is in place, the posts project anteriorly about 2 mm from the skin surface. These posts are covered with silicone obtained from an intravenous infusion set (Deseret Co., Sandy, Utah, Catalog #5310). Liquid acrylic is placed on the ends of the tubing. This hardens and covers the ends of the wire (Figs. 1 and 2).

CASE REPORT

A white female patient was born on 8 December 1983 with a microphthalmic right eye and normal left eye. Figure 3 shows the appearance of the patient at age 3 months before fitting of the first expansion prosthesis. Figure 4 shows the expansion prosthesis in place at age 9 months. Figure 5 is the appearance at age 15 months and Figure 6 shows the patient at age 18 months. Figure 7 is the patient with a conventional ocular prosthesis at age 24 months.

DISCUSSION

Expanders that produce anteroposterior pressure with posts, silicone dipped springs, and bent silicone rods have been suggested by Soll and Asbell [4]. However, the device described here is the first that provides medial and lateral canthal stretching. The ocularist or parents can expand the prosthesis by periodically bending the posts outward when the prosthesis becomes loose. When maximum outward angulation of the posts is obtained and the entire prosthesis becomes loose, another expansion prosthesis is constructed to fit the enlarged socket. Definitive progressive stretching of the medial and lateral canthi is achieved with the pressure produced by the metal posts. The superior and inferior fornices are enlarged by progressive enlargement of the upper and lower margins of the prosthesis itself in the same manner as conventional acrylic expanders. The use of a prosthesis rather than an acrylic expander, combined with expansion posts to stretch the medial and lateral canthi has given encouraging results in the patient presented. Continued evaluation of this technique is suggested.

Note — Since the submission of this manuscript, three additional patients have been successfully treated with the expansion prosthesis.

REFERENCES

1. Kiskadden WS, McDowell AJ, Keiser T: Results of early treatment of congenital anophthalmos. *Plast Reconstr Surg* 1949; 4:426–433.
2. Callahan MA, Callahan A: *Ophthalmic Plastic and Orbital Surgery*. Birmingham, AL, Aesculapius Publishing Co., 1979:33–34.
3. Silverstone PJ, Beyer-Machule CK, Schaefer DP: Treatment of anophthalmos and socket reconstruction. In: Smith BC (ed): *Ophthalmic Plastic and Reconstructive Surgery*, St. Louis, MO, CV Mosby Co., 1987:1329–1331.
4. Soll DB, Asbell RL: Congenital anophthalmos — experimental devices in socket expansion. In: Guibor P, Gouglemann HP (eds): *Problems and Treatment of Contracted Sockets, Exenterated Orbit, Alkali Burns*. New York, Intercontinental Medical Book Corporation, 1973:43–49.

Orbito-Palpebral Reconstruction in Anophthalmos and Severe Congenital Microphthalmos

Serge Morax, M.D. and T. Hurbli, M.D.

ABSTRACT

In patients with congenital anophthalmos and severe microphthalmos, a tiny orbit and socket exist with little eyelids, frequently preventing retention of a standard conformer or prosthesis. Socket expansion is sometimes impossible with microorbitism; the retention of a prosthesis is also difficult when malformations of the eyelids exist.

The treatment of these difficult cases includes three stages. The first stage is orbital expansion that depends on the cephalometric studies of the patient: transverse osteotomy on the maxilla and the zygomatic bone with lateral bar by extracranial route, vertical osteotomy on the roof of the orbit by intracranial route. In some cases, the osteotomy includes expansion in the transverse and vertical diameter with bone grafts in the defects and on the lateral and superior rims. Simultaneously, socket expansion is performed by incision of the conjunctival sac circumferentially, with mucosal or split skin grafts on a conformer.

The second stage includes eyelid reconstruction by different flaps. A third stage is frequently needed for correction of eyelid malposition on the prosthesis: ptosis, entropion surgery.

Two cases of congenital anophthalmos are reported. Methods and indications of treatment are discussed.

INTRODUCTION

Anophthalmos and severe microphthalmos without colobomatous cysts are rare congenital malformations of the ocular area, their treatment is purely cosmetic and often disappointing. The aim of the treatment is to fit an immobile esthetic prosthesis that will often be too small because of the reduction in size of the orbit and its contents.

This goal becomes essential as early as the first months of life, and allows enhancement of the orbital growth by regular and gradual replacement of the prosthesis with a larger one, thereby delaying orbito-palpebral surgery (Fig. 1A and B). In some cases, microorbitism or atresia of the socket will prevent the fitting of a conformer and compel early surgical procedures.

We report two cases of severe anophthalmos that gained benefit from orbito-palpebral reconstructive surgery.

REPORT OF CASES

CASE 1

A 12-year-old Cambodian girl (Fig. 2) presented with a right congenital anophthalmos. No family history. Past history included a ductus arteriosus operated at age 9 and a congenital distichiasis of both lids of the other eye operated at age 2.

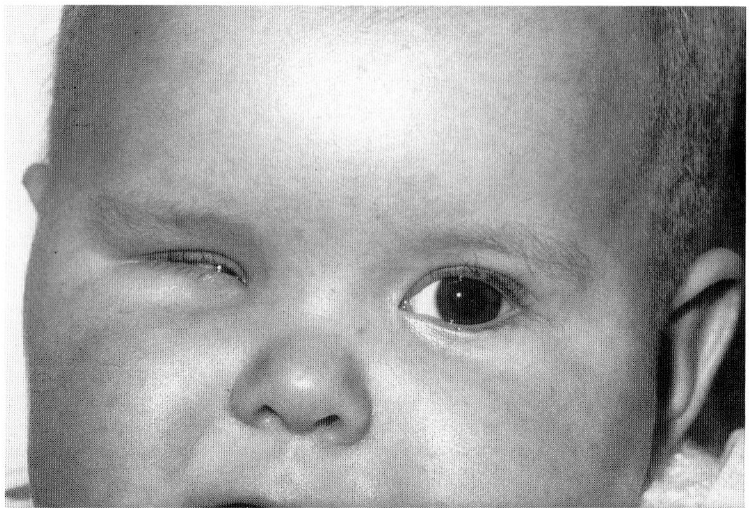

A

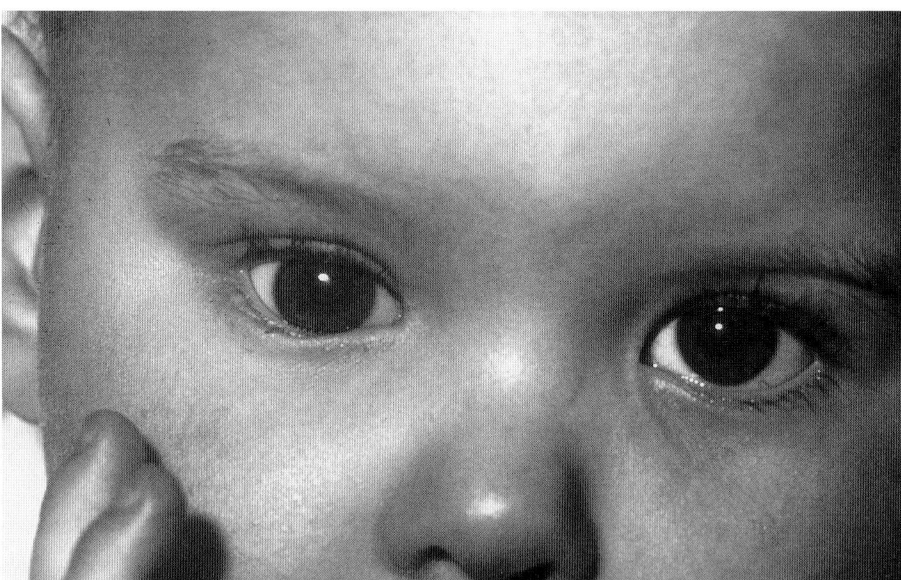

B

Figure 1. (A) Severe congenital microphthalmos at six months of age. (B) Result at one year of life after gradual enlargement of prosthesis.

Upon examination, the right orbital cavity showed atresia of its fundus and fornices. The eyelids were small: microblepharos of the upper eyelid with subnormal ciliary implantation, total ptosis with no levator function; the lower lid was almost nonexistent (Fig. 2A). CT-scan and X-ray investigations showed a microorbitism with important lessening of the transverse orbital diameter by hyperostosis of the maxillary, malar bone, and external pillar of the orbit. The vertical diameter of the orbit was slightly diminished but the roof and the upper orbital rim were only a bit lowered as indicated by the normal eyebrow level as compared to the other side (Fig. 2A). A primary optic nerve and nonfunctional oculomotor muscles were present deep in the orbit. No colobomatous cyst could be found. There were no lacrymal canaliculi. The left eye was normal; the eyelids show scars of the previous distichiasis procedure.

No anomaly could be found on the remaining craniofacial examination: no craniostenosis, no facial cleft or 1st brachial arch syndrome. No other systemic ailment was present except for the operated cardiovascular anomaly. Psychomotor development was excellent but the child was very much affected by her orbital malformation. It was impossible to fit a prosthesis in this tiny socket; a surgical protocol was set up to expand the small anophthalmic socket, including four stages scheduled over a one-year period from May 1984 to June 1985 (Fig. 2B).

First Step. Widening of the bony orbit is completed at the expense of the vertical and transverse diameter by extracranial approach combined with expansion of the socket by labial mucosal graft (Fig. 2C and D).

By extracranial coronal approach, a complete subperiosteal dissection of the orbit is performed. The transverse diameter is widened by mobilization of half of the external orbital rim and grinding of the external wall, infero-external and supero-external angle of the orbit. The vertical diameter is widened by collapsing the orbital floor while preserving the inferior orbital rim. The sagittal diameter is increased by apposition grafts of the newly formed lateral orbital rim. Simultaneously, the conjunctival sac was incised and dissected toward the fornices, expansion of the socket was accomplished by fitting a hollow implant covered by two labial mucosal grafts, the curved surface being externally directed (Fig. 2E and F). A tarsorrhaphy is then performed and left in place two months to ensure consolidation of the socket and its adaptation to the newly formed bony orbit.

Second Step. The tarsorrhaphy is released two months later. The external part of the still narrow socket is enlarged by another labial mucosal graft that is kept in place with a conformer.

Third Step. The almost absent lower eyelid (nearly a case of total ablepharon) that prevented the retention of the conformer is reformed using an orbitonasogenial flap lined with a labial mucosal graft.

Fourth Step. This last step includes the correction of the residual upper eyelid ptosis on a temporary prosthesis by suspension to the frontalis muscle.

After a one year follow-up, the result is considered satisfying, with an almost complete symmetry in the straightforward gaze and static position (Fig. 2G and H).

CASE 2

An 18-year-old Algerian female patient (Fig. 3A) with no family history, presented with a left congenital anophthalmos, as part of a first brachial arch syndrome (Goldenhar's syndrome) as shown by the left preauricular appendix, the right external canthus dermolipoma, and the right limbic dermoid.

Examination of the left orbital and facial areas showed a congenital anophthalmos with

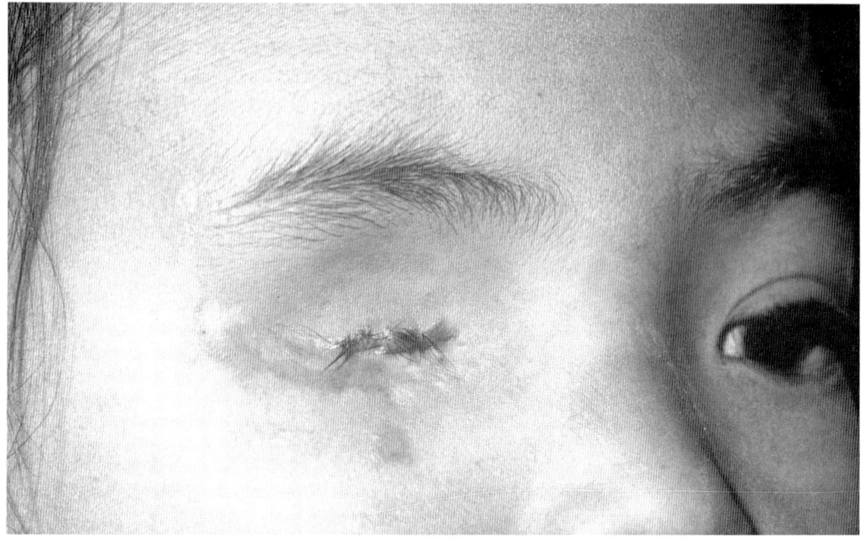

A

B

Figure 2. (A) Right congenital anophthalmos. Tiny socket—Microblepharon and Microorbitism. (B) Tiny socket preventing retention of a standard conformer. (*Figure continued on the following pages.*)

atresia of the cavity. A relative microblepharon was present, the lids being short in length and in height. Although entropion was present, the ciliary margin was present and the upper lid was ptotic; the function of the levator was difficult to assess. There was a malformation and malposition of the eyebrow; on one side there was hypertrichosis with reduction in length, on

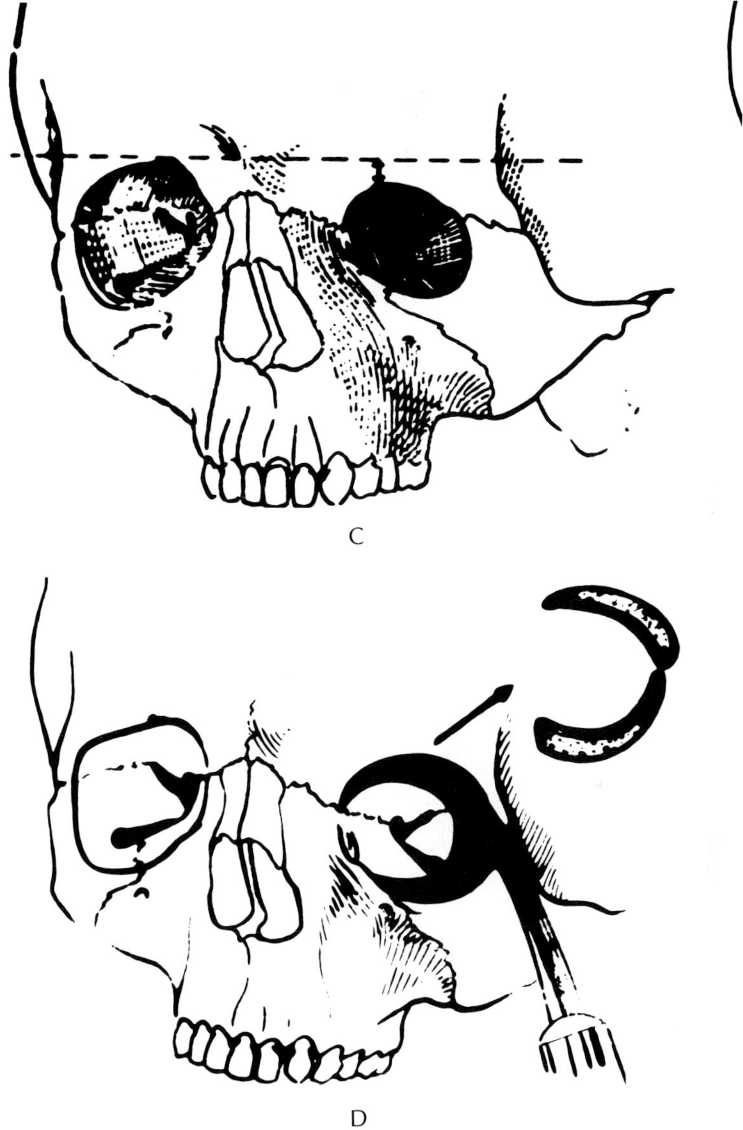

Figure 2 continued. (C) Microorbitism involving vertical and transverse diameters (left side). (D) Microorbitism correction: (left side) according to Tessier's technique, by extracranial route expansion in the vertical and transverse diameters, bone grafts in the defects. (Figures 2C and 2D reproduced with permission from Rougier J, Tessier P, Hervouet F, Woillez M, Lekieffre M, Derome P: *Chirurgie Plastique Orbito-Palpébrale*. Rapport SF (ed), Masson, Paris, 1977.)

the other, a 1 cm level lowering as compared to the other side was explained by the lowering of the roof of the orbit.

Radiological and CT-scan investigations revealed an important (Fig. 3B) microorbitism, with reduction of the vertical (lowering of the supraorbital rim and roof of the orbit) and

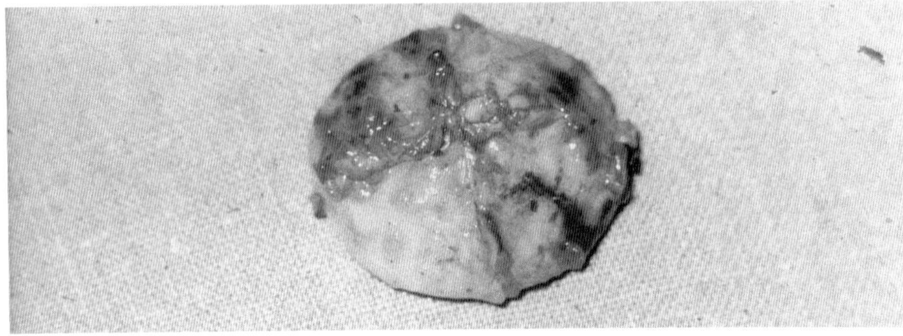

E

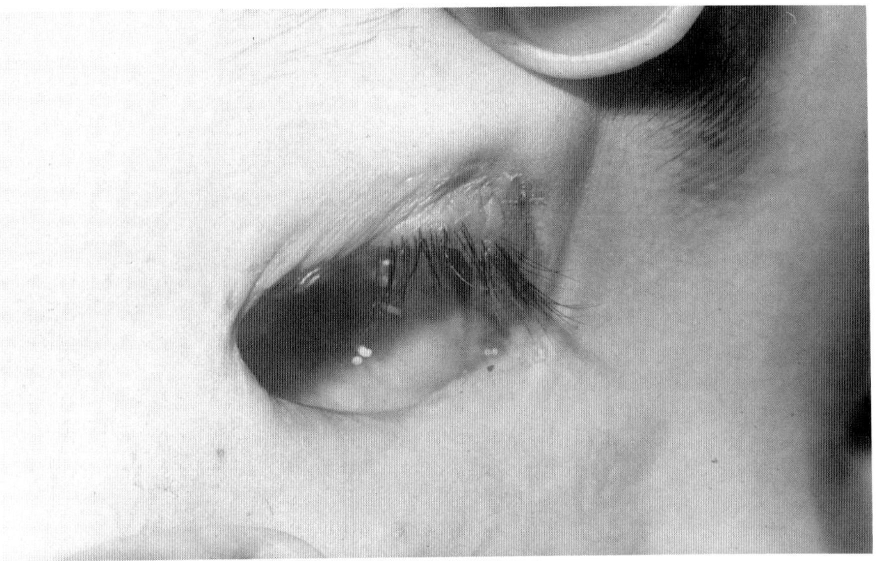

F

Figure 2 continued. (E) Simultaneously, socket expansion is performed with buccal mucosal graft on conformer. (F) Postoperative appearance of the cavity after orbit and socket expansion.

transverse diameter (hyperostosis of the external orbital pillar). In the orbital apex, an embryonic optic nerve and an ocular stump are found. The remainder of the general examination was normal.

The surgical treatment of this left congenital anophthalmos (or severe microphthalmos, because of the presence of an ocular stump) was performed by three successive operations separated by periods of two months.

First Step. This step consisted of correction of the microorbitism by orbital expansion and treatment of the atretic socket by an epithelial inlay (Fig. 3C).

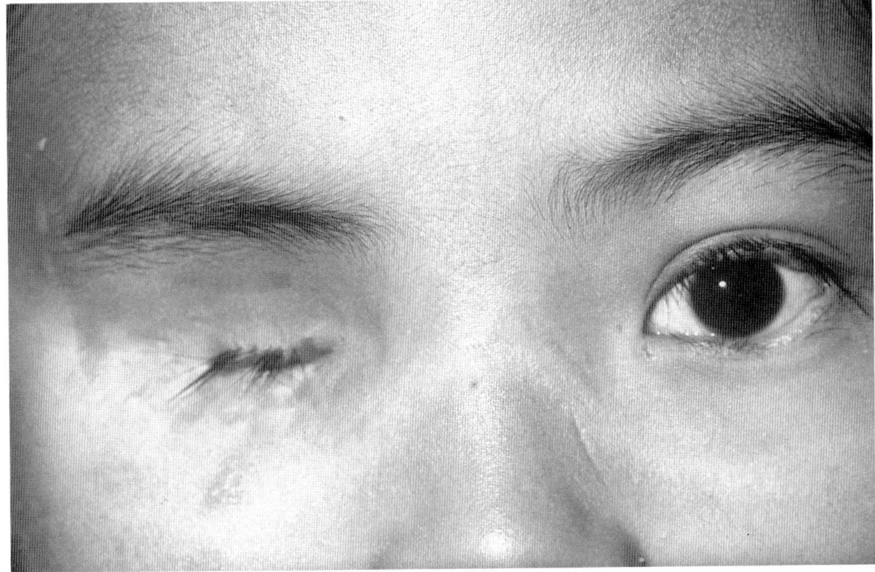

G

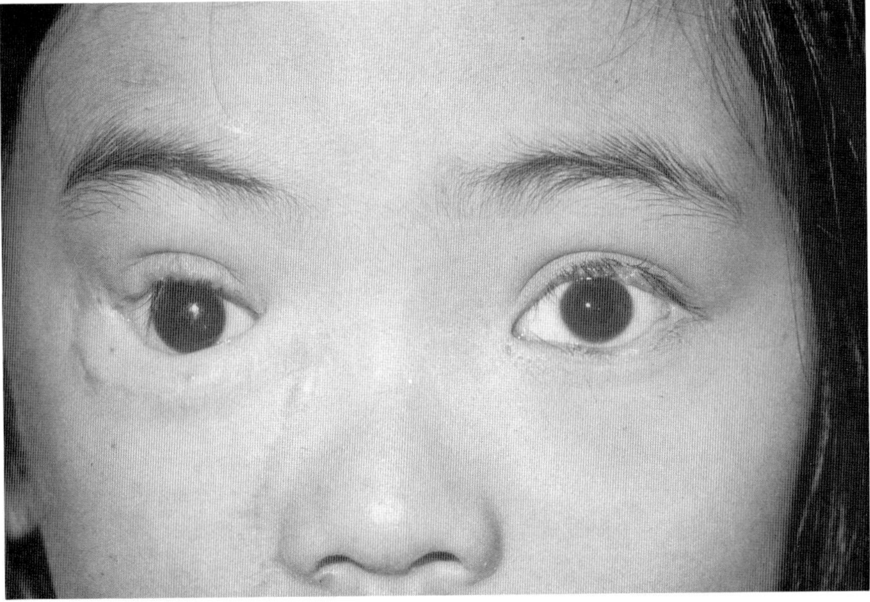

H

Figure 2 continued. (G) Right congenital anophthalmos. Preoperative appearance. (H) Right congenital anophthalmos. Postoperative final result after: orbital and socket expansion; inferior eyelid reconstruction by ONG flap; blepharoptosis correction by frontalis muscle suspension; prosthesis fabrication.

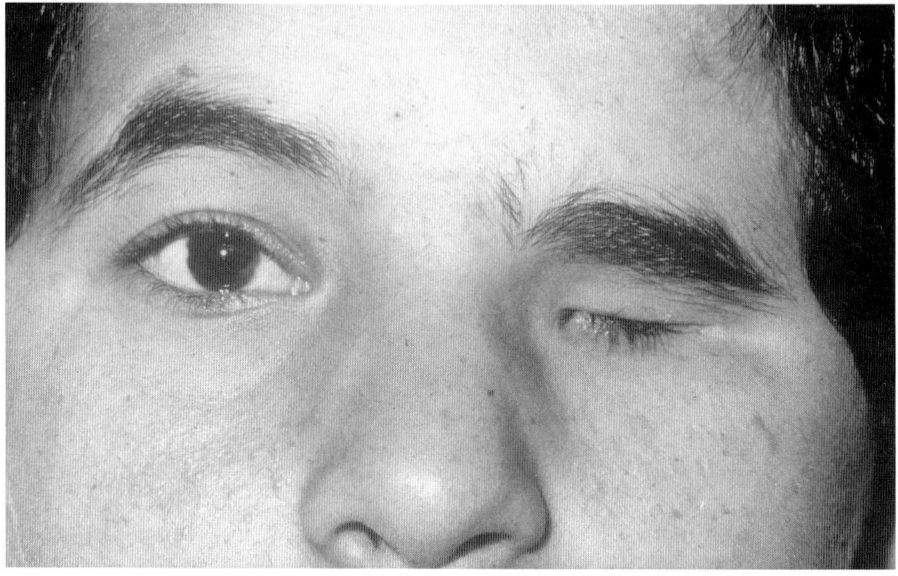

A

Figure 3. (A) Left congenital anophthalmos. Goldenhar syndrome. Tiny socket. Microblepharon and Microorbitism. (*Figure continued on the following pages.*)

The approach was coronal and intracranial, a frontal flap was developed, the base of the brain was reclined, and the orbital roof elevated by 1 cm. The external wall of the orbit was enlarged by reduction of the internal half of the lateral orbital rim and by grinding of the external wall, infero-external angle and supero-external angle of the orbit. The floor was lowered by an infra-orbital approach sparing the infra-orbital rim. The vertical and transverse diameters of the orbit are therefore increased (Fig. 3C).

In the same setting, the socket was enlarged by a deep incision and dissection towards the fornices, then implantation of a thin dermo-epidermal graft (taken from the internal part of the thigh) maintained in place by a hollow implant and a total tarsorrhaphy for a two-month period (Fig. 3D).

Second Step. This step consisted in releasing the tarsorrhaphy, checking the size of the cavity that by now became appropriate (Fig. 3E) and elevating the eyebrow by resection of the hypertrichosis. A temporary prosthesis was fitted in the cavity.

Third Step. This step consisted in adjusting the palpebral malpositions on the prosthesis (Fig. 3F and G). Upper eyelid ptosis was corrected by levator resection technique, straightening the upper ciliary margin by external application and reformation of the palpebral crease. The cicatricial entropion of the lower lid was adjusted with a conchal cartilage graft to correct the shortening of the tarso-conjunctival plane and straightening of the lower ciliary margin.

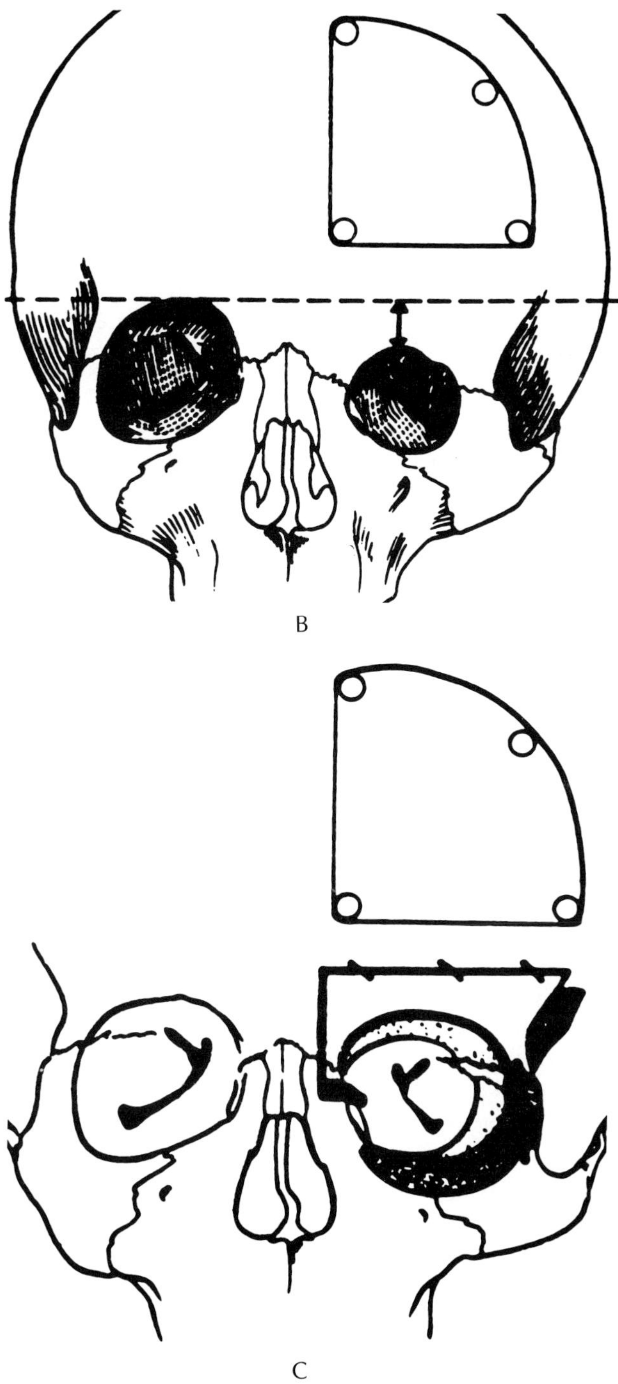

Figure 3 continued. (B) Microorbitism involving vertical diameter. (C) According to Tessier's technique, by intracranial route, orbital roof expansion, bone grafts in the defects. (Figures 3B and 3C reproduced with permission from Rougier J, Tessier P, Hervouet F, Woillez M, Lekieffre M, Derome P: *Chirurgie Plastique Orbito-Palpébrale*. (Rapport SF (ed), Masson, Paris, 1977.)

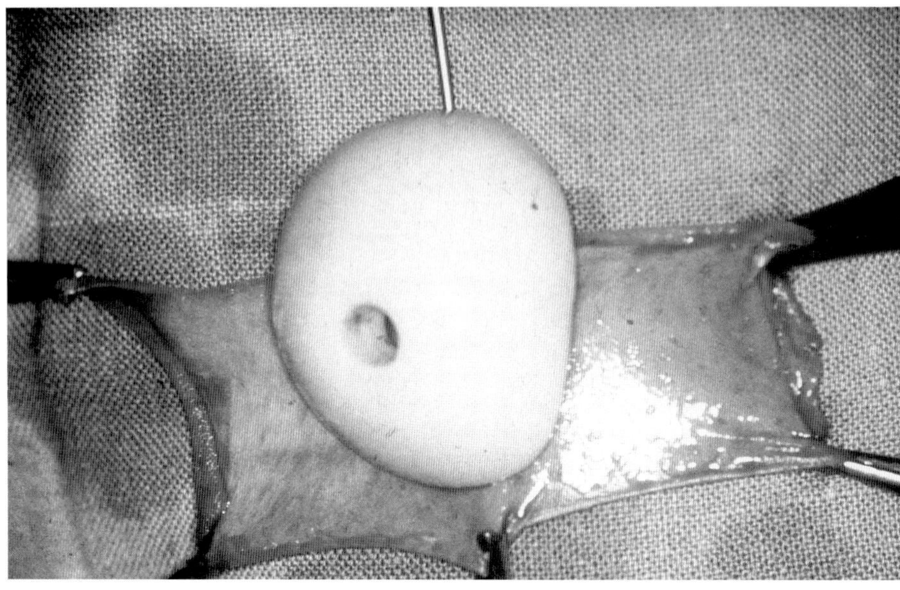

D

Figure 3 continued. (D) Simultaneously, socket expansion is performed with a split-skin graft on conformer.

DISCUSSION

As encountered in the reported cases, congenital anophthalmos is always accompanied by severe orbito-palpebral malformations [1]. The eyelids are short, atrophic, and immobile. The levator muscle is absent. The degree of the anomaly varies, ranging from small but well-formed lids with normal ciliary implantation to complete ablepharon.

The socket is atrophic with no symblepharon, it can easily be subject to expansion if the bony orbit is not too small. If it is too small, the orbit can be investigated radiologically, the atresia can be both transverse and vertical; transverse by hyperostosis of the external orbital wall and vertical by lowering of the orbital roof. Disappearance of the supero-external angle of the orbit may be associated. The internal wall and floor are seldom modified.

Upon examination of a congenital anophthalmos the size of the socket is evaluated and essentially the anomalies of the orbito-palpebral adnexa.

The aim of the treatment is to fit a stable aesthetically acceptable prosthesis. This is only possible if the socket is specially prepared with an enlarged bony orbit and lengthened eyelids.

The first stage of the treatment includes dilatation of the socket by conformers of progressively increasing sizes. This must be started as early as the first months of life, and repeated at regular intervals (every month in the beginning) until age 18 months; most frequently at this age the socket cannot be enlarged any more because of a relative microorbitism.

Surgical treatment is considered when socket enlargement is impossible, either because the conformer treatment was never started or when the expansion is stopped by a small orbit.

It is difficult to estimate the best age to perform the first surgical procedure, especially concerning orbital osteotomies. Opinions are different in various publications. Some authors suggest waiting until the end of facial growth [2,3], others suggest operating at around 6 or 8 years of age. Operated and published cases are too few to be able to draw conclusions. Our two pa-

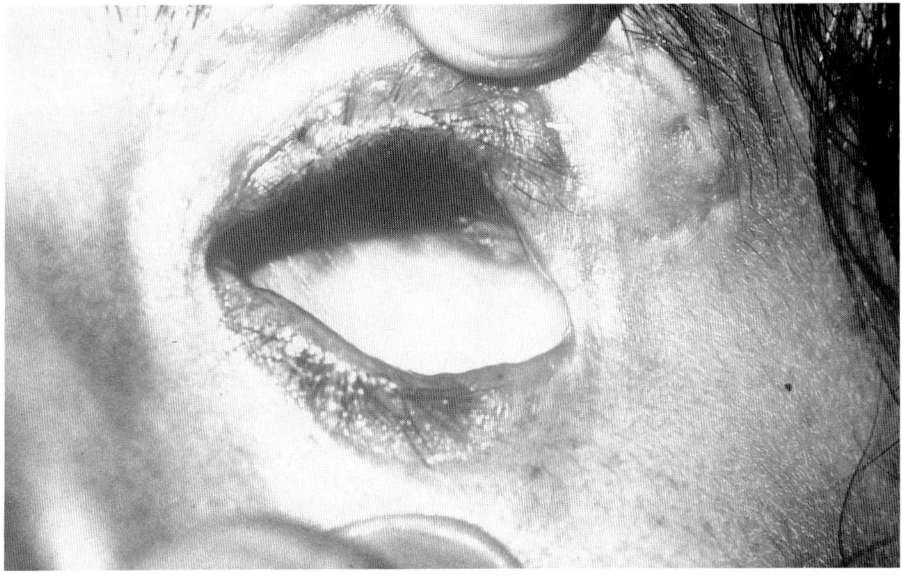

E

Figure 3 continued. (E) Postoperative appearance of the cavity after orbit and socket expansion.

tients were operated upon at ages 12 and 18. In the first case we had to wait until age 12 to obtain good operative conditions (treated congenital cardiopathy); in the second case it was the first consultation of this 18-year-old girl, and no previous treatment was suggested to her until that age.

Because of the advances in craniofacial surgery introduced by P. Tessier [4], there seems to be no objections to start an orbital surgical treatment in early childhood (3 to 4 years); this was done on a recent patient. The procedure, as well as the postoperative course, do not seem more complicated. The short-term results were satisfactory, but time will indicate whether this will persist on long-term follow-up.

Surgical indications depend on several criteria, especially on the inability to enlarge the socket by nonsurgical techniques, on the child's age, on the desire of the surgeon and the family to correct the maximum number of abnormalities as early as possible. In other words, each situation must be individualized.

Because the manifestations are protean, the surgical treatment is difficult to classify. Only general indications can be drawn. Treatment must be aimed on three narrowly linked symptoms: the bony orbit, the socket, and palpebral malformations and malpositions.

First Step. The first surgical step must include expansion of the orbital cavity and socket. If atresia of the transverse orbital diameter exists, expansion of the bony orbit is done by an extra-cranial approach. After subperiosteal dissection of the whole orbit, the transverse diameter is enlarged by resection to the external temporal fossa and by collapsing of the internal orbital wall. A modelling resection of the supero-external angle of the orbit and of the external orbital pillar will allow enlargement of the palpebral aperture and will be used as bony

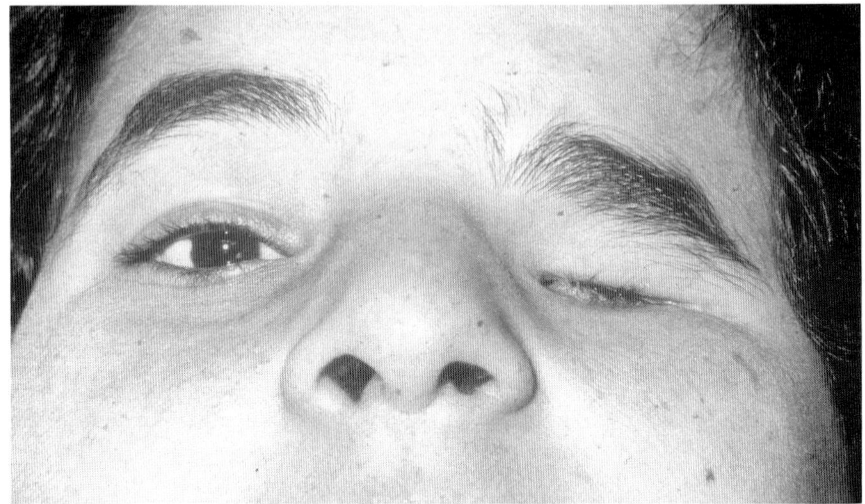

F

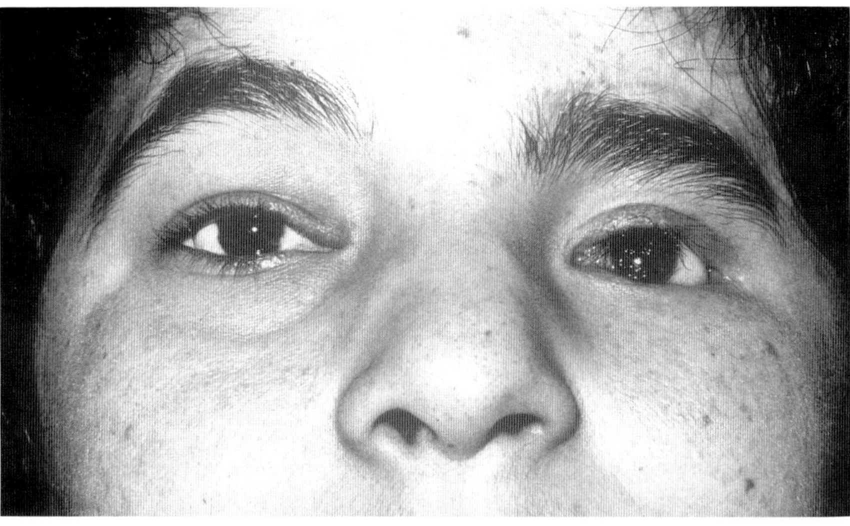

G

Figure 3 continued. (F) Left congenital anophthalmos. Preoperative appearance. (G) Left congenital anophthalmos. Postoperative appearance after: expansion of the orbit and socket; prosthesis fabrication; correction of the palpebral malpositions on prosthesis (entropion, blepharoptosis), and upward eyebrow displacement.

graft to reform the hypoplastic orbital rims. Collapsing of the orbital floor and perforation of the roof may enhance the vertical diameter.

In atresia cases of the vertical diameter of the orbit, an intracranial approach is necessary. It allows elevation of the roof and supra-orbital edge, and resection of the inferior border of the superior orbital rim that will be used as bony graft in remodeling hypoplastic orbital contours. Simultaneously, the other walls will be collapsed or perforated according to the clinical, radiological, and perioperative findings.

This bony orbit expansion aims at enlargement of the socket that must be done in the same setting. Indeed, orbital cavity expansion results in dead space subject to hematomas, infections, and retractions if the socket is not expanded at the same time.

Enlargement of the socket must allow the fitting of an implant that will be adapted to the new orbit. According to the amount of tissue to be grafted, this will be performed either by a labial mucosal graft on a conformer or by a thin dermo-epidermal graft for larger cavities.

A two-month subtotal temporary tarsorrhaphy is essential because it will allow retention of the implant and grafts associated with the orbital expansion and prevent any retraction or early rejection of the implant. There is a natural tendency for exteriorization of the implant if placed behind malformed lids. A partial opening in the tarsorrhaphy allows the drainage of secretions preventing any infection.

During dissection of conjunctival fornices and because of the atrophy of the orbital fat, contact with the periosteum is rapid and must be preserved for protection of the osteotomies and bony grafts.

Second Step. The second surgical step must include the release of the tarsorrhaphy, and verification of cavity and lids. If the cavity is still small, a second cutaneous or labial mucosal graft, again maintained in place by conformer and tarsorrhaphy, might be considered; this was done in the first case. If the lids are small or prevent the retention of the conformer, palpebral reconstruction is a must, according to well-known principles. Doubling the upper eyelid length by transfer of the lower eyelid and reconstruction of the latter by a temporo-jugal flap was proposed [2,4]. In the first case reconstruction of the lower lid and Tessier's orbito-naso-genial flap were put in place towards the external angle [5].

Third Step. The third step and other complementary procedures are directed towards adjusting the eyelids on a temporary prosthesis. The lower lid is often too short and subject to cicatricial entropion that may be corrected by lengthening of the posterior lamella (chondro-mucosal graft, cartilage graft) and repositioning of the ciliary implantation; this was done in the second case. The upper lid may be subject to several malformations: cicatricial entropion with shortening of the posterior lamella, cutaneous deficiency giving an appearance of ptosis of the eyebrow (often associated), lack of palpebral fold, ptosis because of an atrophic and nonfunctional levator. Palpebral exploration by a cutaneous approach, as was done in both cases, will deal with these palpebral disorders by allowing ptosis correction by a large full-thickness resection of the levator or in cases of nonfunctioning levators by suspension to the frontalis muscle. Repositioning of the ciliary implantation on the prosthesis, correction of the palpebral fold, lengthening of the posterior lamella by a composite graft, lengthening of the anterior lamella by a cutaneous graft, can all be associated in one or more settings as we did in both our cases.

CONCLUSION

Rougier et al. [1] noted that treatment of anophthalmos and severe congenital microphthalmos is one of the most difficult in orbito-palpebral surgery. Nevertheless, an acceptable result in the primary position may be obtained if expansion of the socket by mucosal or skin graft on a conformer is combined with expansion of the bony orbit by osteotomy at the same sitting and followed by palpebral reconstruction at a later date: either palpebral reconstruction in cases of partial or total ablepharon, or palpebral repositioning on the temporary prosthesis. At least three surgical steps are necessary to obtain this result, that can certainly be ameliorated over the long-term by further repositioning procedures and by calling for the co-operation of an excellent prosthetist that will be able to modify the prosthesis and enhance the expansion of the socket.

REFERENCES

1. Rougier J, Tessier P, Hervouet F, Woillez M, Lekieffre M, Derome P: *Chirurgie Plastique Orbito-Palpébrale.* Rapport SF (ed). Paris, Masson, 1977:261–268.
2. Tessier P, Callahan A, Mustarde JC, Salyer K (ed): *Symposium on Plastic Surgery in the Orbital Region.* St. Louis, MO, C V Mosby Co, 1976.
3. Tessier P: Réflexions sur la chirurgie cranio-faciale d'aujour-d'hui et son avenir chez l'enfant. *Ann Chir Plast* 1979; 24(2):109–119.
4. Mustarde JC: *Repair and Reconstruction in the Orbital Region.* Edinburgh, Scotland, Churchill, Livingstone, 1980.
5. Tessier P: Blépharopoïèses inférieures. *Bull Mem Soc fra Ophthalmol* 1960; 73, 231–254.

Orbito-Palpebral Reconstruction in Two Cases
of Incomplete Cryptophthalmos

S. Morax, M.D., M. L. Herdan, M.D., and T. Hurbli, M.D.

ABSTRACT

Two cases of congenital symblepharon (variant of cryptophthalmos) are reported. Cryptophthalmos is a very rare congenital defect, with incomplete or complete failure in the development of one or both eyelids with skin recovering the anterior segment. Surgical treatment is described including expansion of the conjunctival fornix with eyeball conservation if possible. At the same time or later, the upper eyelid is reconstructed by inferior eyelid flap. The ophthalmic features of cryptophthalmos and its systemic associations are reviewed.

INTRODUCTION

Cryptophthalmos is a rare and congenital anomaly in which the skin passes continuously from forehead to cheek, inducing a complete ablepharon. Zehender [1] and Manz [2] presented the first case in 1872. The ophthalmic features, systemic associations, and reconstructive surgery in two cases of incomplete cryptophthalmos are reported here.

CASE REPORTS

CASE 1

A full-term boy of healthy parents presented with an incomplete cryptophthalmos (Fig. 1A).

On the right side, there was an incomplete superior ablepharon involving the medial two-thirds of the lid, the skin of the forehead covered the eyeball completely; the latter, on palpation was small, of normal consistency, and moved spontaneously in a normal orbit. The lower eyelid, fornix, and lacrimal punctum showed no anomaly.

On the left side, the cornea was keratinized in its superior two-thirds; note a coloboma of the medial half of the upper lid, an ectropion of the lower lid, and a partial symblepharon of the lower fornix.

Other facial deformities were also found: depression of the temporal regions, downward sweep of the frontal hairline, bilateral colobomas of the medial two-thirds of the eyebrows that are continuous with the palpebral colobomas.

There was no other evidence of facial and systemic anomalies (fingers and toes and urogenital system were normal). The psychomotor development was perfect.

The surgical procedure was divided in several steps. On the left side, at the age of six

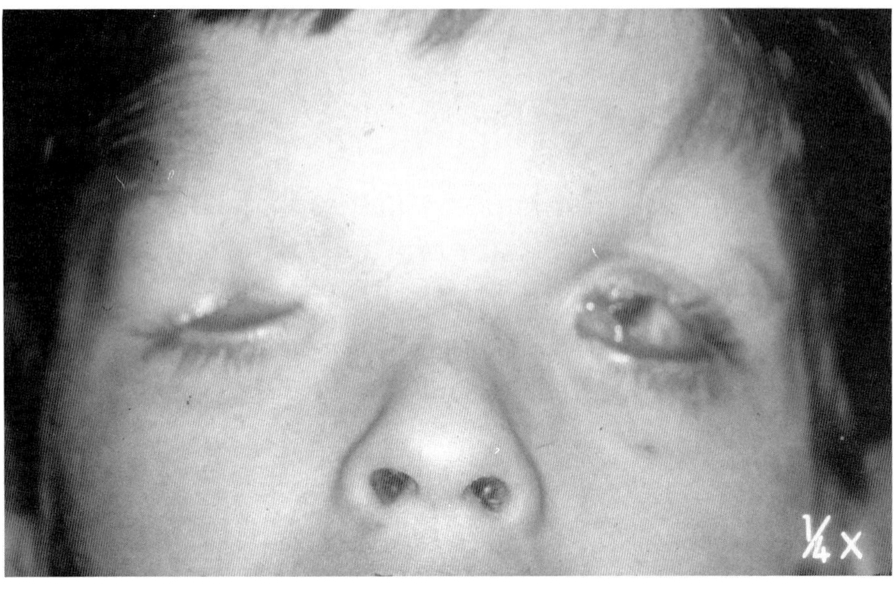

Figure 1. (A) Right and incomplete congenital cryptophthalmos (congenital symblepharon) with left eyeball malformation. (*Figure continued on the following pages.*)

months, the superior eyelid coloboma responsible for corneal exposure of that eye was treated with a full-thickness inferior lid flap. After lateral cantholysis, the donor site was closed by suturing the skin, edge to edge. At 12 months of age, the left eye was protected by proper lid position, and an optic iridectomy was performed allowing a visual acuity of 1/50.

On the right side, where cryptophthalmos was incomplete, a three-step surgical procedure was managed when the boy was 11 years old.

First Step. On the whole, excision of the microphthalmic, functionless and useless eyeball, and of the skin adherent to the superior palpebral coloboma was completed (Fig. 1B). Reconstruction of the defects was managed with labial mucosal grafts to reline the new orbital cavity and the superior fornix and with a full-thickness medial pedicle inferior lid flap to correct the upper lid coloboma (Fig. 1C).

Second Step. Three weeks later the flap pedicle was cut, and the flap correctly adjusted. The lower fornix was lined with a labial mucosa graft large enough to provide a posterior lamella for the new lower lid. Reconstruction of the lower lid was performed with an orbito-nasal-genial (ONG) flap (Figs. 1D and E). A temporary prosthesis was fitted.

Third Step. During the third stage we proceeded to palpebral revision and correction with the conformer in place. Blepharoptosis is treated with levator resection and eyelid fold reformation. This child is now fourteen and has a well-tolerated cosmetic prosthesis.

Upon histologic examination of the enucleated eye Dr. P. Dhermy confirmed the cryptophthalmos. The anterior segment was disorganized or absent; there was a fibrous adherence between the ciliary processes and the skin. Microphthalmos was present with retinal detachment and glial proliferation.

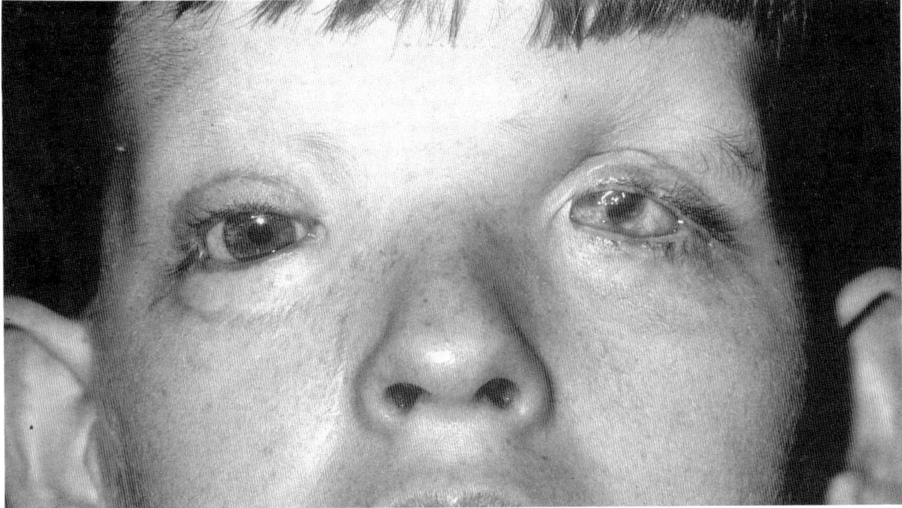

B

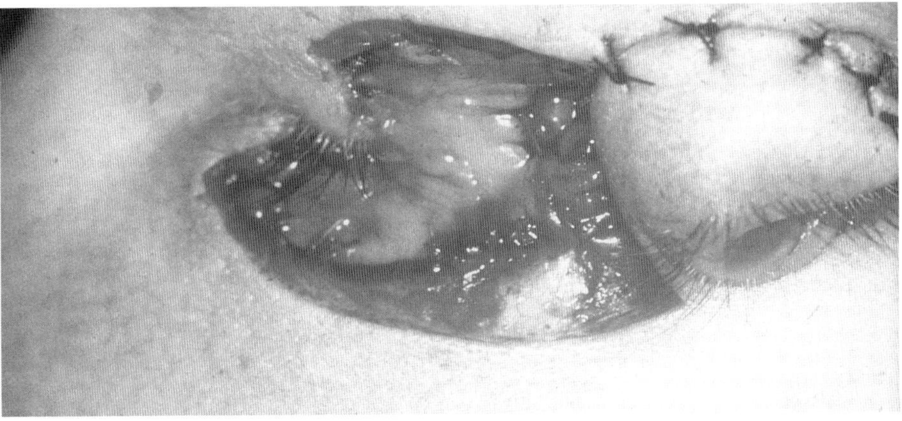

C

Figure 1 continued. (B) Postoperative appearance six months later; surgical treatment included: enucleation; reconstruction of the superior eyelid with a full-thickness inferior lid flap; reconstruction of the lower lid with an ONG flap; prosthesis fabrication. (C) Removal of the "skin curtain" that sticks to the eyeball, and enucleation. Socket expansion performed with buccal mucosal graft on conformer. Superior eyelid reconstruction (ablepharons with a full-thickness medial pedicle inferior lid flap).

CASE 2

A full-term boy of healthy parents was born with an incomplete and moderate cryptophthalmos first seen at the age of 20 (Fig. 2A). There was no anomaly on the right side, visual acuity was 4/10 with a horizontal pendular nystagmus. On the left side, complete superior ablepharon was noted; a sheet of skin from the forehead was adherent to the eyeball. Through the skin, an eyeball of normal size with hypertropia and normal ocular movements could be palpated. The lower lid was present but short; the lid margin was in correct position. Lower

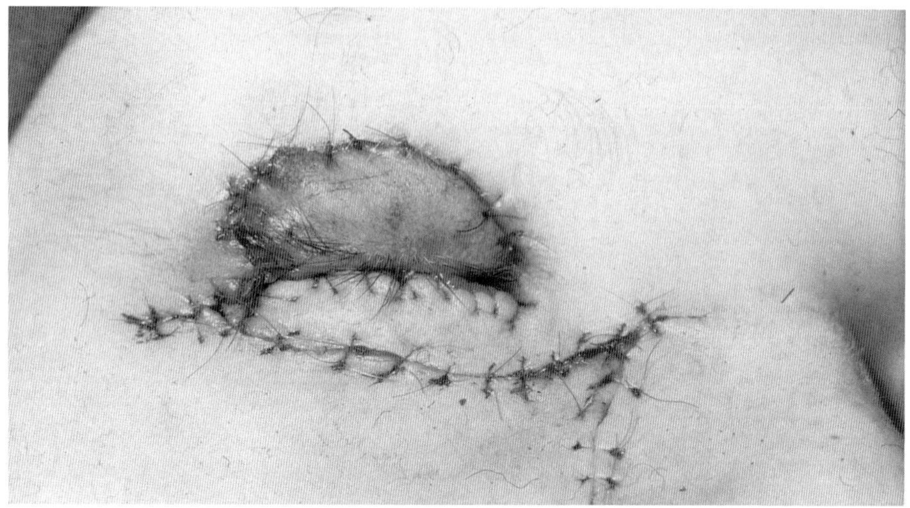

D

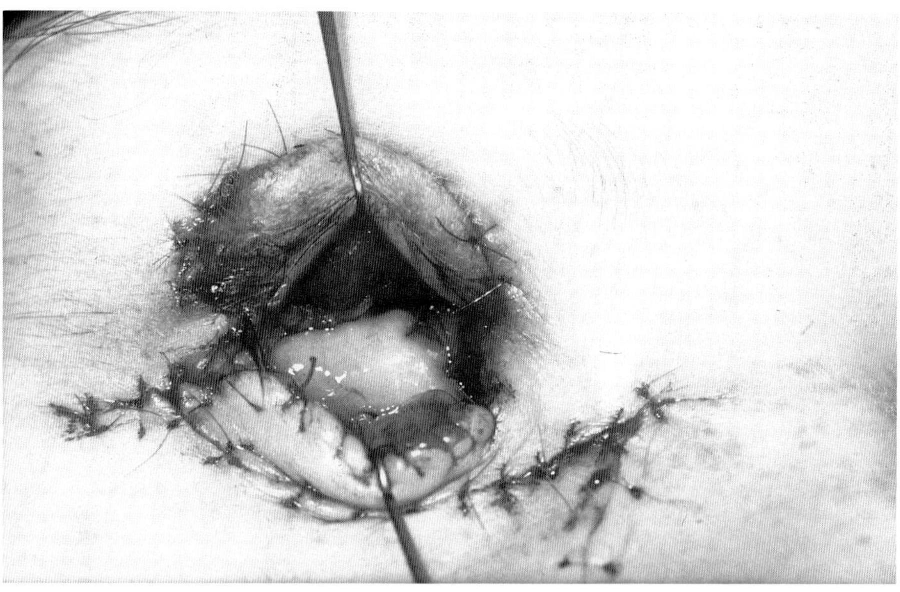

E

Figure 1 continued. (D) Division of the flap. Reconstruction of lower lid with an orbito-nasal-genial (ONG) flap. (E) Simultaneous expansion of the conjunctival fornices is performed with a new buccal mucosal graft.

fornix and lacrimal punctum were normal. Hair was absent on the lateral two-thirds of the eyebrow. As in the first case no other systemic anomalies were found.

CT scans showed left sided microorbitism; the globe was of normal size and the oculomotor muscles were present. The surgical procedure was developed in three main stages.

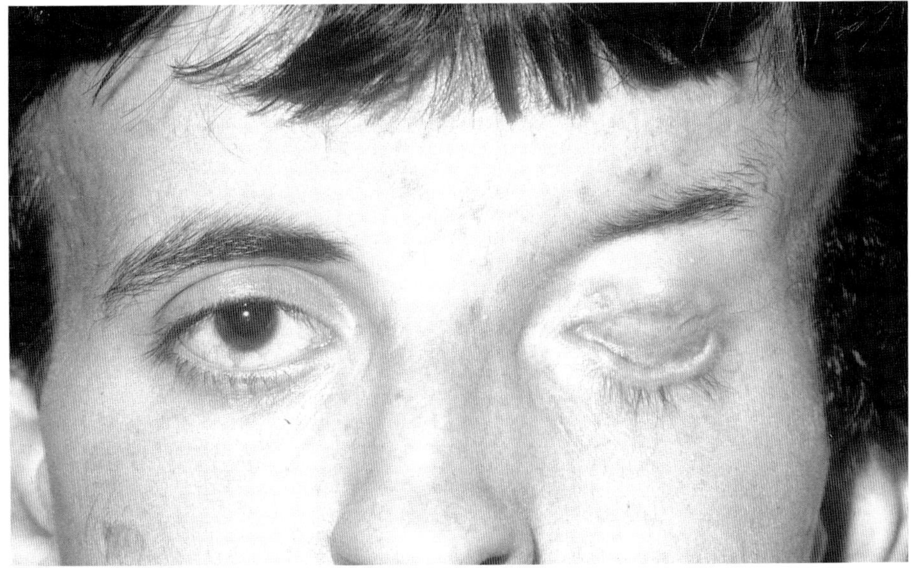

A

Figure 2. (A) Left incomplete unilateral congenital cryptophthalmos (congenital symblepharon). Superior eyelid is a "skin curtain" that sticks to the anterior part of the cornea (superior ablepharon). (*Figure continued on the following pages.*)

First Stage. Initially the skin adherent to the eyeball was resected allowing a precise dissection of the different tissue planes, for preservation of the globe. The oculomotor muscles and a rudimentary levator muscle were found, but there was no available soft tissue socket, especially no upper fornix (Figs. 2B, C and D). Reconstruction of the socket and the fornices was performed using two large labial mucosal grafts, which were also used to cover the globe. The upper lid was reconstructed with a broad laterally pedicled lower lid Abbe flap (Figs. 2E, F and G). A temporary prosthesis was then fitted.

Second Stage. The second stage was performed four weeks later; the pedicle of the flap was incised and the flap adjusted (Figs. 2H and I). The socket was revised and a new labial mucosal graft was applied to further deepen the fornix. The lower lid that had been used to reconstruct the upper lid was then itself reconstructed. The posterior lamella and inferior fornix were reformed using a buccal mucosal graft. The anterior lamella was reconstructed with an ONG flap (Fig. 2J and K).

Third Stage. During the third stage, we adjusted the ONG flap and made a one-third medial brow graft with a flap pedicled on the superficial temporal artery.

During the final surgical procedure we cut the pedicle of the temporal flap and revised the ONG flap. A temporary prosthesis was then fitted.

The cosmetic results of Case 2, fitted with a prosthesis, were acceptable, giving a good appearance in primary gaze (Fig. 2L).

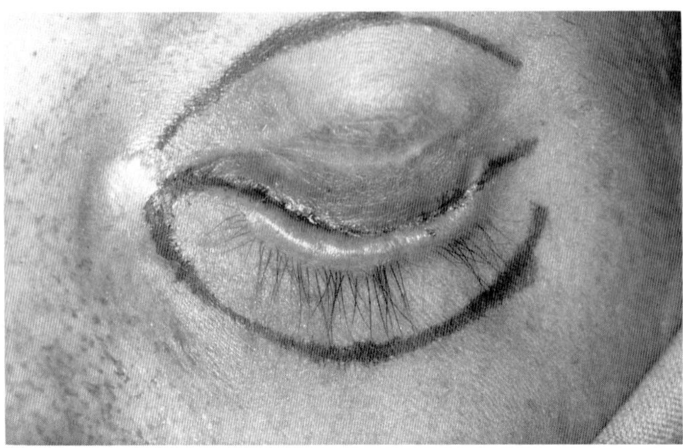

B

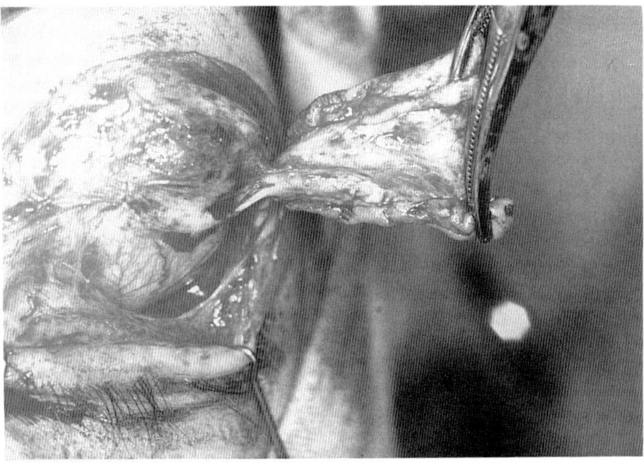

C

Figure 2 continued. (B) Drawing of the superior eyelid excision and of the full-thickness inferior eyelid flap. (C) Excision of the "skin curtain" sticking to the eyeball. (D) Anomalies of the eyeball are shown. Levator muscle is normal. Recti are present.

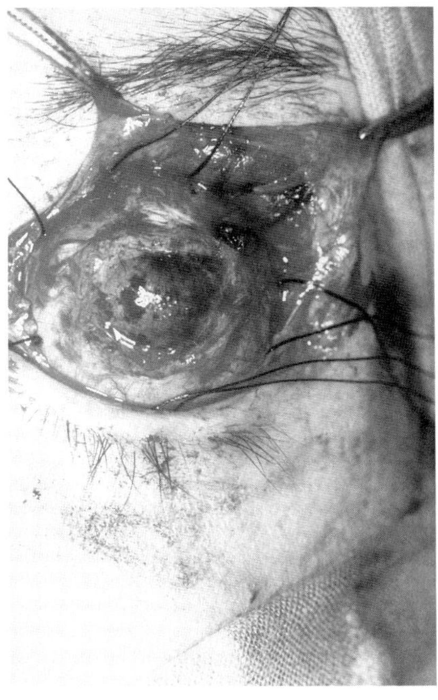

D

DISCUSSION

Since the first description by Zehender and Manz [1,2], most cases of cryptophthalmos have been reported. François [3] divided the ophthalmic malformations into three groups:

1. Complete cryptophthalmos,
2. Incomplete cryptophthalmos,
3. Congenital symblepharon.

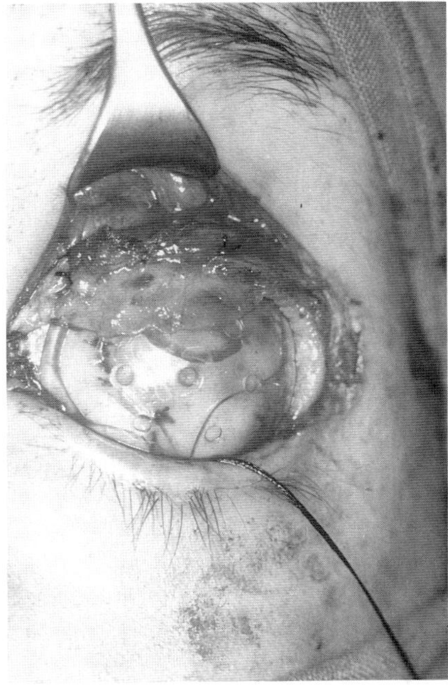

E

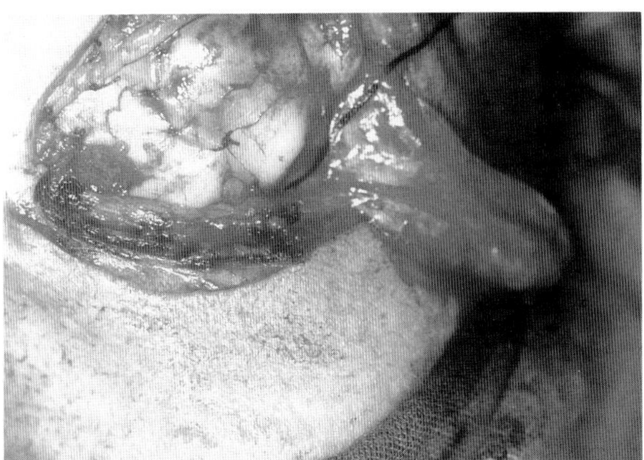

F

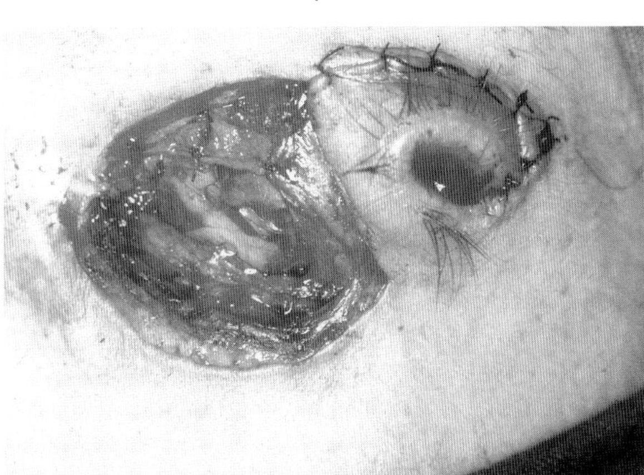

G

Figure 2 continued. (E) Reconstruction of the socket is performed with buccal mucosal graft on the eyeball. (F) Dissection of the lateral pedicle full-thickness inferior lid flap. (G) Adjustment of this flap.

Complete cryptophthalmos is the most common form. The lids are replaced by a sheet of skin running from forehead to cheek, covering the globe. The skin is adherent to the underlying cornea, the conjunctival sac is absent. Neither lashes, nor gland structures, nor eyebrows are identified.

In the case of incomplete cryptophthalmos, rudimentary lids and conjunctival sac are identified in the lateral third; the medial two-thirds are covered by a sheet of skin adherent to the cornea. The eyeball is not seen.

In congenital symblepharon, the upper lid is a real sheet of skin, without a defined margin, adherent to 75% of the upper cornea. The inferior part of the cornea is often keratinized and opaque. The superior fornix and lacrimal punctum are absent. Most of the time a microphthalmos is associated. The lower lid is quite normal.

The two reported cases are identical to the congenital symblepharon described by François [3] and Sugar [4], with some variations. In these cases, the globe was completely covered with skin, and no part of the cornea was visible.

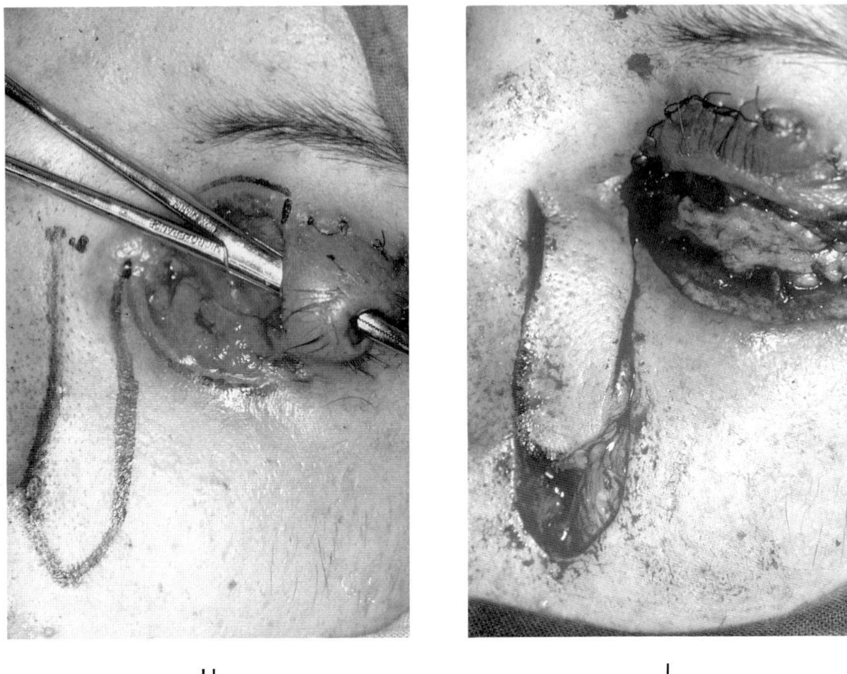

H   I

Figure 2 continued. (H) Appearance of the flap, three weeks later. Drawing of the orbito-nasal-genial (ONG) flap for the future inferior eyelid reconstruction. (I) Resection of the flap and adjustment to the superior eyelid. Dissection of the orbito-nasal-genial (ONG) flap.

Most of the time, cryptophthalmos is bilateral. The malformation may be complete and symmetric. The asymmetric forms consist of about 33% of the cases and are of a great variety: complete cryptophthalmos on one side, incomplete cryptophthalmos, congenital symblepharon, upper lid coloboma or epibulbar dermoid on the other side.

The first case was a bilateral and asymmetric form with a congenital symblepharon on one side, an upper lid coloboma with disorganization of the anterior segment on the other side. The second case was an isolated congenital symblepharon.

Cryptophthalmos may stay purely isolated or be accompanied by other systemic malformations [3,5]. An important number of associated lesions have been described: syndactyly of feet and hands, anomalies of the genito-urinary tract, anomalies of the controlateral eye (dermoids, upper eyelid coloboma, microphthalmos, coloboma of the eyebrow), facial clefts, flattening of the frontotemporal bone, anomalies of the nose and ears, mental retardation, meningo-encephalocele, atresia of the larynx, cleft palate, umbilical hernia, renal aplasia, atresia of the bladder and anus.

François [3], has classified the encountered lesions into isolated malformations and cryptophthalmic syndrome combining in different degrees four more or less important components: cryptophthalmos, dyscephaly, syndactyly, and genito-urinary tract malformations.

Histological examination of 12 cryptophthalmic eyes has been reported in the literature [3] and shows that the skin covering the eyeball possesses a keratinized and stratified squamous

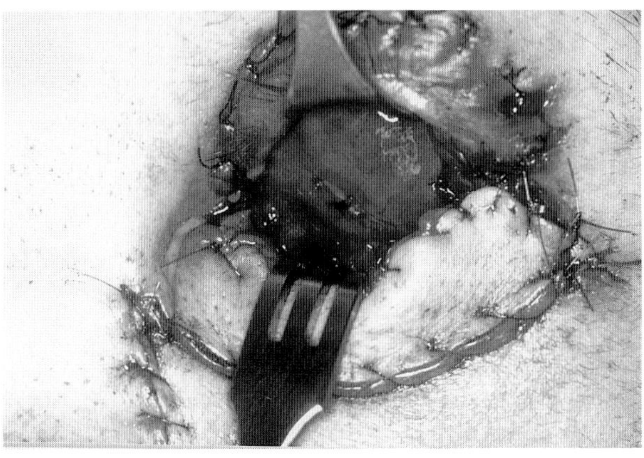

J

Figure 2 continued. (J) Mobilization of the orbito-nasal-genial (ONG) flap and adjustment to the inferior eyelid. (K) Superior eyelid is reconstructed with a full-thickness inferior eyelid flap. Inferior eyelid is reconstructed with a composite graft: buccal mucosal graft covered with an orbito-nasal-genial (ONG) flap. The ONG defect zone is reconstructed by a cheek rotation flap.

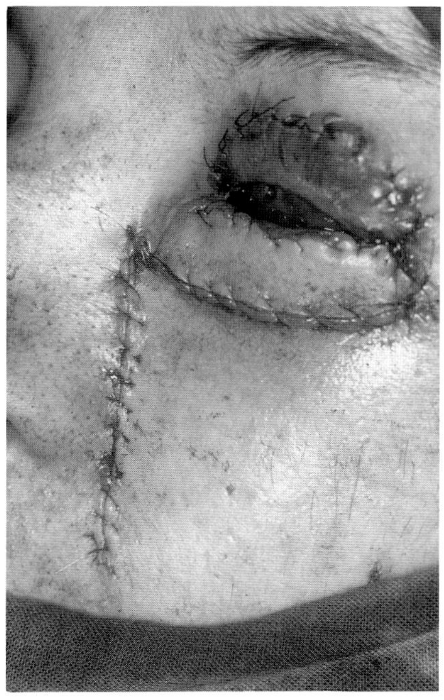

K

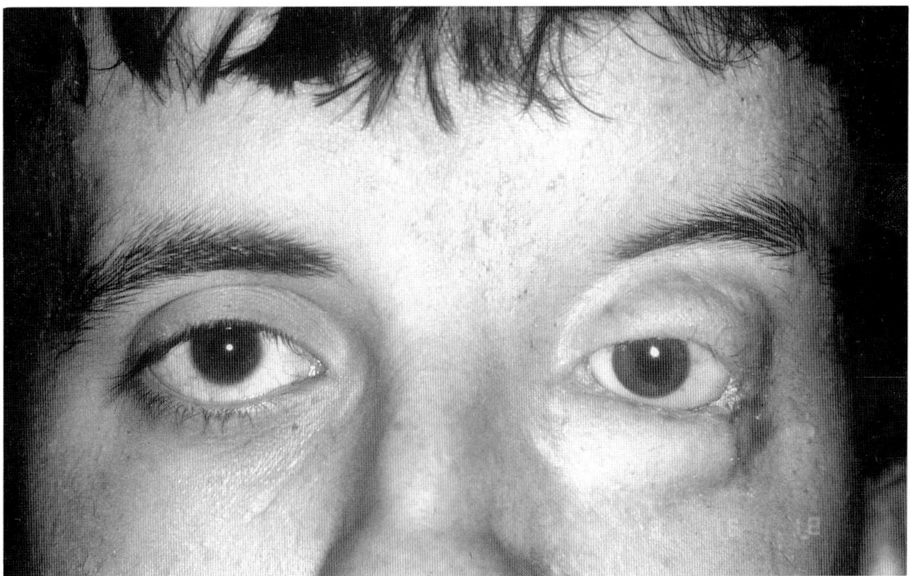

L

Figure 2 continued. (L) Postoperative appearance following: socket expansion with buccal mucosal graft; superior eyelid reconstruction by an inferior lid Abbe-Mustardé flap; inferior eyelid reconstruction by an orbito-nasal-genial (ONG) flap; prosthesis fabrication.

epithelium. The choroid merges with a fibrovascular tissue that replaces the cornea. The eye is usually microphthalmic, rarely buphthalmic. Pilous and glandular systems are absent. The orbicularis and levator muscles are present as in Case 2. The anterior chamber is shallow or absent, the lens often nonexistent, the iris either absent or totally adherent to the posterior corneal surface, whereas the ciliary body is atrophic. The choroid and retina are either normal or totally disorganized.

According to Ehlers [6] one-fifth of cases are associated with microphthalmos and colobomatous cysts. In Case 1, the eye showed anomalies that were consistent with those described in the literature. The cornea was metaplasic, covered with a keratinized epithelium, the anterior segment including the lens was absent, the whole posterior segment modified, pilous, and glandular adnexa were missing whereas oculomotor and palpebral muscles were preserved. The conjunctival fornix facing the symblepharon was absent.

Complete cryptophthalmos seems to occur at the embryonic stage, caused by failure of eyelid development [7]. The ectoderm covering the cornea is transformed into skin and the conjunctival fornix cannot be formed. Congenital symblepharon could be explained by failure of development of the upper eyelid (upper eyelid is derived from the fronto-nasal bud whereas lower eyelid originating from the maxillary bud is normal). From the genetic point of view, an autosomal recessive inheritance was found in 15% of cryptophthalmos cases, especially those from consanguineous parents. The disease can affect either sex equally and no chromosomic abnormality has been reported. Recently Zhang [8], reported a cryptophthalmic syndrome affecting three siblings of the same family. Until lately, too little reference has been made in the literature to the surgical treatment of the cryptophthalmos syndrome [3,7]. Because of the severe disorganization of the cryptophthalmic eyeball as described in all histological studies, no functional surgery can be attempted. In unilateral forms with oculopalpebral malformations involving the contralateral eye (coloboma, symblepharon, anterior segment abnormality), surgical treatment of this functional eye is essential to improve vision and to further protect the anterior segment. Nevertheless, the presence of multiple abnormalities can prevent re-establishment of satisfactory visual function. In Case 1 (congenital symblepharon), the contralateral eye gained benefit from correction of the upper palpebral coloboma using a lower eyelid flap; this was followed by an inferior optic iridectomy.

Concerning the nonfunctional cryptophthalmic eye, the only aim of the treatment was to fit an esthetic prosthesis on the ocular stump if the globe could be spared or in the orbital cavity in case of enucleation. Because of the great variety of anatomic conditions, treatment is difficult to standardize. Surgery must be aimed towards the two principal symptoms and must seek two goals: on one hand reconstruction of the conjunctival fornix, and palpebral reconstruction on the other.

In the two cases of congenital symblepharon, reconstruction involved the whole conjunctival fornix and the upper eyelid (subtotal ablepharon); several surgical stages were necessary.

First Step. The first surgical stage included the reconstruction of the conjunctival fornix according to classical cavity reconstruction techniques using buccal mucosal grafts, and the reconstruction of the upper eyelid. The conjunctival symblepharon was delicately separated from the anterior surface of the cornea. The eyeball was then explored. Although nonfunctional, it was nevertheless preserved as it was used as a support for the future prosthesis. This was not possible in Case 1. In both cases the skin covering the cornea was not preserved. It could have served as an anterior layer to a later reconstructed upper lid, but this would have necessitated several procedures and yielded an incomplete result (absence of a palpebral unit, absence of a lid margin). We preferred to sacrifice this cutaneous flap and reconstruct the upper ablepharon using a full-thickness lower eyelid flap [9].

Labial mucosal grafts must line the future cavity (in contact with the eyeball if it has been preserved) and the upper fornix; the graft must be secured as high as possible towards the supraorbital rim to avoid any secondary shallowness of the upper fornix that is a cause of malposition of the prosthesis when it is fitted later. Retention of the conjunctival fornix is done by placing a temporary conformer.

It is advisable to reconstruct the upper eyelid at the same time, after creating the new conjunctival fornix, because this will allow the retention of the conformer that is impossible in the absence of palpebral support. This palpebral reconstruction may call for all described flap techniques [9]. A lower lid full-thickness graft that has the advantage of providing a complete lid unit with its ciliary margin is advocated.

Second Step. The second surgical step allows the section of the flap pedicle, the adjustment of the upper palpebral flap, and the reconstruction of the inferior fornix and lower lid (deficient because of its transposition to the upper lid). For this, an orbito-naso-genial (ONG) flap [10] has been used that will be thick enough to need only a mucosal graft as its deep layer and long enough to be secured on the lateral canthus. A large labial mucosal graft stabilized by a conformer will be used to reconstruct the inferior part of the cavity, the lower fornix and the deep layer of the future lower lid.

Complementary procedures are often necessary, as they were in the two cases presented, including adjustment and correction of the palpebral ptosis with the prosthesis in place. These procedures must be done six months after the conjunctival fornix and palpebral reconstruction, after healing of tissues has been completed. In some cases an important retraction of the fornices calls for a repeated expansion by mucosal grafts on a conformer.

Congenital symblepharon is an incomplete variety of cryptophthalmos associating an ocular malformation (nonfunctional eye) and a partial upper ablepharon, the upper lid being replaced by a sheet of skin adherent to the cornea.

The surgical treatment combines reconstruction of the conjunctival fornices and lids. In the two cases reported, after two important procedures and some complementary operations, an acceptable result has been obtained.

REFERENCES

1. Zehender VW: Eine missegeburt mit hautüberwachscnen Augen oder Kryptophthalmus. *Klin Monatsbl Augenheilkd* 1872; 10:225.
2. Manz: Ein Missegeburt mit hautüberwachsenen Augen oder Kryptophthalmus. *Anatomische beschreibungder Augen Klin Montasbl* Augenheilkd, 1872; 10:234.
3. Francois J: Syndrome malformatif avec cryptophthalmie. *Acta Genet Med Gemellol* 1969; 18:18.
4. Sugar HS: The cryptophthalmos–syndactyly syndrome. *Amer J Ophthal* 1968; 66:897–899.
5. Idec CH, Wollschlaeger PB: Multiple congenital abnormalities associated with cryptophthalmos. *Arch Ophthalmol* 1969; 81:638–644.
6. Ehlers M: Cryptophthalmos with orbito-palpebral cyst and microphthalmos. *Acta Ophthalmol* 1966; 44:84.
7. Brazier DJ, Hardman L, Collin JRO: Cryptophthalmos: Surgical treatment of the congenital symblepharon variant. *Brit J Ophthal* 1986; 70:391–395.
8. Zhang H: Cryptophthalmos: a report on three sibling cases. *Brit J Ophthalmol* 1986; 70:72–74.
9. Mustarde JC: *Repair and Reconstruction in the Orbital Region.* Edinburgh, Scotland, Churchill, Livingstone, 1980.
10. Tessier P: Blépharopoïèses inférieures. *Bull Mem Soc Fr Ophthalmol* 1960; 73:231–254.

The Myofibroblast and the Anophthalmic Socket

Sara A. Kaltreider, M.D.

ABSTRACT

One of the greatest advances in the understanding of wound healing was the identification and characterization of the myofibroblast by Gabbiani in 1971. Since that time this contractile cell has been found in the early stages of wound healing and in many pathologic states. In a recent study, the myofibroblast was found in healing and contracting anophthalmic sockets.

HISTORY OF THE MYOFIBROBLAST

The myofibroblast, a modified fibroblast, has been identified in granulation tissue and has been implicated as the agent causing wound contraction [1]. Gabbiani et al. reported several cellular features distinguishing the myofibroblast from the fibroblast: 40–80 Angstrom cytoplasmic microfilaments, nuclear indentations, and surface differentiations called hemidesmosomes and maculae adherens [1].

Later, the origin of the myofibroblast from the fibroblast rather than from the vascular smooth muscle component of granulation tissue was proposed [2,3]. Many studies revealed the myofibroblast not only in experimental animals, but also in human granulation tissue [4,5]. The myofibroblast was discovered in open skin wounds, around breast implants, in the nodules of Dupuytren's contracture, and in a multitude of other fibrocontractive diseases [4–6]. The myofibroblast has not been seen consistently in small, linear wounds where contraction was not necessary for closure of the wound [7].

In experimental models, several factors have been suggested to influence the differentiation and activity of myofibroblasts. Tissue loss, inflammation, and cell mediators may play a role in fibroblast transformation into a contractile cell [6]. Contraction of myofibroblasts has been stimulated in vitro with smooth muscle agonists — angiotensin, vasopressin, norepinephrine, bradykinin, epinephrine, and 5-hydroxytryptamine [5]. Anoxia has been noted to inhibit its contraction, as well as the drugs papaverine and thiphenamil (Trocinate) [5].

An experiment by McGrath and Hundahl in 1982 quantified myofibroblasts in granulation tissue by immunoperoxidase staining techniques and determined the distribution of myofibroblasts over time [8]. Myofibroblasts were most abundant between days 10 and 21 of wound healing, when the rate of clinical wound contraction was the greatest [8]. Myofibroblasts were

Supported in part by a grant to the Medical College of Virginia from Research to Prevent Blindness, Inc.

found in highest concentration near inflammatory foci suggesting a relationship between inflammatory cells and the differentiation of the myofibroblast from the fibroblast [8].

RECENT ADVANCES

In recent research of the anophthalmic socket, myofibroblasts were identified in healing sockets, both contracting and noncontracting [9]. Eight enucleated cynomolgus monkey sockets and biopsies from two human anophthalmic sockets were studied. Two of the eight monkey sockets were caused to contract using croton oil. One of the human sockets was clinically contracted and the other was not contracted, but required a secondary sphere implant. In this study, myofibroblasts were identified by immunoperoxidase staining of actin for light microscopy and myosin subfragment-1 staining of actin for electron microscopy. Myofibroblasts were present in the normally healing (noncontracted) monkey sockets, but only in those specimens containing active granulation tissue. Myofibroblasts were also seen in the contracting monkey socket specimens in areas with active granulation tissue. Immunoperoxidase staining for actin identified myofibroblasts in the specimen from the human contracted socket, but not in the specimen from the human noncontracted socket. Myosin subfragment-1 staining revealed myofibroblasts in the human noncontracted socket, but not in the contracted socket, perhaps because of a lack of active granulation tissue in the small tissue sample (Figs. 1A and 1B). Cytoplasmic actin occurred in arterioles, venules, capillaries, myoepithelial cells associated with lacrimal gland acini, smooth muscle, and skeletal muscle, as well as in myofibroblasts [9]. As in open wound healing, the myofibroblast is apparently present in the socket during normal healing and during pathologic contraction.

DISCUSSION

The presence of the myofibroblast in healing and contracting sockets is only circumstantial evidence of a link between this cell type and clinical contraction. Discovery of a direct quantitative relationship between the myofibroblast concentration and loss of socket depth or volume would indicate that the myofibroblast is indeed responsible for socket contraction. Once such a relationship is established, then experimental investigations could be directed toward finding clinically useful smooth muscle antagonists or other agents to inhibit the differentiation or activity of the myofibroblast in socket contraction.

Wound geometry, size, loss of tissue, inflammation, humoral and cellular elements have been suggested factors determining the differentiation and activity of the myofibroblast in open skin wounds [4–6,8,10–12]. Do these same factors influence the myofibroblast in the contracting socket? The socket is a unique three-dimensional structure with intricately arranged soft-tissue structures in a rigid bony support. Presumably, some of the same principles of open wound healing apply to socket healing with formation of granulation tissue, healing of epithelial surface defects, scarring and, in certain circumstances, contraction.

The contraction process has been shown to involve the anterior tissues of the socket, particularly the subconjunctival area consisting of Tenon's capsule, that is, in the vicinity of the surgical site [9]. Other structures, extraocular muscles for example, may be pulled into the contractile tissue by fibrous bands [9]. Clinical problems arise in particular when the socket structures become distorted because of contraction, and a prosthesis cannot be retained in the socket.

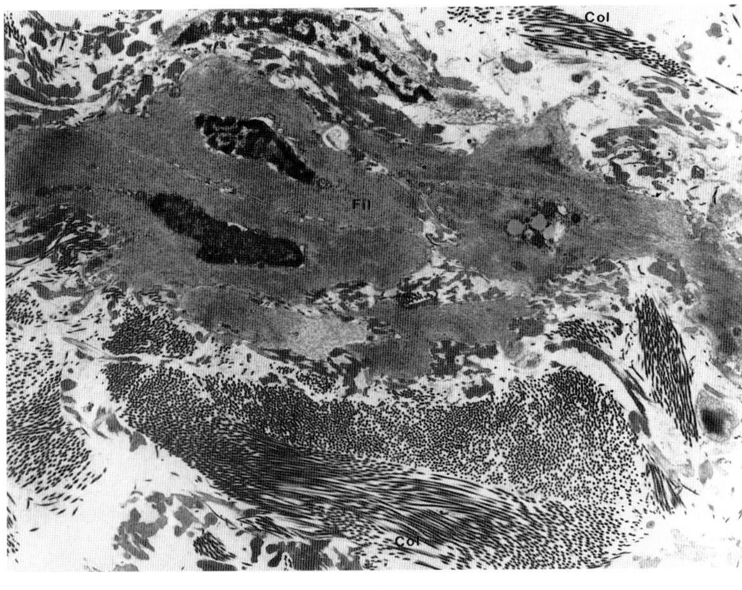

A

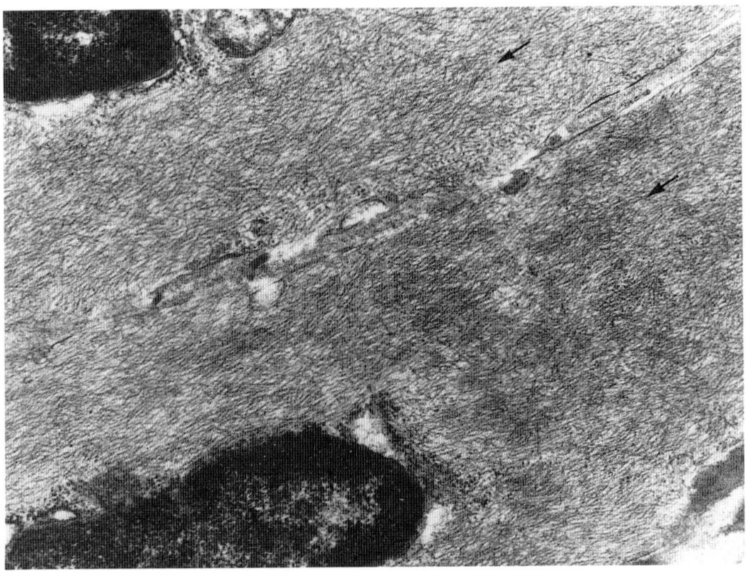

B

Figure 1. (A) A representative myofibroblast surrounded by bundles of collagen fibrils (Col) was found in the human noncontracted socket. Densely packed microfilaments (Fil) are seen in the cytoplasm of these cells. (B) In a higher magnification of Figure 1A, note the "herringbone" pattern of the microfilaments caused by decoration with myosin subfragment-1. (Reprinted with permission from Kaltreider SA, Wallow IHL, Gonnering RS, Dortzbach RK: The anatomy and histology of the anophthalmic socket — Is the myofibroblast present? *Ophthal Plast Reconstr Surg* 1987; 3(4):207–230.)

Several anatomical problems may prevent successful prosthetic wear including lower lid laxity and ectropion, soft-tissue deficit, and contraction of the socket. Progressive lower lid laxity and ectropion may result in loss of the structural support of the prosthesis [13,14]. A soft-tissue deficit necessitating a bulky, globular prosthesis — for example, when no implant is present, or the implant is too small — may cause difficulty in retaining the prosthesis. Localized or generalized socket contraction may prevent prosthetic wear by obliterating the fornices and the potential space between the lids and posterior surface of the socket [9,13,15,16]. In the latter situation, the myofibroblast may be the agent responsible for the loss of the "normal" anophthalmic contour and configuration of the fornices, and consequent loss of socket volume and depth. Understanding the behavior and life history of the myofibroblast may facilitate the search for more effective means to prevent, control, and treat the contracting socket.

REFERENCES

1. Gabbiani G, Ryan GB, Majno G: Presence of modified fibroblasts in granulation tissue and their possible role in wound contraction. *Experientia* 1971; 27:549–550.
2. Ryan GB, Cliff MB, Gabbiani G, Irle C, Statkov PR, Majno G: Myofibroblasts in an avascular fibrous tissue. *Lab Inves* 1973; 29(2):197–206.
3. Schurch W, Seemayer TA, Lagace R, Gabbiani G: The intermediate filament cytoskeleton of myofibroblasts: An immunofluorescence and ultrastructural study. *Virchows Arch Pathol Anat* 1984; 403:323–336.
4. Montandon D, Gabbiani G, Ryan GB, Majno G: The contractile fibroblast — Its relevance in plastic surgery. *Plast Reconstr Surg* 1973; 52(3):286–292.
5. Guber S, Rudolph R: The myofibroblast. *Surg Gyn Obstet* 1978; 146:641–649.
6. Gabbiani G: The role of contractile proteins in wound healing and fibrocontractive diseases. *Meth Achiev Exp Pathol* 1979; 9:187–206.
7. Ryan GB, Cliff WJ, Gabbiani G, Irle C, Montandon D, Statkov PR, Majno G: Myofibroblasts in human granulation tissue. *Human Path* 1974; 5(1):55–67.
8. McGrath MH, Hundahl SA: The spatial and temporal quantification of myofibroblasts. *Plast Reconstr Surg* 1982; 69(6):975–985.
9. Kaltreider SA, Wallow IHL, Gonnering RS, Dortzbach RK: The anatomy and histology of the anophthalmic socket — Is the myofibroblast present? *Ophthal Plast Reconstr Surg* 1987; 3(4):207–230.
10. Majno G: The story of the myofibroblast. *Am J Surg Path* 1979; 3(6):535–542.
11. Rudolph R: Contraction and the control of contraction. *World J Surg* 1980; 4:279–287.
12. McGrath MH, Simon RH: Wound geometry and the kinetics of wound contraction. *Plast Reconstr Surg* 1983; 72(1):66–73.
13. Soll DB: The anophthalmic socket. *Ophthalmol* 1982; 89(5):407–423.
14. Vistnes LM, Iverson RE, Laub DR: The anophthalmic orbit — Surgical correction of lower eyelid ptosis. *Plast Reconstr Surg* 1973; 52(4):346–351.
15. Vistnes LM, Iverson RE: Surgical treatment of the contracted socket. *Plast Reconstr Surg* 1974; 53(5):563–567.
16. Putterman AM, Scott R: Deep ocular socket reconstruction. *Arch Ophthalmol* 1977; 95:1221–1228.

Reconstruction of the Partially Contracted Ocular Socket or Fornix

James W. Karesh, M.D. and Allen M. Putterman, M.D.

ABSTRACT

Foreshortening of the conjunctival fornices by symblepharon or scar formation can result in a variety of cosmetic and functional abnormalities both for the anophthalmic and the sighted patient. To correct this problem, a technique has been modified for the management of totally contracted ocular sockets. Unlike the procedure for total socket reconstruction, which uses a custom-designed conformer wrapped with a full-thickness mucous membrane graft, partial socket reconstruction uses a 0.5 mm thick mucous membrane graft sutured to the resected socket conjunctiva and splinted in place by a custom-designed conformer. Seventeen patients with a variety of underlying pathologic conditions associated with both trauma and prior surgery underwent successful ocular fornix reconstruction using this technique.

INTRODUCTION

Scarring and foreshortening of the ocular cul-de-sacs can result in a variety of problems, including decreased ocular motility, entropion, and an inability to retain a prosthesis or scleral shell. An important aspect of the surgical management of the compromised fornix is its reformation both vertically and posteriorly so that it can closely approximate the form and function of the normal fornix. Although correction of severe degrees of socket contracture requires considerable scar excision and conjunctival dissection in conjunction with extensive mucosal grafting and fornix reconstruction, moderate degrees of contracture can be approached more simply. This technique has been modified and simplified for the reconstruction of severely contracted sockets [1,2] and has been applied to the correction of mildly to moderately foreshortened conjunctival fornices. This report describes this modified approach and our surgical experience with it over a 10-year period.

PATIENTS AND METHODS

Between 1975 and 1985, 10 consecutive anophthalmic sockets with moderately foreshortened conjunctival fornices and seven eyes with moderate symblepharon formation underwent partial socket reconstruction. Patients were selected for reconstruction based on several cri-

Reprinted with permission from *Arch Ophthalmol* 1988; 106:552–556. Copyright 1988, American Medical Association.

This work was supported in part by core grant EY1972 from the National Eye Institute, National Institute of Health, Bethesda, MD.

teria, including an inability to be fitted with or retain an ocular prosthetic device, ocular motility disturbances, and cicatricial entropion. In addition to conjunctival shrinkage and subconjunctival fibrosis, eyelid retraction was also present in many cases. In all cases, both the socket and fornices had been stable for at least six months before partial socket reconstruction.

Anophthalmic patients were evaluated preoperatively and postoperatively in consultation with an experienced ocularist, who ruled out treatment by alteration of the prosthesis. The various large C-shaped conformers used in the reconstructive technique were custom-designed (Fig. 1). In addition, preoperative evaluation included complete ophthalmic history and a careful examination of the eyelids, conjunctiva, bony orbit, globe (when present), and ocular socket. Specific attention was directed towards the condition of the oral mucosa, the adequacy of the fornices and the extent of symblepharon formation, as well as other cicatricial eyelid changes.

There were 12 male and five female patients, ranging in age from 7 to 50 years (average, 31 years). Postoperative follow-up was six to 76 months (average, 30 months) after removal of the conformer. The underlying pathologic processes in these cases included penetrating and blunt trauma (seven cases), chemical injuries (three cases), pterygium surgery, trachoma, congenital anophthalmos, retinoblastoma, and Stevens-Johnson syndrome (one case each) (Table 1). In two cases, the clinical history was unknown. Four patients had undergone previous reconstructive procedures to their fornices and sockets (Table 1). These included mucous membrane grafting (two cases), symblepharon lysis (two cases), removal of an extruding orbital implant (one case), and scleral grafting (one case).

SURGICAL TECHNIQUE

The procedure was modified from the one previously described [1,2] for the reconstruction of the totally contracted socket. Many of the operative steps have appeared in previous publications [1,2] and therefore will not be reproduced here. The modified procedure will be described here.

Although local infiltrative anesthesia can be used, general anesthesia with nasotracheal intubation is preferred, both for patient comfort and facilitation of the surgical approach to the oral mucosa.

When the globe is absent, scissors are used to create a horizontal incision through the conjunctiva lining the posterior aspect of the socket, which is then dissected from all underlying cicatricial tissue up to the upper and lower tarsal borders. If a globe is present, a peritomy is performed to carefully separate the conjunctiva from the underlying scar tissue. Meticulous dissection is required to prevent any damage to either the levator complex or the extraocular muscles and to preserve the integrity of the conjunctiva. To recreate adequate fornices, the dissection must be carried out both posteriorly and inferiorly under the roof and over the floor of the orbit.

After deep cul-de-sacs have been formed and all cicatricial tissue lysed, a custom-designed large C-shaped conformer (Figs. 1 and 2) is chosen for stenting a partial-thickness oral mucous membrane graft within the reconstructed fornices. (Custom-designed conformers for partial socket reconstruction are available from Robert B. Scott, Chicago, IL.) Two separate types of conformers are used, one for the anophthalmic socket (Fig. 1) and one when there is a globe present (Fig. 2). These differ both in thickness and size as well as in the dimensions of the central drainage aperture. Both types of conformers feature large vertical and posterior dimensions as well as drill holes for fixation to the orbital rims. Incisions approximately 2 cm long

Table 1. Clinical History, Prereconstruction Socket Intervention, and Follow-up
in Patients Undergoing Partial Socket Reconstruction

Patient/Age/Sex	History	Previous therapy	Follow-up, mo
1/11/M	Congenital anophthalmos	Expansion conformer, lateral canthoplasty, mucous membrane grafting	76
2/20/M	Stevens–Johnson syndrome following phenytoin (Dilantin) therapy	None	59
3/24/M	Unknown	Enucleation	18
4/45/M	Penetrating injury/phthisis	None	6
5/48/M	Alkali burn	Scleral graft, upper eyelid recession, upper eyelid coloboma repair symblepharon lysis	72
6/25/F	Alkali burn	None	6
7/33/M	Unknown	Enucleation removal of migrated implant	70
8/24/F	Motor vehicle accident/phthisis	None	8
9/47/F	Penetrating injury	Enucleation	8
10/47/M	Penetrating injury	Enucleation, excision of basal cell carcinoma, lower eyelid reconstruction	18
11/20/M	Gunshot wound	Enucleation, partial socket reconstruction	35
12/7/M	Retinoblastoma	Enucleation	6
13/50/M	Motor vehicle accident	Enucleation	12
14/32/M	Trachoma	Enucleation	73
15/53/M	Motor vehicle accident	Enucleation	6
16/28/M	Chemical injury	None	12
17/53/M	Ptergium	Multiple pterygium excisions and symblepharon lysis	20

are made over the central superior and inferior orbital rims that are then exposed with blunt dissection. The periosteum is elevated from both the orbital rims and the orbital floor and roof. With a pneumatic drill, two holes are made approximately 6 mm apart in both the superior and inferior rims. These holes exit approximately 8 mm posterior to the rims from the orbital floor and roof. If a globe is present, a malleable retractor is used to protect it while the holes are being drilled. A 2-0 polyfilament (Supramid, S. Jackson, Alexandria, VA) suture is passed in a mattress fashion through the holes in the superior rim and a similar suture is passed through the holes in the inferior rim. A large, slightly curved surgical needle is used to pass the suture ends through periosteum into the newly created fornices. If a globe is present, the surgeon's finger protects it during the passage of the needle. An appropriate custom-designed conformer is selected that is snug-fitting but allows the eyelids to be closed over it. The suture ends are placed through the most peripheral of the conformer's suture holes in an external-to-internal direction. Then the supramid is placed through the central holes in an internal to external direction. The conformer is not placed into position until the mucous membrane graft is harvested and sutured in place.

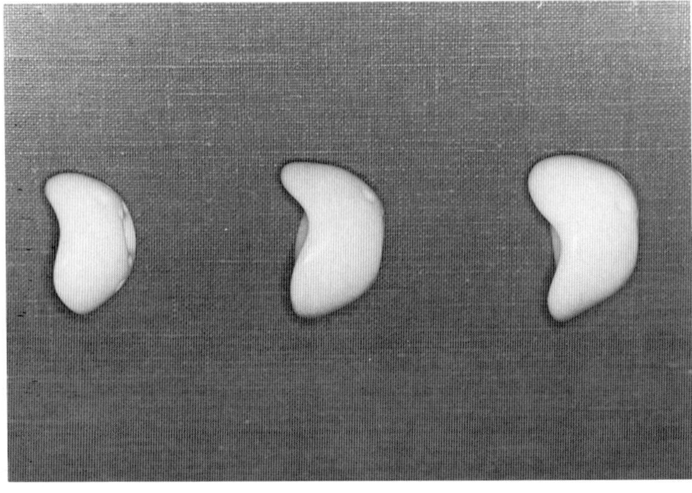

A

B

Figure 1. Large C-shaped conformer used in partial reconstruction of anophthalmic socket as viewed from side (A) and front (B).

The oral mucosa of the lips and cheeks are used for harvesting graft material. The inside of the lower lip provides the most expeditious location for obtaining mucosa. Several milliliters of 1% lidocaine with 1:100,000 epinephrine are initially injected submucosally for hemostasis. Then approximately 20 mL of sterile saline are injected submucosally until the mucosal surface is very rigid. Towel clamps placed through the lip and cheek facilitate exposure and stabilization of the donor site. A Castroviejo mucotome (Storz Instrument, Inc., St. Louis, MO) or Steinhaeuser orotome (Walter Lorenz, Surgical Instruments, Inc., Jacksonville, FL) set to 0.5 mm thickness is placed parallel to the mucosa and slowly pushed across its rigid sur-

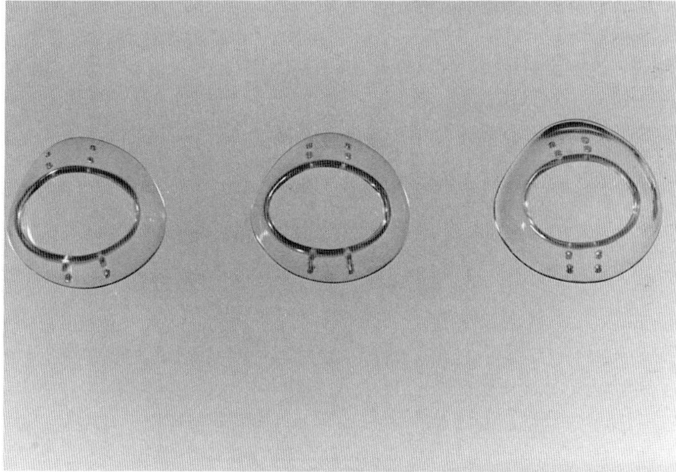

Figure 2. Large C-shaped conformer used for socket reconstruction in presence of globe.

face. The graft is gently grasped with forceps as it comes through the head of the mucotome and pulled onto a moist metal ruler. (This prevents the graft from twisting and bunching and keeps it oriented with the external surface upward.) If necessary, additional mucosa can be obtained from the cheeks or upper lip. The donor site is allowed to spontaneously heal over several weeks.

Using 6-0 polyglactin (Vicryl, Ethicon, Somerville, NJ) sutures, the graft is sutured with its raw surface inward to the remaining palpebral and bulbar conjunctiva in the socket (Fig. 3). The conformer is placed behind the eyelids and the polyfilament sutures are adjusted and tightened so that the conformer's central position is located in the midaspect of the socket. The

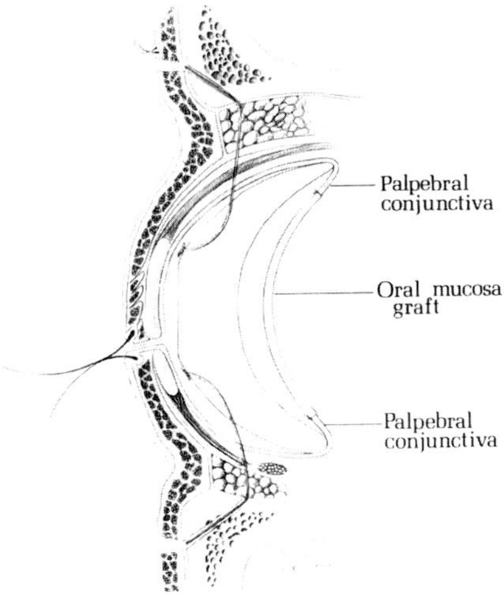

Figure 3. Socket reconstructed with large C-shaped conformer sutured to orbital rims.

sutures are tied with several knots, and, to prevent slippage, the cut ends are melted into bulbous tips using disposable cautery. The eyelids are united over the conformer with suture tarsorrhaphies of 4-0 silk and the incisions over the orbital rims closed in layers. Prophylactic antibiotics are given intravenously during surgery and for 48 hr after surgery. Skin sutures are removed in one week, tarsorrhaphy sutures in six weeks, and the conformer and polyfilament sutures in three months.

RESULTS

Seventeen patients underwent partial socket reconstruction between 1975 and 1985. Nine of these patients were anophthalmic, one had congenital anophthalmos, and the remaining seven had intact globes with extensive symblepharon formation. In the anophthalmic cases, surgery was performed to facilitate the fitting and retention of a cosmetically acceptable ocular prosthesis. In the others, surgery was performed to allow for the fitting of a cosmetic scleral shell (two cases) and to improve ocular and eyelid motility and symmetry with the opposite normally functioning eye (five cases).

Although a variety of underlying conditions accounted for the loss of the ocular fornices in our patients (Table 1), blunt and penetrating trauma and chemical injuries were the etiologic factors in 10 of the 17. In 12 patients, a variety of surgical interventions may also have contributed to the occurrence of cicatricial changes within the fornices and socket. Nine patients had undergone enucleation, and five had undergone some form of socket or eyelid reconstruction.

At the time of conformer removal, a variety of problems remained uncorrected in 7 of 15 cases (Table 2). These included cicatricial entropion, blepharoptosis, eyelid crease-fold disparity, cosmetically significant enophthalmos, narrowing of the horizontal fissure, and diplopia. Additional surgical intervention to correct these problems included transmarginal rotation, blepharoptosis repair using a fascia lata sling, eyelid crease reconstruction, dermis-fat grafting, and lateral canthoplasty [3].

There were several postoperative complications of partial socket reconstruction. Two patients had infraorbital anesthesia that resolved spontaneously; one patient had a streptococcal infection of the socket that was successfully treated with oral (ampicillin) and topical

Table 2. Residual Problems and Interventions Existing Following Partial Socket Reconstruction in 7 out of 15 Patients

Problem	No. of patients	Management	No. of patients
Cicatricial entropion	5	Transmarginal rotation	3
Blepharoptosis	2	Unilateral facia lata sling	2
Eyelid crease-fold disparity	2	Eyelid crease-fold reconstruction	2
Enophthalmos	3	Removal of orbital implant and dermis-fat grafting	1
Horizontal fissure disparity	1	Lateral canthotomy and reconstruction of temporal upper and lower eyelids	1
Diplopia	1	None	1

(gentamicin) antibiotics; and two patients developed mucous membrane granulomas, that were excised at the time of conformer removal.

The postoperative success of partial socket reconstruction was based on at least six months of evaluation following conformer removal. In all cases, stable and spacious ocular cul-de-sacs were the minimum requirements for a successful result. Over an average follow-up of 32 months, all ten anophthalmic patients were able to be fitted with and retain a cosmetically acceptable ocular prosthesis (Figs. 4 A–D). Similarly, over an average follow-up of 26 months, deep and stable fornices were formed in all seven sockets containing globes. In addition, all these showed improvement in ocular motility, widening of the palpebral fissure, and improved symmetry with the opposite normal eye.

COMMENT

Foreshortening of the conjunctival fornices and partial contracture of the ocular socket can result from a variety of factors, such as trauma, surgery, infection, chemical injury, and systemic disease. Various surgical techniques have evolved to solve these problems. When a small symblepharon is present, a Z-plasty or the use of a local conjunctival flap may be adequate [3–6]. For more extensive symblepharon formation or deficiencies in the fornices, either split-thickness mucosal grafts or full-thickness conjunctival grafts are necessary [3–8]. In general, if the socket is only partially compromised and some normal conjunctiva remains, split-thickness mucosal grafts or dermis-fat grafts are adequate for reconstruction [3–7]. When total reconstruction is necessary due to a severely compromised socket, more extensive surgery with full-thickness mucosal grafts is required [1–7].

The seventeen patients in this report represent a distinct group that is separate from those with total contracture. In partial contracture of the socket, the fornices are only moderately foreshortened by underlying scar tissue and a fair amount of normal conjunctiva is still present. Because less dissection and undermining is required to reconstruct these sockets, there is also a reduced propensity for recurrent scarring as compared to those sockets that are severely contracted with extensive underlying scar tissue. This situation permits the use of partial thickness mucous membrane grafts. These grafts are more cosmetically pleasing than full-thickness grafts and are more easily harvested with less trauma to the patient. However, they are more susceptible to shrinkage and contracture. Therefore, they can only be used when the area to be grafted is not susceptible to extensive scar formation. In addition, the presence of residual normal conjunctiva within the partially contracted socket obviates the need for extensive resurfacing with a full-thickness mucous membrane wrapped conformer. Rather, the graft needs only to be stented in place by the conformer which at the same time reforms the reconstructed fornices that remain surfaced by the residual normal socket conjunctiva.

The surgical procedure for partial socket reconstruction differs from total socket reconstruction in the type of mucous membrane used, the amount of dissection required to reform the fornices, and the size of the area needing resurfacing. However, both procedures use custom-designed conformers. The normal ocular fornices extend posteriorly above the orbital floor and below the roof, as well as vertically and horizontally. Previous approaches to fornix reconstruction have used thin symblepharon rings or prostheses with adequate vertical and horizontal dimensions. However, these procedures have paid little attention to the normal posterior dimension of the fornix. The use of a large C-shaped custom conformer, which is fixated to the orbital rims, not only reestablishes the vertical and horizontal dimensions of the

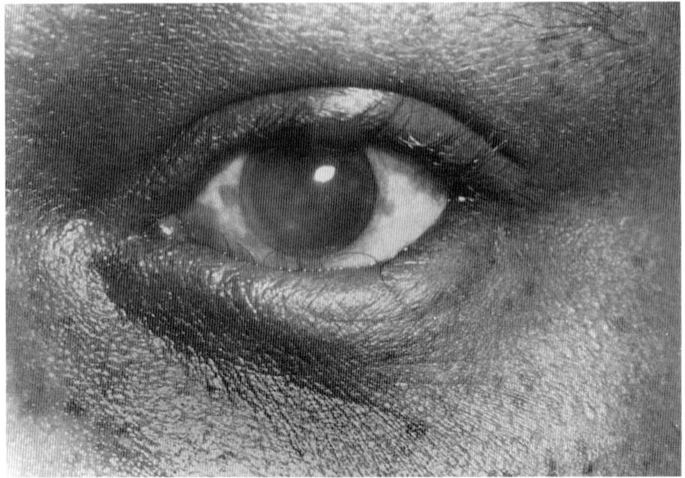

A

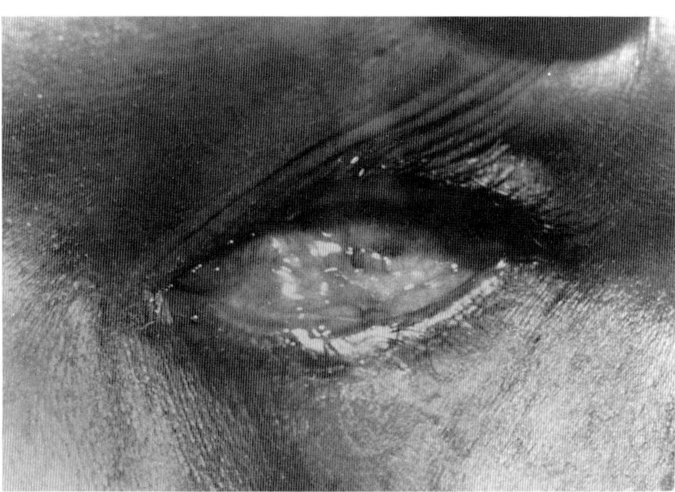

B

Figure 4. Case 9. (A) Preoperative view of partially contracted left socket showing cicatricial entropion of lower eyelid and poor inferior fitting of prosthesis. (B) Preoperative view of partially contracted left socket showing shallowing of inferior fornix. (*Figure 4 continued on facing page.*)

conjunctival fornices, but also is able to re-form the normal posterior conformation of these fornices through the exertion of posterior force by the conformer. (Figs. 3 and 5).

All the patients undergoing partial reconstruction achieved successful surgical results. The re-formed cul-de-sacs were deep and spacious; anophthalmic patients were able to retain a cosmetically acceptable ocular prosthesis, and patients with globes demonstrated improvement in ocular motility as well as an improved symmetry with the opposite normal eye. Surgical

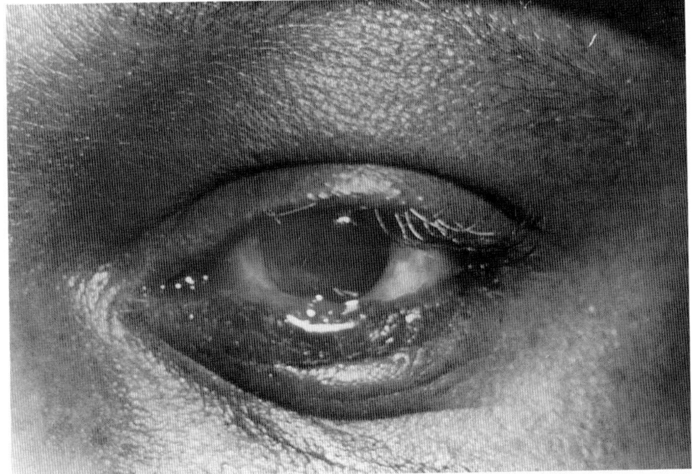

C

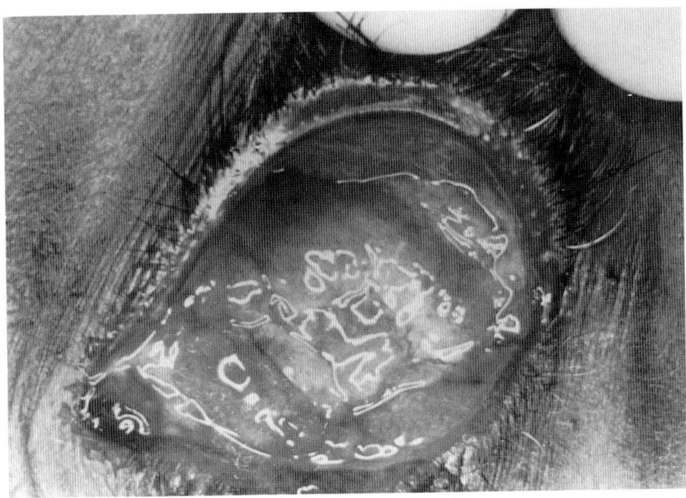

D

Figure 4 continued. (C) Postoperative view of left socket with ocular prosthesis following partial socket and transmarginal rotation. (D) Postoperative view of left socket showing deep and spacious cul-de-sacs.

complications of the procedure were few and easily treated. All reconstructed fornices remained stable after conformer removal for at least six months and in several cases for over five years. We feel that partial socket reconstruction with split-thickness mucous membrane grafts stented in place by a large custom-designed C-shaped conformer is a successful procedure for re-forming contracted ocular fornices and is a useful addition to the ophthalmic surgical armamentarium.

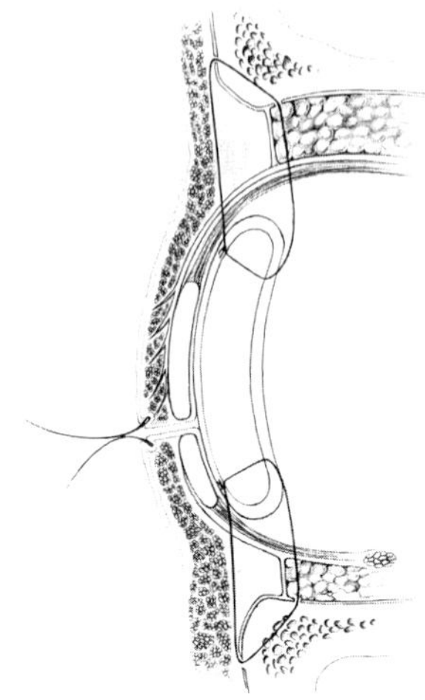

Figure 5. Socket reconstructed with standard-sized conformer sutured to orbital rims.

REFERENCES

1. Putterman AM, Scott R: Deep ocular socket reconstruction. *Arch Ophthalmol* 1977; 95:1221–1228.
2. Putterman AM, Karesh JW: A surgical technique for the successful and stable reconstruction of the totally contracted ocular socket. *Ophthalmic Surgery* 1988; 19:193–201.
3. McCord CD Jr, Tanenbaum M (eds): *Oculoplastic Surgery* ed 2. New York, Raven Press, 1987:327–349.
4. Baylis H, Shorr N, Tanenbaum M, McCord CD Jr: The anophthamic socket: Evaluation and management of surgical problems. In: McCord CD Jr, Tanenbaum M (eds): *Oculoplastic Surgery* ed 2. New York, Raven Press, 1987:425–449.
5. Callahan A: Contracted and deformed sockets. In: Soll DB (ed): *Management of Complications in Ophthalmic Plastic Surgery*. New York, Aesculapius Publishers Inc, 1976:345–359.
6. Putterman AM: Basic oculoplastic surgery. In: Peyman GA, Saunders DR, Goldberg MF (eds): *Principles and Practice of Ophthalmology*. Philadelphia, PA, WB Saunders Co, 1980:2321–2328.
7. Callahan A: Correction of abnormal soft tissue sockets. In: Silver B (ed): *Ophthalmic Plastic Surgery*. San Francisco, CA, American Academy of Ophthalmology and Otolaryngology, 1977:314–319.
8. Vastine DW, Stewart WB, Schwab IR: Reconstruction of the periocular mucous membrane by autologous conjunctival transplantation. *Ophthalmol* 1982; 89:1072–1081.

A Surgical Technique for the Reconstruction
of the Totally Contracted Ocular Socket

Allen M. Putterman, M.D. and James W. Karesh, M.D.

ABSTRACT

The successful and stable reconstruction of 47 severely contracted sockets over a 10-year period is described. The surgical technique used in all these cases was a large custom-designed C-shaped conformer wrapped with a full-thickness oral mucous membrane graft. After all cicatricial tissue within the socket was excised, the wrapped conformer was sutured at its mid-periphery to the inferior and superior orbital rims. In contrast to other procedures using flatter conformers, which direct their force in a vertical dimension, this uniquely designed conformer directs its force both vertically and deeply posteriorly within the socket. A somewhat modified but similar conformer can also be used for sockets compromised by total symblepharon formation. Excluding six patients with inadequate follow-up, we were able to successfully reform spacious and stable fornices in 40 of 41 severely contracted sockets. The average postoperative follow-up after reconstruction in these cases was 23.9 months. This technique represents an effective approach to successfully reconstruct and maintain stable ocular cul-de-sacs in cases of severe socket contracture or total symblepharon formation.

INTRODUCTION

The totally contracted ocular socket is a particularly difficult problem to manage. The progressive nature of the fibrotic process and the conjunctival shrinkage associated with multiple surgical interventions make reconstructive techniques prone to failure. Successful reconstruction requires the formation of a postoperatively stable and spacious socket that can retain a cosmetically acceptable conformer. In 1977 Putterman and Scott described a new technique for the reconstruction of the severely contracted socket [1]. This involved wrapping a large custom-designed C-shaped conformer with a full-thickness mucous membrane graft and suturing the entire unit to the orbital rims. Over the past 10 years this technique has been used to manage a variety of severely contracted sockets. This paper reviews our experience and long-term results with this procedure and describes modifications of the original procedure for reforming the ocular cul-de-sacs in cases of total socket contracture or symblepharon formation.

Reprinted with permission from *Ophthalmic Surg* 1988; 19(3):193–201.

This work was supported in part by core grant #EY1792 from the National Eye Institute, National Institute of Health, Bethesda, Maryland.

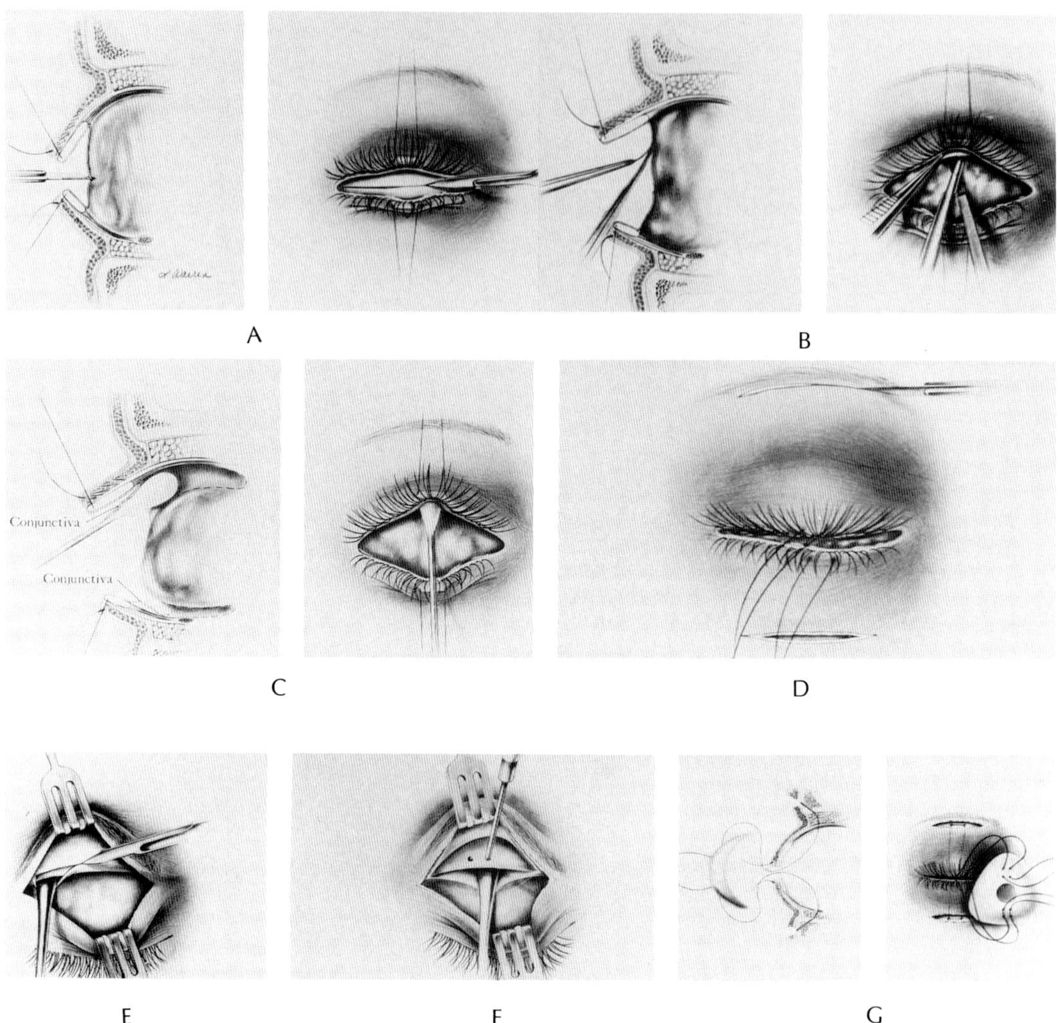

Figure 1. Procedure for total socket reconstruction. (A) Horizontal incision of central conjunctiva is made within contracted socket. (B) Conjunctiva is dissected from underlying scar tissue. (C) Cul-de-sac is recreated with blunt dissection using cotton-tipped applicators. (D) Incisions are made over superior and inferior orbital rims. (E) Periosteum is incised and elevated. (F) Holes are drilled in orbital rim, while periosteal elevator retracts periosteum. (G) Custom-designed large C-shaped conformer is sutured to orbital rims. (*Figure continued on facing page.*)

PATIENTS AND METHODS

The records of 39 patients from the private practice of one of the authors (AMP) and eight patients from the Oculoplastic Clinic at the University of Illinois Eye and Ear Infirmary were retrospectively examined. Between 1974 and 1986 all patients underwent reconstruction of a totally contracted socket or ocular fornices compromised by total symblepharon formation using the technique described herein. Preoperatively and postoperatively, patients were evaluated in consultation with an experienced ocularist who fabricated the custom-designed

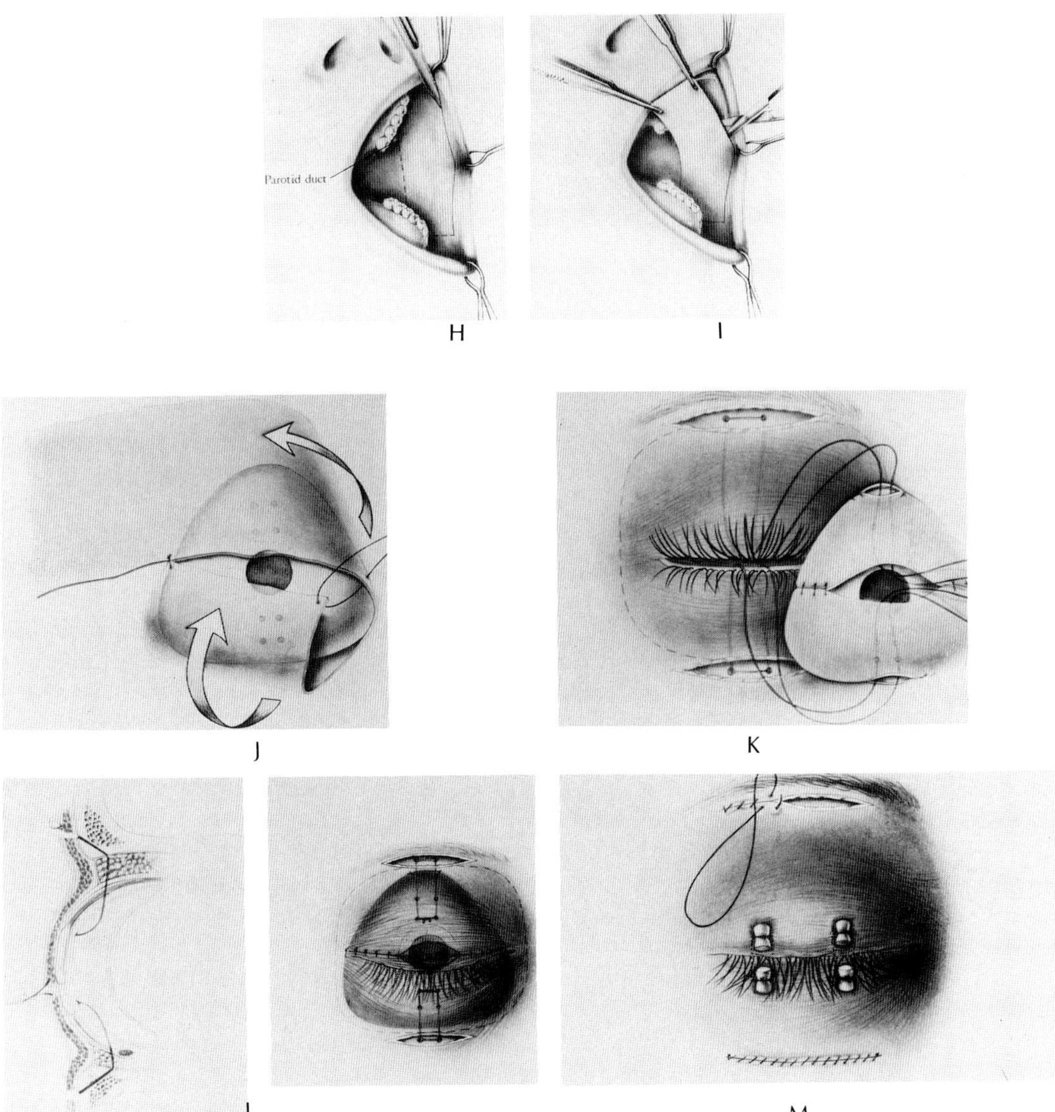

Figure 1 continued. (H) Incision is made for oral mucous membrane graft. (I) Oral mucous membrane graft is excised. (J) Conformer wrapped with mucosal graft in "P" shape configuration, raw surface outward. (K) Conformer wrapped with mucosal graft. (L) Conformer and graft are placed within reformed socket, sutures are tied and knotted. (M) Skin incision is closed; tarsorrhphy is in place.

C-shaped conformer used as part of the reconstructive technique. In some cases this ocularist was also present during surgery to aid in the intraoperative fitting of this conformer.

Patients were selected for total socket reconstruction based on an inability to retain a cosmetically acceptable prosthesis within an anophthalmic socket, or an unsuccessful effort by the ocularist to fashion a cosmetically acceptable artificial eye that would fit over a nonfunctioning globe. In all cases these failures were related to extensive fibrosis and conjunctival shrinkage within the socket, as evidenced by extensive anklyoblepharon and symblepharon formation, extensive foreshortening of the ocular cul-de-sacs, and severe cicatricial entropion. Other associated problems included absent or poor levator function, traumatic disruption of the eyelid margins, and scarring of the eyelid skin. Patient evaluation included a complete ophthalmic history, as well as a careful examination of the ocular socket and its contents, eyelids, bony orbit, and periorbital tissue. Particular attention was directed toward the adequacy of the ocular cul-de-sacs and conjunctiva, presence or absence of an orbital implant globe, cicatricial eyelid changes, levator function, and integrity of the superior and inferior orbital rims. The oral mucosa was also examined to determine its adequacy for grafting.

SURGICAL TECHNIQUE

The procedure (Figs. 1 and 2) can be performed using either local or general anesthesia, however, the latter is preferred for patient comfort. The eyelids are separated with traction sutures and the conjunctiva remaining in the socket is incised horizontally from the lateral to medial canthus. Thorough undermining is performed until the conjunctiva is released from all underlying scar and connective tissue up to the tarsus of the upper and lower eyelids. A medial or lateral cathotomy may also need to be performed if the palpebral fissure is decreased. To create an adequate space for the new ocular fornices, further dissection and excision of scar tissue is carried superiorly under the orbital roof and inferiorly over the orbital floor. This may also need to be performed medially and laterally if there is cicatrization of these areas.

One of three differently sized prefabricated custom-designed C-shaped conformers is then chosen to act as a stent for the new ocular fornices. These conformers have a 5 mm central drainage hole, as well as several suture holes, to facilitate fixation to the inferior and superior orbital rims. It is ideal to choose a conformer that fits snugly within the socket while allowing the eyelids to easily close. The size and posterior extent of the conformers is essential to the reformation of deep and spacious cul-de-sacs, as well as to the long-term maintenance of a stable postoperative result.

Incisions over the central inferior and superior orbital rims are made and the bone in these areas exposed. After the periosteum is elevated from the rims and orbital floor and roof, two drill holes are made through the central area of both rims. These holes begin several millimeters from the inferior and superior rims and exit through the orbital floor and roof. A 2-0 polyfilament (Supramid, S. Jackson, Alexandria, VA) suture is then inserted into the superior drill holes, and using a large curved needle, the suture material is passed through the bony opening exiting into the newly created superior fornix. Similarly, suture material is passed into the inferior fornix from the drill holes in the inferior rim. These sutures are then placed through the midperipheral holes in the conformer.

A full-thickness mucous membrane graft is taken from the oral mucosa of the cheek and lips. The submucosal injection of lidocaine with epinephrine is helpful for both hemostasis and the free-hand dissection of the mucosa. A number 15 Bard-Parker blade (Storz, St. Louis, MO) is used to incise the mucosa 3 mm from its junction with the lip across the entire extent of the lip and cheek. Incisions are then made down to the gingival mucosa from each end of the initial incision and these are connected approximately 3 mm distal to the gingiva and parallel to the lip incision. The full-thickness oral mucosal graft is then excised using blunt and

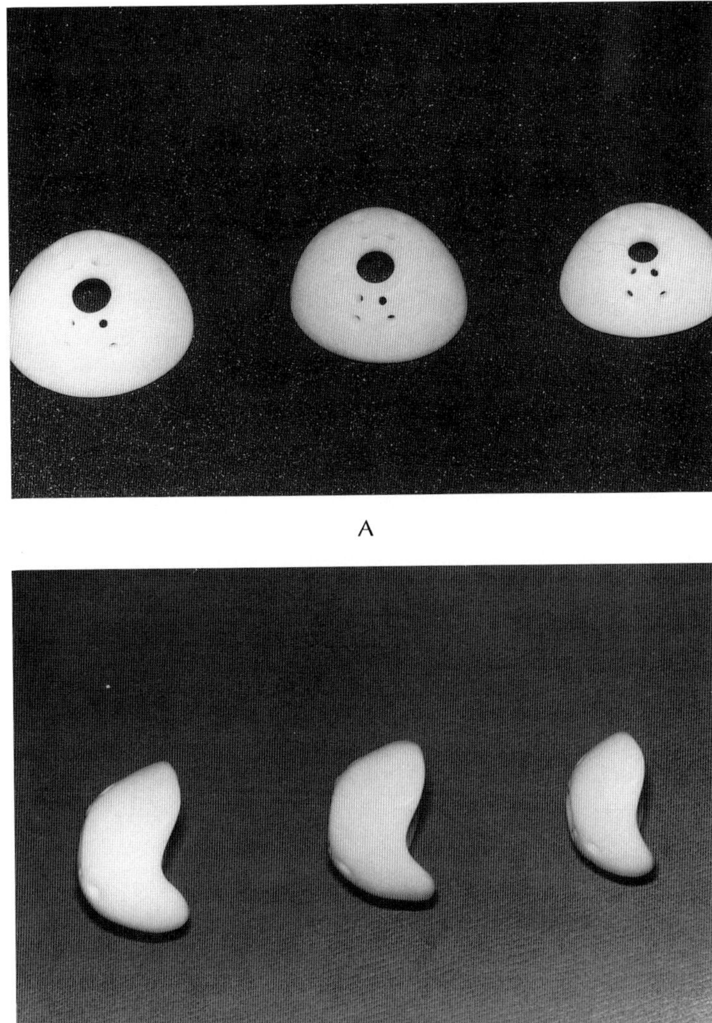

Figure 2. Custom-designed large C-shaped conformer used in total socket reconstruction. (A) Anterior view; (B) lateral view.

sharp dissection with a Wescott scissors (Storz, St. Louis, MO). Commonly, the graft measures 6 to 8 cm by 2.5 cm. After trimming submucosal tissue from the graft, it is wrapped around the conformer, raw surface outward, and sutured to itself with 6-0 polyglactin 910 (Vicryl, Ethicon, Somerville, NJ) sutures. The conformer is completely covered with graft material except centrally where the Supramid sutures are passed through the central drainage opening. It is essential to completely cover the conformer to successfully resurface the socket and obtain a stable postoperative result. The graft-covered conformer is then placed behind the eyelids and into the socket. The Supramid sutures are drawn tight and tied so that the conformer is centered within the socket. The eyelids are closed over the conformer with suture tarsorrhaphies of 4-0 silk. The incisions over the superior and inferior rims are sutured in a standard fashion. The skin sutures are removed in one week and the tarsorrhaphies in six to nine weeks.

TOTAL SYMBLEPHARON RECONSTRUCTION

The same procedure can be performed for total symblepharon. In such cases added care is taken to avoid injury to the globe during blunt and sharp dissection around the eye during passage of the Supramid sutures with the large curved surgical needles. The ocularist makes three C-shaped symblepharon rings (Fig. 3). These are thinner than the conformers used for total socket contracture and have a large central opening, not only for drainage but to prevent pressure on the cornea. The shape of the rings and placement of the midperipheral and central suture holes are similar to those of the socket conformers. The procedure is otherwise the same described for total socket reconstruction, including the complete wrapping of the oral mucous membrane graft around the symblepharon ring.

RESULTS

Between 1974 and 1986 a total of 47 patients with severely contracted ocular sockets underwent total socket reconstruction. Six anophthalmic patients (three male and three female) are not included in the final results because of inadequate follow-up (less than six months) following socket reconstruction. The underlying pathologies in these patients included trauma (four patients), glaucoma (one patient), and chemical injury (one patient). However, none of

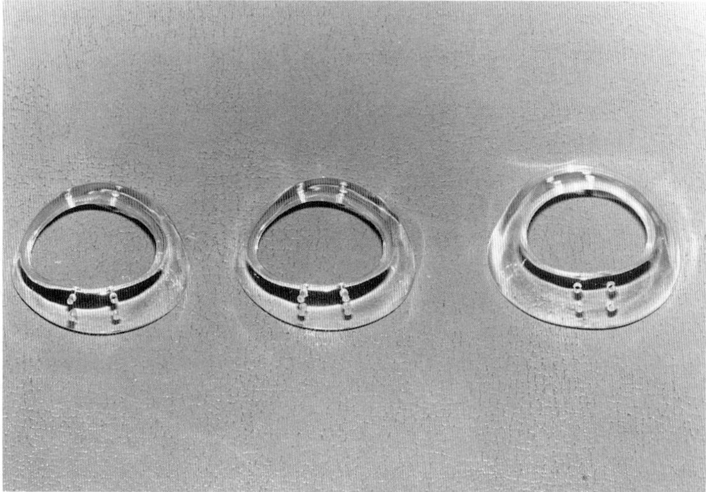

Figure 3. Custom-designed symblepharon rings for total symblepharon reconstruction.

these six patients developed any evidence of recurrent socket contracture during the short time they were followed postoperatively. Among the other patients, there were 22 female and 19 male patients, ranging from 7 to 88 years (average, 36 years). Follow-up was from seven to 115 months (average 23.9 months after conformer removal). At the time of socket reconstruction 36 sockets were anophthalmic and five sockets had nonfunctioning globes. Among the anophthalmic sockets underlying pathologies included trauma (12 patients), tumors (13 patients), chemical injuries (four patients), glaucoma (two patients), and one case each of cryptophthalmos, microphthalmos, congenital anophthalmos, facial paralysis, and Sjogren's syndrome (Table 1). Among the other cases, socket contracture was associated with chemical injuries (two patients), and cicatricial pemphigoid, cryptophthalmos, syndrome, and thermal injury (one patient each) (Table 1).

Prior to socket reconstruction, 10 patients had undergone radiation therapy for malignant tumors. A variety of surgical procedures had been performed on an additional 20 sockets (Table 2). These included various attempts at symblepharon lysis and socket reconstruction with oral mucous membrane or skin grafts (17 sockets), open reduction and repair of orbital and facial fractures (three sockets), and multiple surgeries to replace extruded orbital implants (one socket). Multiple infections were a factor in five cases.

At the time of conformer removal, six months following mucous membrane grafting, all sockets and eyelid margins required some revision to remove excess mucosa and granulation tissue. A variety of additional problems developed in 33 patients over the period of postsurgical follow-up (Table 3). The most frequent of these were oral cicatrix formation, cicatricial entropion, upper eyelid coloboma, upper eyelid retraction, blepharophimosis and anklyoblepharon, socket infection, granuloma formation, and blepharoptosis. In 24 patients some intervention was needed to correct these problems. This included transmarginal rotation (eight patients), blepharoptosis surgery (six patients), canthal reconstruction (five patients), granuloma excision or steroid injection (seven patients), recession of upper eyelid retractors (two

Table 1. Clinical History of 47 Patients Requiring Total Socket Reconstruction

Underlying pathology	No. of patients
Retinoblastoma	6
Gunshot wound	5
Childhood tumor	4
Childhood trauma	4
Alkali burn	4
Acid burn	3
Glaucoma	3
Thermal burn	3
Auto accident	3
Anophthalmia/microphthalmia	2
Rhabdomyosarcoma	2
Cryptophthalmos syndrome	2
Firecracker injury	1
Sjogren's syndrome	1
Ocular pemphigoid	1
Rodent bite	1
Meningioma	1
Facial paralysis	1

Table 2. Intervention Before Total Socket Reconstruction ($n = 47$)

	No. of procedures	No. of patients
Enucleation only	17	17
Enucleation plus additional interventions	41*	23*
1. Radiation therapy	(9)	(9)
2. Partial socket reconstruction	(11)	(7)
3. Total socket reconstruction		
A. with skin	(3)	(3)
B. with mucous membrane	(5)	(5)
4. Orbital floor reconstruction	(3)	(3)
5. Subperiosteal implant	(1)	(1)
6. Lower eyelid reconstruction	(1)	(1)
7. Expansion conformers	(1)	(1)
8. Removal of extruding orbital implant	(5)	(4)
9. Replacement of extruding orbital implant	(2)	(1)
Radiation therapy alone	1	1
Symblepharon lysis alone	2	2
Socket reconstruction alone	6*	3*
1. with skin	(2)	(2)
2. with mucous membrane	(4)	(3)
No intervention	1	1

*Ten patients had more than one intervention performed prior to total socket reconstruction.

Table 3. Problems Occurring Postoperatively in Patients Undergoing Total Socket Reconstruction ($n = 41$)[+]

	No. of patients	No. of patients requiring intervention
No surgical problems	12	0
Postsurgical problems	29*	24**
Oral cicatrix	(16)	(9)
Upper eyelid retraction	(7)	(2)
Blepharoptosis	(8)	(6)
Socket infection	(6)	(6)
Cicatricial entropion	(10)	(8)
Blepharophimosis/anklyoblepharon	(5)	(5)
Socket granuloma	(8)	(7)
Cicatricial ectropion	(2)	(2)
Infraorbital anesthesia	(1)	(0)
Lower eyelid retraction	(1)	(1)
Deep supratarsal sulcus	(1)	(1)
Upper eyelid coloboma	(1)	(1)
Suture abscess	(1)	(1)
Naso-orbital fistula	(1)	(0)

*Eighteen patients had more than one postsurgical problem.
**Fifteen patients underwent more than one intervention.
[+]Excluding six patients inadequate postoperative follow-up.

patients), skin grafting (two patients), and upper eyelid composite grafting with lower eyelid scleral grafting (one patient). Cicatrix formation of the oral mucosa was the most common postoperative problem associated with full-thickness oral mucous membrane grafting, occurring in 16 patients. To successfully treat this condition, six patients required submucosal steroid injections, one patient needed a mucosal Z-plasty, and two patients had both steroid injections and a mucosal Z-plasty [2]. Socket infections occurred in six patients and were successfully treated with oral antibiotics (ampicillin, erythromycin, or cephalexin) and topical antibiotics (gentamicin).

Criteria for good results following total socket reconstruction included both the development of a stable and spacious ocular cul-de-sac and the ability to be fitted with and retain a cosmetically acceptable ocular prosthesis. These results depended in part upon a minimum postoperative follow-up of seven months (i.e., one month after conformer removal). Stable and spacious cul-de-sacs were created in 40 of the 41 sockets undergoing total socket reconstruction (Figs. 4–5). In only one case, a patient with severe cicatricial pemphigoid, foreshortening of the ocular fornix following reconstruction was present. This patient developed a mild loss of both the superior and inferior cul-de-sacs associated with severe cicatricial entropion. The other 36 anophthalmic sockets and the four patients with nonfunctioning globes have been able to retain a cosmetically acceptable artificial eye and have maintained spacious sockets for seven to 113 months, postoperatively.

COMMENT

Total socket with severe cul-de-sac loss and inability to retain a cosmetically acceptable ocular prosthesis can result from a variety of factors, including socket infection, orbital radiation, severe chemical or thermal injury, orbital trauma, multiple socket surgeries, ill-fitting and roughened artificial eyes, and failure to wear an artificial eye [3,4]. The inability to wear a cosmetically acceptable artificial eye is not only physically disfiguring but can be a psychological burden. Many of these patients resort to wearing a black patch, often an unacceptable solution to the problem.

Successful socket reconstruction is related to both the extent of the underlying cicatricial process and the shrinkage of conjunctival tissue. Partially contracted sockets can be successfully repaired through a variety of techniques. Dermis-fat grafting is an excellent procedure for the anophthalmic socket with minimal contracture or in cases of implant extrusion or migration [5]. Partial-thickness oral mucous membrane grafting is a procedure of choice in cases with more extensive socket contracture [6–8]. Total obliteration of the ocular fornices either by symblepharon formation or through extensive socket contracture is the most difficult of socket problems to reverse and often recurs after apparently successful surgical intervention. A variety of surgical techniques have been developed to treat severely contracted sockets. Mustarde [4] advocates the use of split-thickness skin grafts draped over a normally shaped conformer that has been enlarged. An external splinting device is then used to direct pressure against the conformer and prevent its extrusion. Another method for reconstructing severely contracted sockets uses a full- or partial-thickness oral mucous membrane graft or a split-thickness skin graft to reline the sockets [3,6,7]. A cranioplastic cast or other similar conformer wrapped with this mucous membrane or skin is sutured to the orbital rim and remains in place for three to six months. Vistnes and Iverson [9] have developed a technique whereby

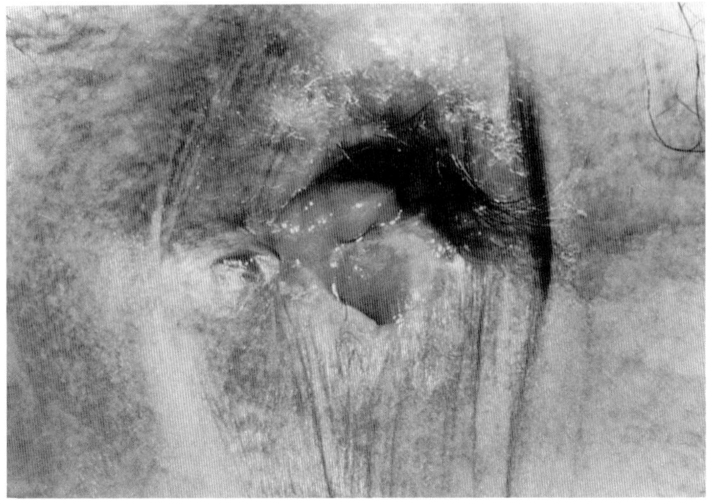

A

B

Figure 4. Patient 18. (A) Preoperative view of severely contracted left socket. (B) Postoperative view showing deep and spacious inferior cul-de-sac. (*Figure continued on facing page.*)

Kirschner pins fastened to the orbital walls are used in conjunction with RTV silicone to stent a partial-thickness oral mucous membrane in the reconstructed socket.

The technique for total socket reconstruction described herein was developed to overcome the problems of recurrent socket contraction following conventional reconstructive surgery [1]. It can also be adapted to the reconstruction of partially contracted sockets or ocular fornices moderately compromised by symblepharon formation [8]. The basis for this technique is in the anatomy of the normal ocular fornix, which has a significant posterior component

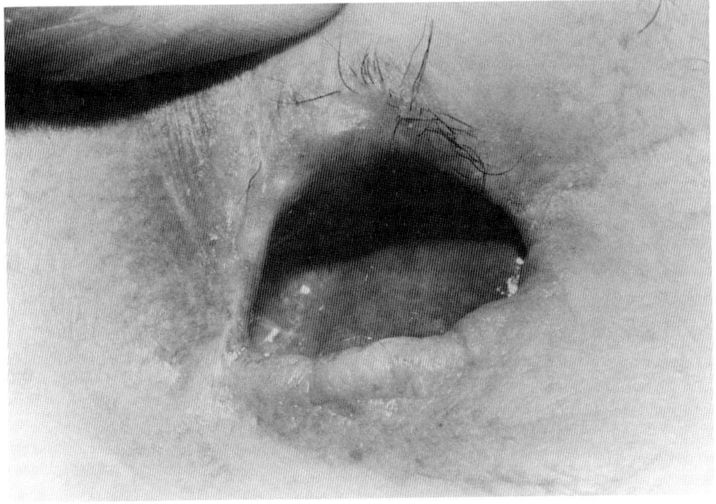

C

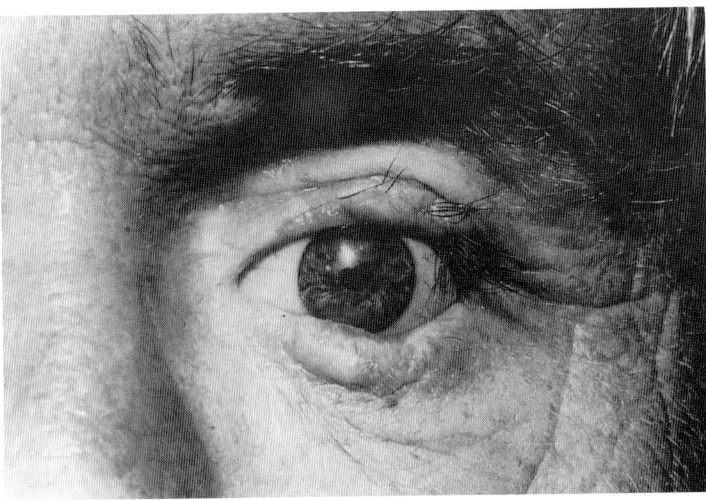

D

Figure 4 continued. (C) Postoperative view showing deep and spacious superior cul-de-sac. (D) Postoperative view with ocular prosthesis.

in addition to its horizontal and vertical components. The large C-shaped conformer was designed to develop this posterior dimension to the greatest possible extent. Other reconstructive techniques use conformers that are relatively flat, concentrating their force vertically. In contrast, the large C-shaped conformer directs its force both vertically and posteriorly to achieve a more normal socket structure. When this conformer is fixated at its mid-periphery to the orbital rims, its posterior portion is pushed much more deeply into the reformed ocu-

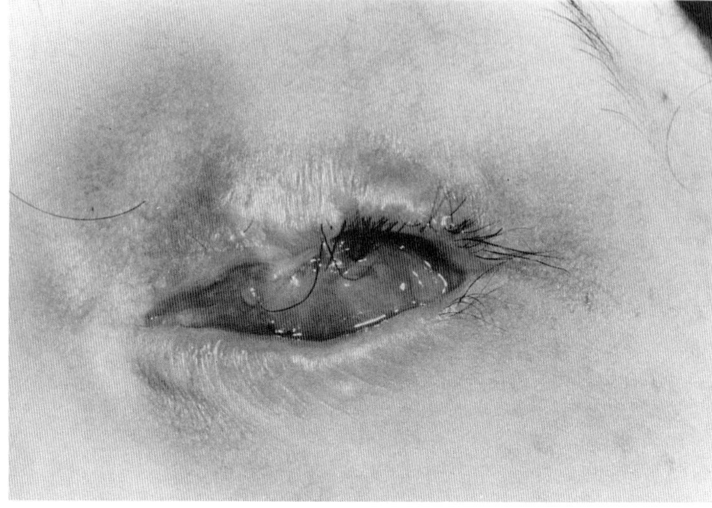

A

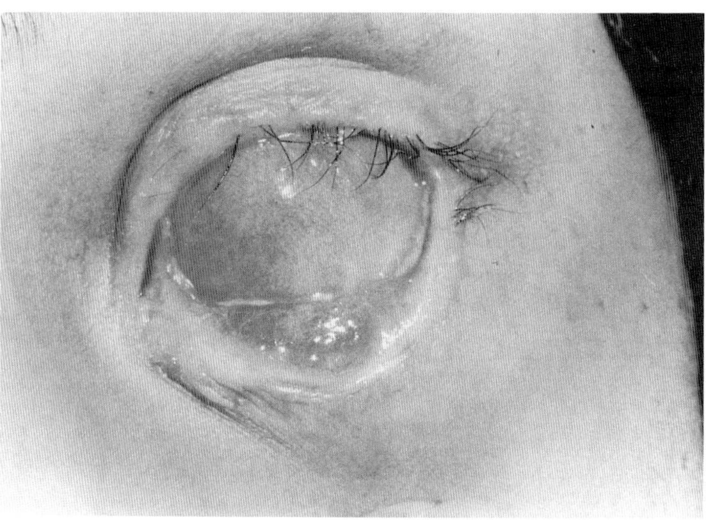

B

Figure 5. Patient 21. (A) Preoperative view of total left ocular symblepharon. (B) Postoperative view showing deep and spacious inferior cul-de-sac. (*Figure continued on facing page.*)

lar fornices than previously described conformers. These two major features of our technique contributed to the successful and stable results we achieved. The large conformer was essential for creating a spacious socket and the fixation of this conformer to the orbital rims for an extended period was essential for ensuring the prolonged stability of the surgical result.

Although excellent postoperative results were achieved with the surgical technique, surgical revision including a variety of postoperative changes involving the socket and the eyelids

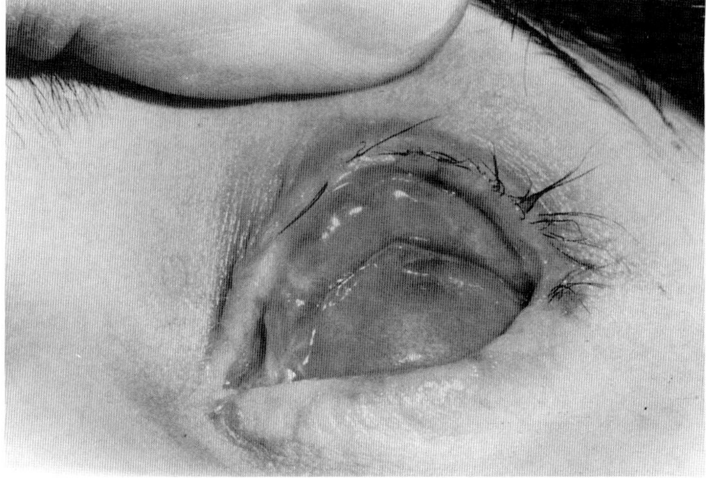

C

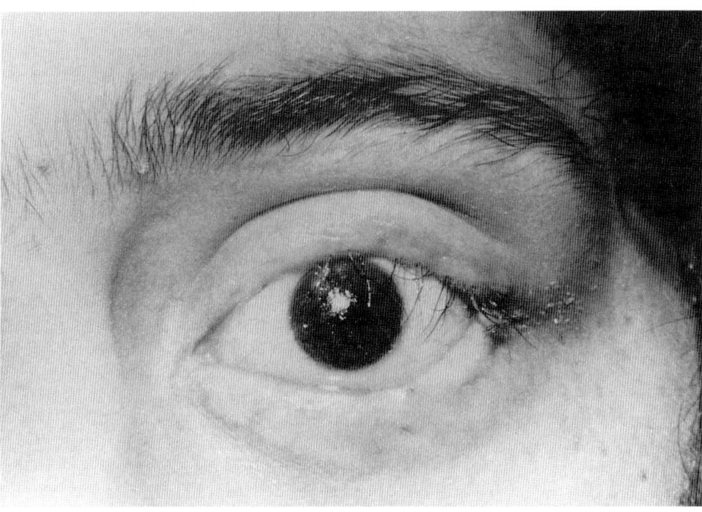

D

Figure 5 continued. (C) Postoperative view showing deep and spacious superior cul-de-sac. (D) Postoperative view with ocular prosthesis.

was often required after conformer removal. Removal of excess oral mucosa, excision of socket granulomas, and division of ankyloblepharons were common. Blepharophimosis, secondary to eyelid fusion, was easily treated by dividing the eyelids and suturing excess conjunctiva to the raw surfaces of the eyelid margins. Minor socket infections occurred infrequently and were easily managed with oral and topical antibiotics. Cicatricial entropion was managed with a transverse blepharotomy, whereas blepharoptosis treatment depended on residual levator function. Both a conjunctiva-Muller's muscle excision and levator aponeurosis surgery were successfully used to correct this problem. Although some complications of socket reconstruction cannot be avoided, careful surgical dissection is essential to prevent trauma to structures such as the levator aponeurosis, orbital nerves, and the thin bone of the orbital floor and medial wall, resulting in blepharoptosis, facial anesthesia, and sinus-socket fistulae.

To avoid postoperative complications involving the oral mucosa, patients were instructed in mouth stretching exercises. These consisted of opening the mouth widely while pushing the involved cheek and lip inwardly and outwardly six times per day for several months. This was helpful in preventing scar contracture at the donor site. Nonetheless, several patients required the injection of steroids into the scar and three patients needed Z-plasties of the oral mucosa [2].

Using this surgical technique spacious and stable sockets were achieved in 40 of 41 severely contracted sockets. These reformed sockets maintained their enlarged dimensions over an average follow-up of more than two years. Only one patient developed a recurrent foreshortening of the inferior cul-de-sac. The remaining forty patients achieved excellent surgical results and were able to be fitted with a cosmetically acceptable ocular prosthesis.

At one time severely contracted ocular sockets were not considered to be candidates for surgery and were relegated to treatment with a black patch. Our procedure for total socket reconstruction provides a successful and stable alternative to this. The excellent surgical results achieved make this procedure for total socket reconstruction an important addition to the armamentarium of the ophthalmic surgeon.

REFERENCES

1. Putterman AM, Scott R: Deep ocular socket reconstruction. *Arch Ophthalmol* 1977; 95:1211–1228.
2. Newhaus RW, Baylis HI, Shorr N: Complications at mucous membrane donor sites. *Am J Ophthalmol* 1982; 93:643–646.
3. Callahan A: Contracted and deformed sockets. In: Soll DB (ed): *Management of Complications in Ophthalmic Plastic Surgery*, Birmingham, AL, Aesculapius Publishing Co., 1976:345–358.
4. Mustarde JC: *Repair and Reconstruction in the Orbital Region*, ed 2. New York, Churchill, Livingstone, 1980:215–244.
5. Gurberina C, Hornblass A, Metzler MA, Soarez V, Smith B: Autogenous dermis-fat orbital implantation. *Arch Ophthalmol* 1983; 101:1586–1590.
6. Callahan A, Dortzbach RK: Socket reconstruction advances. In: Mustarde JC, Jones L, Callahan A (eds): *Ophthalmic Plastic Surgery Up-To-Date*. Birmingham, AL, Aesculapius Publishing Co., 1970:125–138.
7. Baylis H, Shorr N: Correction of problems of the anophthalmic socket. In McCord CD Jr (ed): *Oculoplastic Surgery*. New York, Raven Press, 1981:327–347.
8. Karesh JW, Putterman AM: Reconstruction of the partially contracted ocular socket or fornix. *Arch Ophthalmol* 1988; 106:552–556.
9. Vistness LM, Iverson RE: Surgical treatment of the contracted socket. *Plast Reconstr Surg* 1974; 53:563–567.

Temporalis Muscle Transfer in the Treatment of the Severely Contracted Socket

Giulio Bonavolontà, M.D.

ABSTRACT

The treatment of severely contracted sockets represents one of the most difficult situations in ophthalmic plastic and reconstructive surgery. In particular, the treatment of the postirradiated socket has been considered "hopeless surgery." In recent years a modified approach to this problem has been tried, in which the use of the temporalis muscle provided a well-vascularized bed for delayed reconstructions.

INTRODUCTION

The treatment of severely contracted sockets represents one of the most difficult situations for the ophthalmic plastic surgeon [1]. Failure in these cases occurs because of incorrect assumptions that all cases include similar clinical entities. This false assumption leads to incorrect surgical approaches to the problem [2].

In recent years we have tried to differentiate the contracted socket in five main categories, in relation to their clinical presentation, dividing them as follows:

1. Mild superficial contracted socket (contraction of conjunctival fornix)
2. Severe superficial contracted socket (contraction of lids and conjunctival fornix)
3. Mild deep contracted socket (contraction of conjunctival fornix and orbital fat)
4. Severe deep contracted socket (absence of conjunctival fornix and severe contraction of orbital fat)
5. Total contracted socket (all the previous situations plus developmental bone abnormalities)

Stage five of this classification represents the most difficult to manage, because the absence of a well-vascularized bed is always the cause of failure of traditional techniques [3–4]. This paper discusses the surgical approach to this problem, which has given the best results after long-term follow-up.

MATERIALS AND METHODS

Because the indications for such a technique are fortunately quite rare, during the last five years we have operated on three patients. In the same period of time, among a large number of contracted sockets observed in our institution, only six cases were classified in category five.

 G. BONAVOLONTÀ

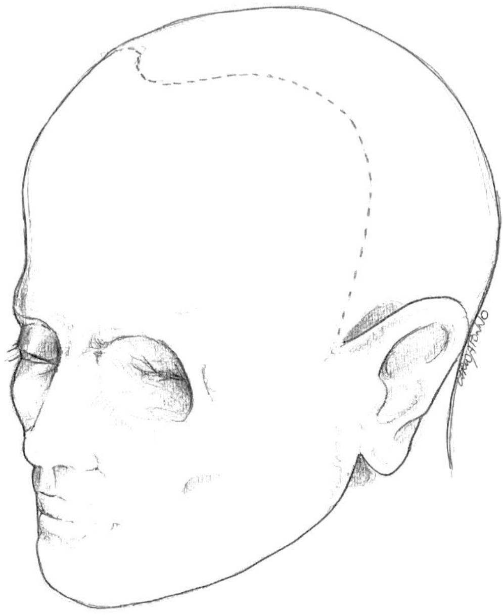

Figure 1. The orbit is exposed with a bicoronal flap.

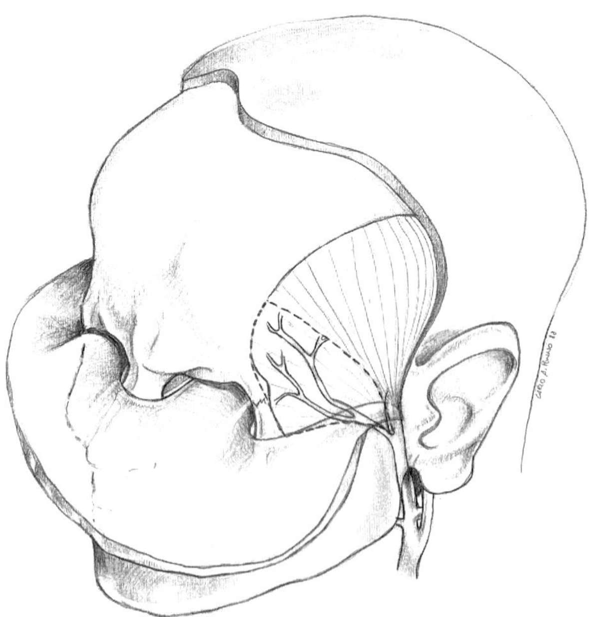

Figure 2. The temporalis muscle is incised vertically, separating its anterior one-third from its posterior two-thirds.

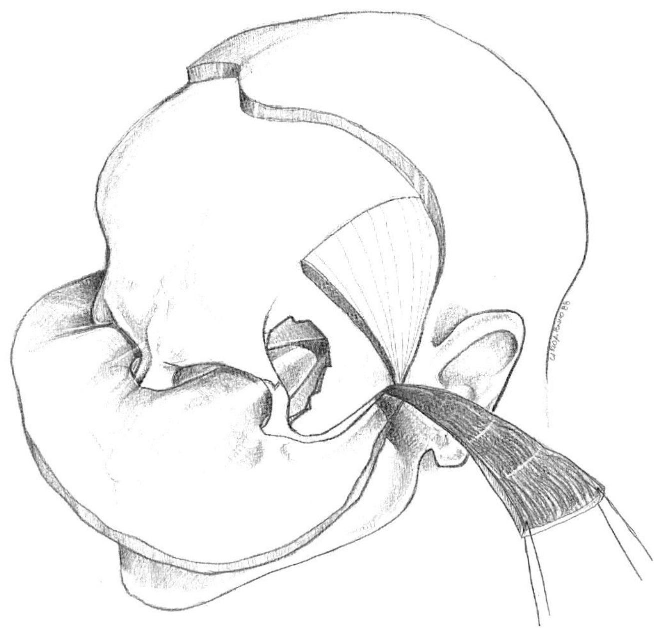

Figure 3. A large lateral floor and lateral wall osteotomy is performed.

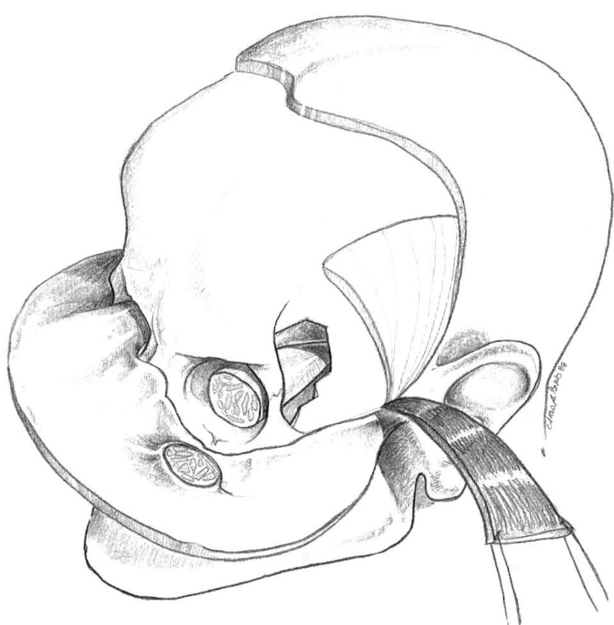

Figure 4. The orbital contents, previously completely released from the periorbita, are trans-sected. The anterior portion is left adherent to the bicoronal flap and the posterior portion is left attached to the orbital apex.

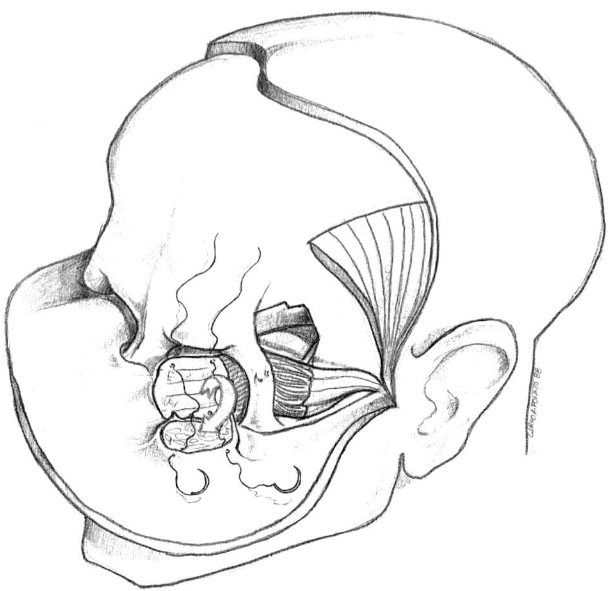

Figure 5. The temporalis muscle flap is transposed into the orbit through the lateral osteotomy. The temporalis fascia is sutured to the anterior orbital periosteum.

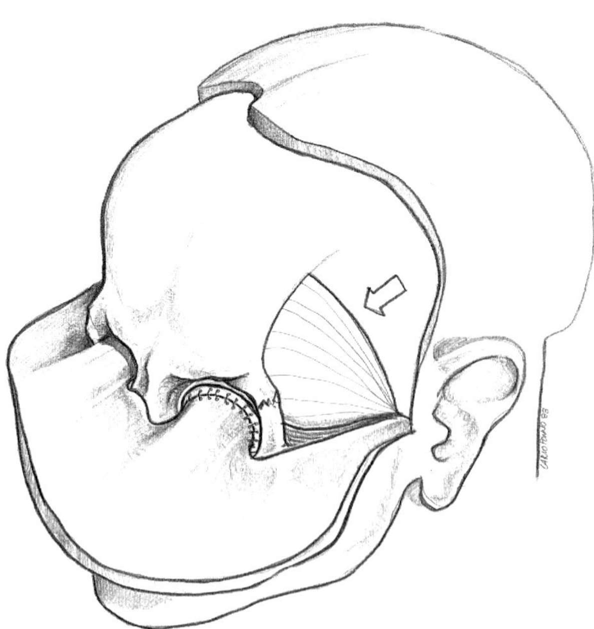

Figure 6. The posterior two-thirds of the temporalis muscle are shifted anteriorly to reduce postoperative depression of the temporalis fossa.

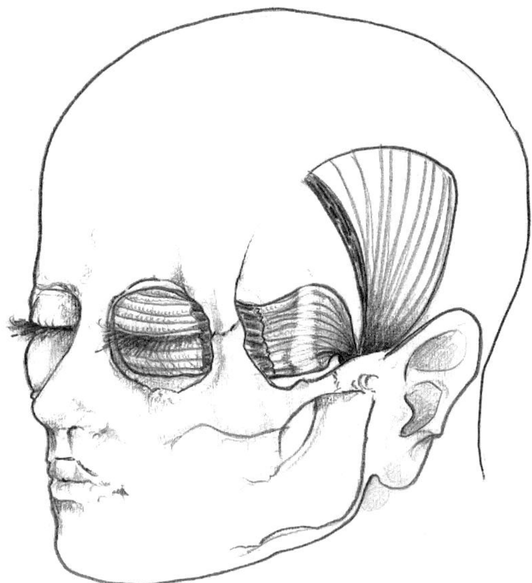

Figure 7. The orbit is filled with temporalis muscle and fascia.

Three of them refused any treatment and were unable to be followed-up. The other three patients were included in our protocol. Their treatment consisted of a first stage, in which we tried to solve the problem of the deep contraction by providing a new well-vascularized bed, with the temporalis muscle transfer (TMT), and a second stage (six months later), in which we completed the reconstruction of the anterior socket. Data and results are summarized in Table 1.

SURGICAL TECHNIQUE

STAGE 1

The surgery is performed under general anesthesia. The orbit is exposed through a coronal incision. The intraorbital contents are totally released, for 360°, from the overlying orbital bones (Fig. 1).

The anterior third of the temporalis muscle is cut with a vertical incision from its insertion to the temporal bone to its deep insertion behind the zygomatic arch, taking care to preserve the blood supply that is provided by the anterior branch of the deep temporal artery (Fig. 2). A large osteotomy is performed in the lateral orbital wall and in the lateral third of the orbital floor up to the infraorbital fissure (Fig. 3).

The coronal flap dissection is extended. The remaining intraorbital contents are incised in a coronal plane parallel to the orbital rims, leaving the inner part attached to the orbital apex and the outer part attached to the skin and leaving a space between the trans-sected orbital stumps (Fig. 4).

The temporalis muscle flap is transposed into the orbital cavity through the lateral osteotomy: the temporalis fascia is turned towards the anterior part of the orbit (Fig. 5).

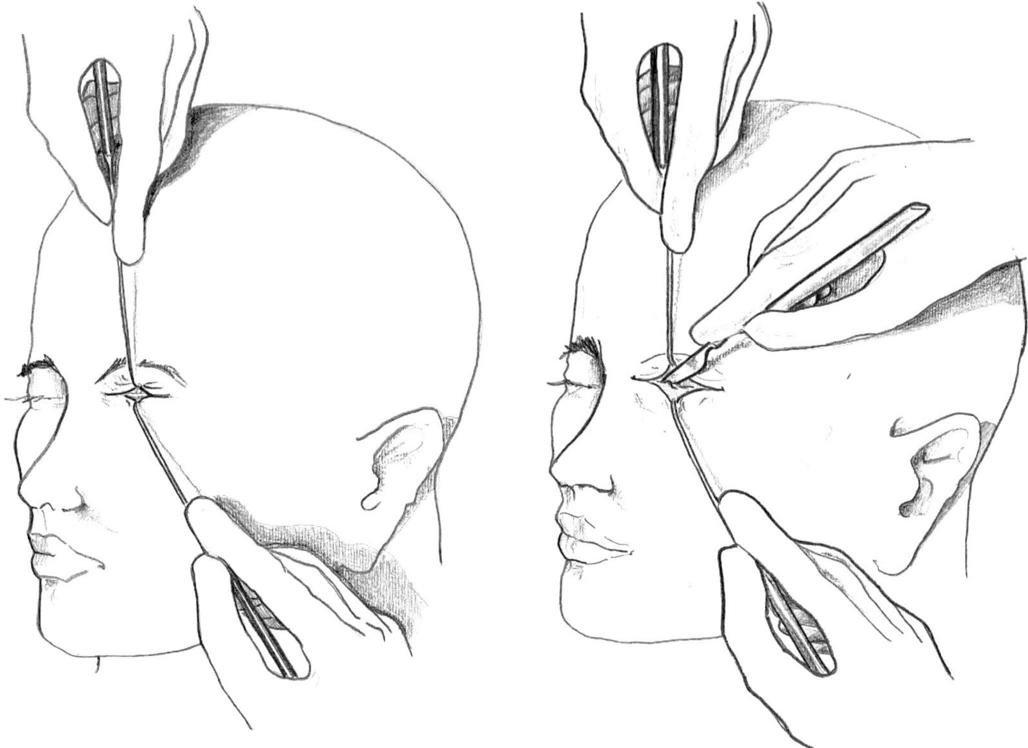

Figure 8. To begin the second stage of the reconstruction of the anterior socket the lids are carefully opened between the lid margins.

Figure 9. The lids are freed from the anterior surface of the temporalis flap.

To keep the temporalis muscle in a good position between the two stumps, it is necessary to suture the muscular fascia all around the periorbital fascia overlying the anterior stump (Fig. 5).

The posterior two-thirds of the temporalis muscle, which were left in their original anatomic position, are shifted anteriorly to reduce the postoperative depression in the temporalis fossa. The subcutaneous and skin layers are closed with vicryl 4-0 and prolene 3-0 sutures (Fig. 6).

At the end of surgery the muscular flap will lie behind the two lids, giving a more "bulky" appearance to the orbit with less of a superior sulcus deformity (Fig. 7).

STAGE 2

Once the physiological shrinkage of the muscular flap is over, which is the main reason for failure of the "one step" traditional techniques, the reconstruction of the anterior socket can be planned.

The lids are carefully opened through the lid margin (Fig. 8). The dissection is carried out, looking for the exposure of the deep temporalis muscle fascia (Fig. 9). When the temporalis fascia is well-exposed it will represent the posterior part of the new socket (Fig. 10).

The fornices and the posterior lid lamella will be restored with free skin or mucous mem-

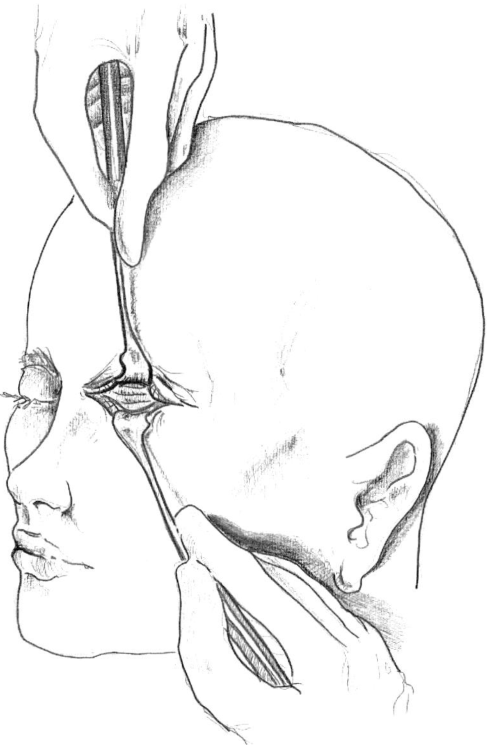

Figure 10. The deep temporalis muscle fascia forms the posterior part of the new socket.

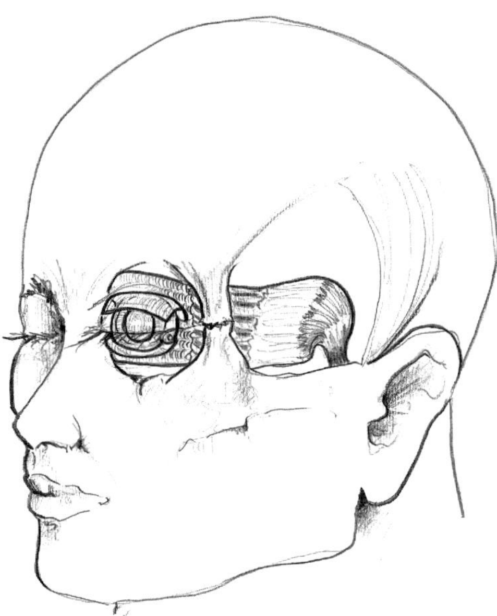

Figure 11. A fornix conformer maintains the fornices and keeps the skin or mucous membrane grafts in proper apposition to the posterior surface of the eyelids.

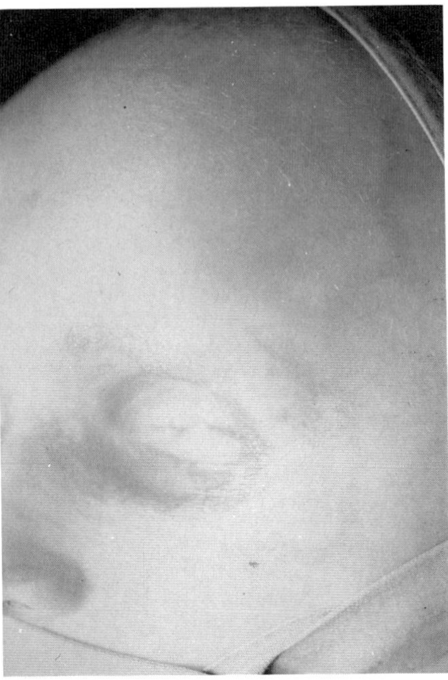

Figure 12. A patient with severely contracted socket in which the lids are attached to the orbital bones and the fornices are totally obliterated.

brane grafts, using a conformer to keep the graft in a good position (Fig. 11). A temporary tarsorrhaphy is necessary for at least 30 days. One lateral hole will allow the washing out of the cavity. Once the tarsorrhaphy has been opened, the conformer can be exchanged for a permanent prosthesis.

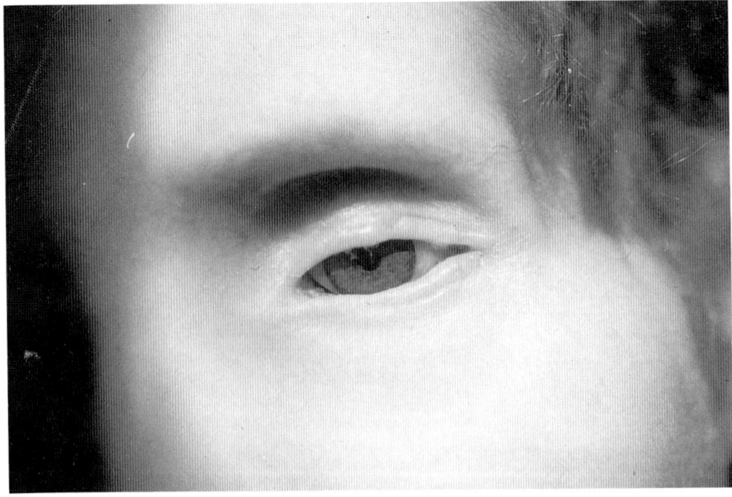

Figure 13. The same patient one year after the second stage of the described surgical technique.

CONCLUSION

Surgery of the severely contracted socket is difficult because of the unpredictability of the scarring process. The best results are obtained with a good understanding of the contraction process and use of appropriate surgical techniques. With our technique, the posterior and anterior orbital contractions are managed with separate surgical approaches. Using a muscle flap, which provides a well-vascularized bed, and a delayed two stage reconstruction follows this principle and explains the good results obtained (Figs. 12 and 13).

REFERENCES

1. Iliff CE, Iliff WJ, Iliff NT: *Oculoplastic Surgery*. Philadelphia, PA, W.B. Saunders, 1979:217–221.
2. Mustardé JC, Lester TJ, Callahan A: *Ophthalmic Plastic Surgery Up-to-Date*. Birmingham, AL, Aesculapius Publishing Company, 1970:128–130.
3. Rougier J, Tessier P, Hervouet F, Woillez M, Lekieffre M., Derome P: *Chirurgie Plastique Orbito-Palpébrale*. Paris, Masson, 1977:47–53.
4. Tessier P, Krastinova D: La trasposition du muscle temporal dans l'orbite anophtalme. *Ann Chir Plast* 1982; 3:213–220.
5. Naquin HA: Orbital reconstruction (utilizing temporalis muscle). *Am J Ophthalmol* 1956; 41:519–521.
6. Reese AB, Jones IS: Exenteration of the orbit and repair by transplantation of the temporalis muscle. *Am J Ophthalmol* 1961; 51:217–227.

Dermis-Fat Orbital Implantation and Complex Socket Deformities

Stephen L. Bosniak, M.D., F.A.C.S.

ABSTRACT

Autogenous dermis-fat grafts implanted within the orbit survive best, with little loss of volume, when they are placed within Tenon's capsule immediately following the removal of the globe; when the rectus muscles (and anterior ciliary arteries) are anastomosed to the dermal edge of the graft; when no cautery has been applied to the recipient bed; and when the anterior diameter of the graft is no larger than 22 mm. Primary grafting in patients without systemic vascular disease is more effective than secondary procedures, performed on patients with fibrotic, compromised recipient beds and without direct apposition of the rectus muscles to the graft.

CONTRACTED SOCKETS

I assume that these grafts are nourished by the anterior ciliary arteries, vascular ingrowth, and conjunctival migration over the anterior dermal surface, and vascular ingrowth along the posterior borders of the graft. Chemically or thermally burnt sockets, as well as scarred and contracted sockets cannot support an autogenous dermis-fat graft. The grafts will undergo rapid and complete resorption. However, the establishment of a vascular bed can and will support additional autogenous grafting, allowing for socket volume augmentation.

A convenient method for re-establishing a vascular bed within the socket is temporalis muscle transfer through a window in the lateral wall of the orbit [1,2]. The pedical flap will augment the orbital soft-tissue volume and provide support and nourishment for a dermis-fat graft (Figs. 1–4). This can be accomplished by a coronal scalp flap or a direct incision. The external aspect of the lateral wall of the orbit is exposed.

A pneumatic drill is used to fashion a bony window of sufficient dimensions to accommodate the bulky muscle flap. The transposed temporalis muscle flap is fixated to the posterior of the medial orbit wall. A free dermis-fat graft is implanted on the anterior surface of the muscle pedicle flap during the same operation; however in cases of severe socket deformity the dermis-fat graft may be implanted secondarily 6 to 8 weeks after stabilization of the muscle flap.

In sockets that are mildly contracted with slight compromise of the fornices, a recession of the fornices with a dermis-fat graft may be adequate. If however, insufficient forniceal depth is the result, mucous membrane grafting techniques may be combined with dermis-fat implantation or performed at a second stage.

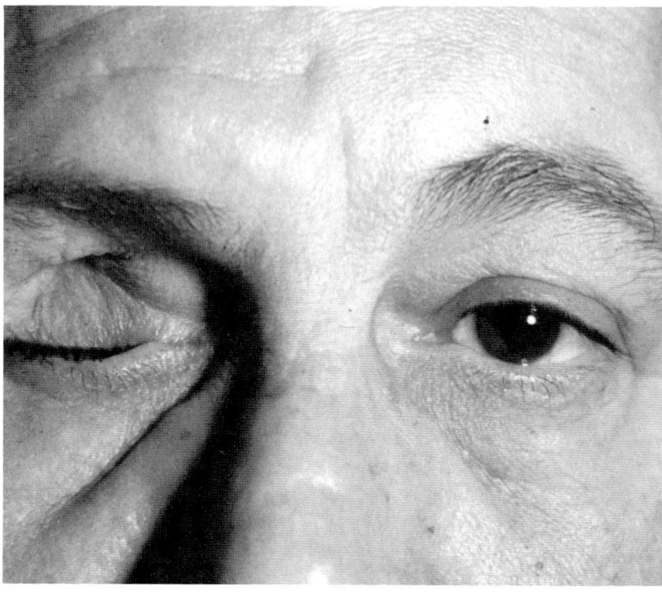

Figure 1. A 49-year-old man suffered a contracted anophthalmic socket with obliterated fornices following an alkali burn. (From Bosniak et al, 1985. Published courtesy of *Ophthalmology* 1985; 92:292–296.)

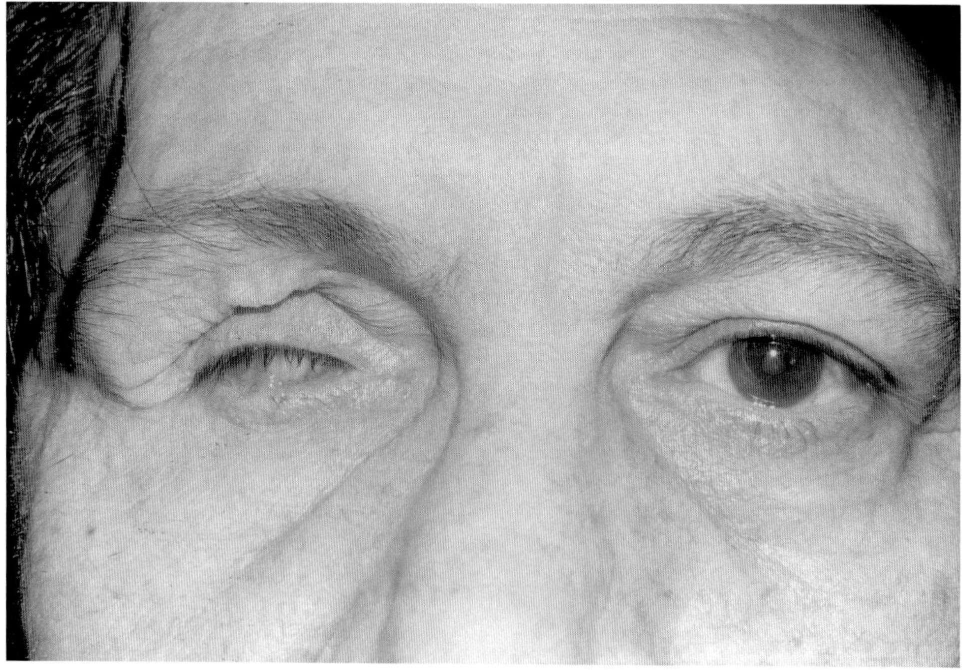

Figure 2. Augmentation of his contracted socket volume was accomplished following autogenous dermis-fat implantation on a vascular bed of temporalis muscle.

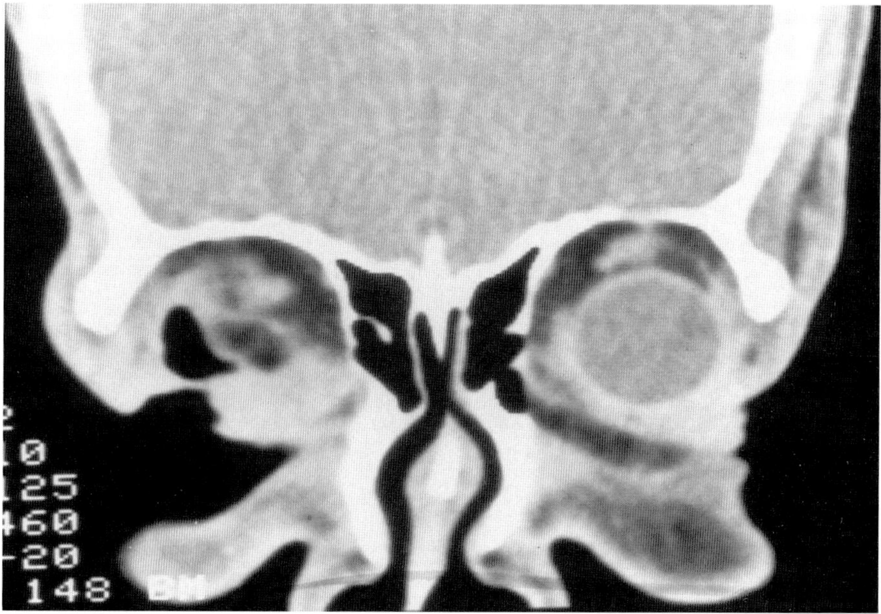

Figure 3. An orbital CT scan of the 49-year-old patient demonstrates the dermis-fat graft on a vascular pedicle flap six months following implantation.

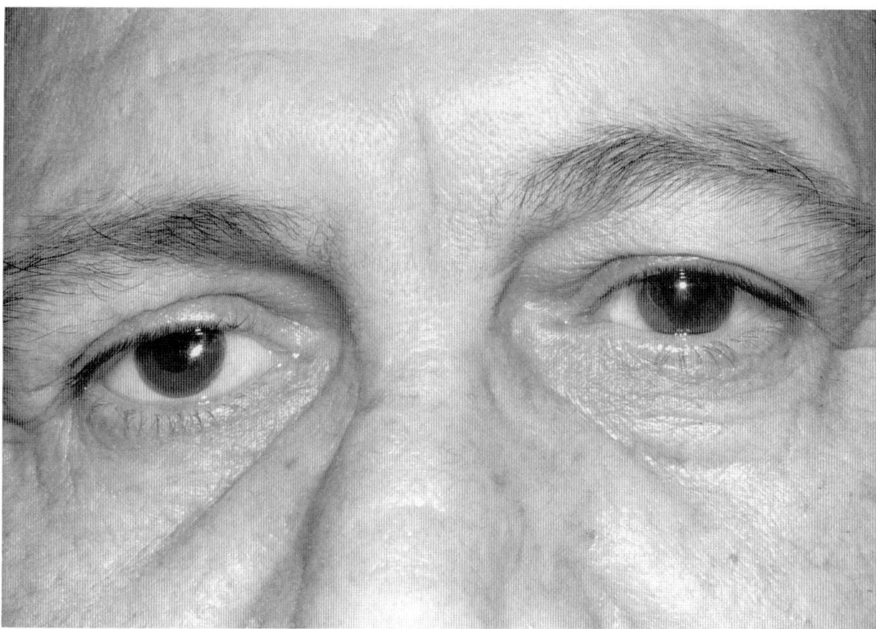

Figure 4. The same patient was able to wear a prosthesis after the temporalis muscle transposition and dermis-fat implantation.

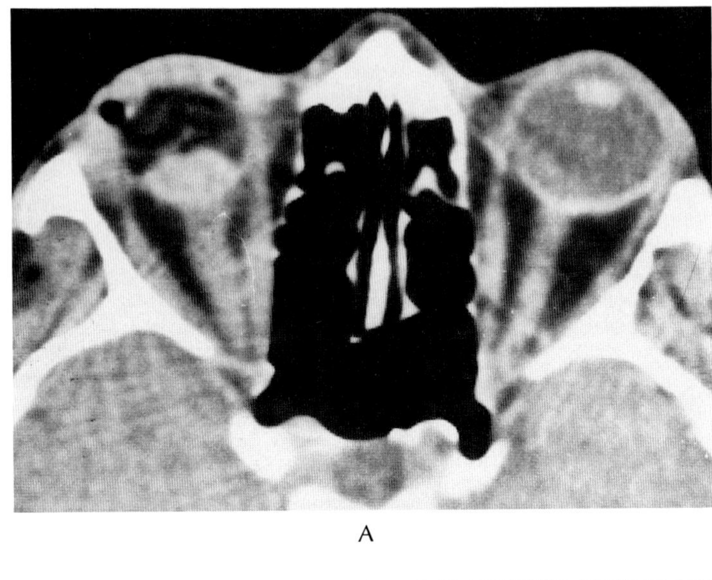

A

B

Figure 5. (A) and (B) These CT scans demonstrate a phthisical globe supporting an autogenous dermis-fat graft.

Although skin-lined sockets require more rigorous daily toilet than mucous-lined sockets, historically these techniques have been used to correct severe deformities when sufficient mucous membrane was not available. If a dermis-fat graft is used to augment orbital volume or enhance the fornices of a skin-lined socket, it need not be de-epithilialized. If additional skin is required, the epidermal component of the graft may be enlarged when the graft is being harvested.

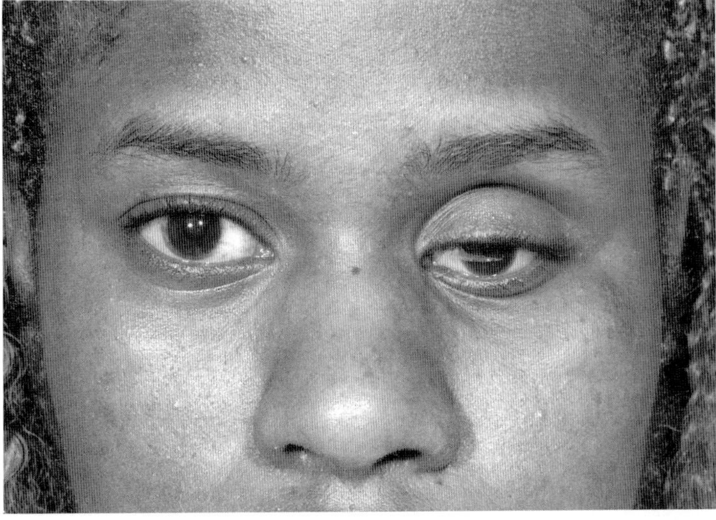

A

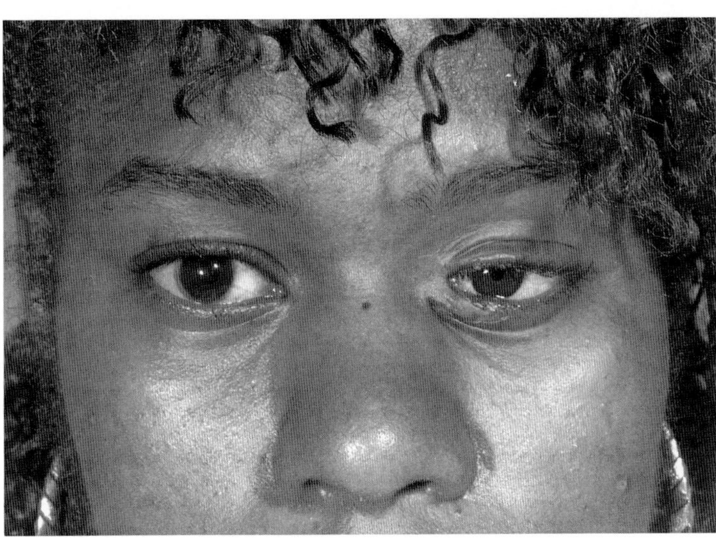

B

Figure 6. (A) A phthisical globe produced a marked superior sulcus deformity. (B) Following autogenous dermis-fat implantation supported by a phthisical globe, a medial canthoplasty and additional subperiosteal volume augmentation by the attending and resident staffs of the Manhattan Eye, Ear, and Throat Clinic, her superior sulcus deformity was improved.

MARKED SUPERIOR SULCUS DEFORMITIES

Correction of severe sulcus deformities is difficult. Phthisical globes or shrivelled postevisceration scleral shells without implants may be used as platforms to support dermis-fat grafts and to supplement orbital soft-tissue volume. Removing these ocular remnants is counter-

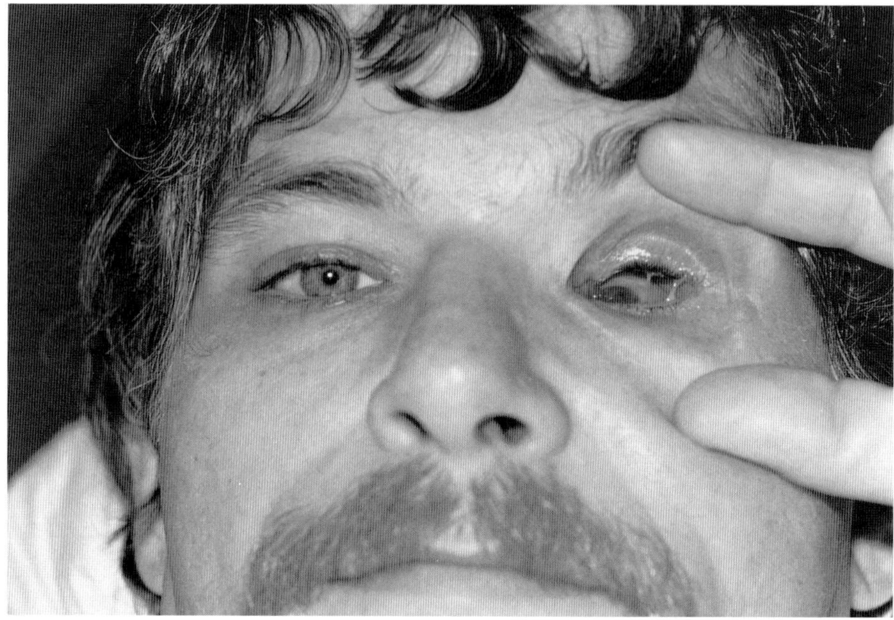

Figure 7. Traumatic cryptophthalmos followed an auto accident, leaving this 34-year-old man with a phthisical globe deep within his socket.

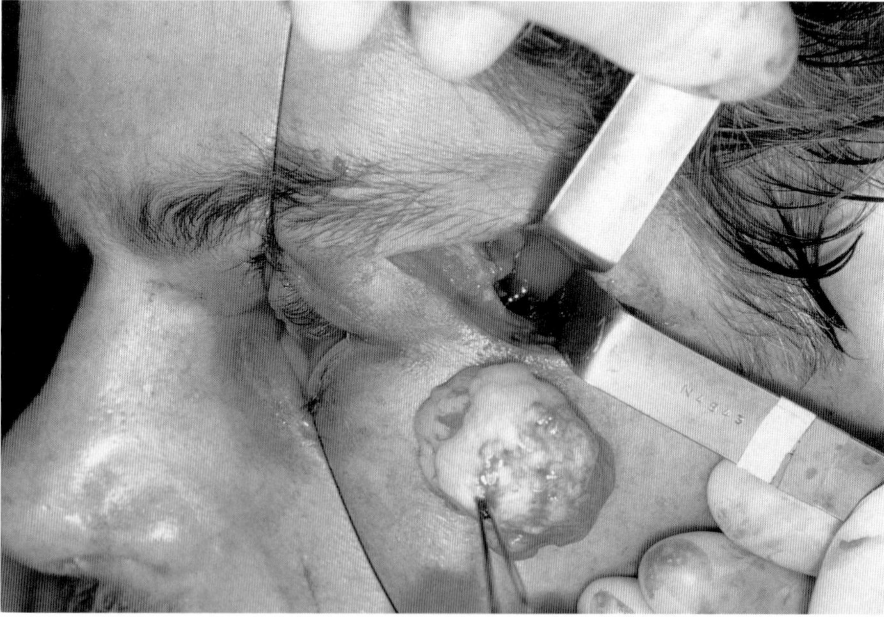

Figure 8. A dermis-fat graft was placed behind the phthisical globe through a window in the lateral orbital wall. Photograph courtesy of Samuel Amstutz, M.D.

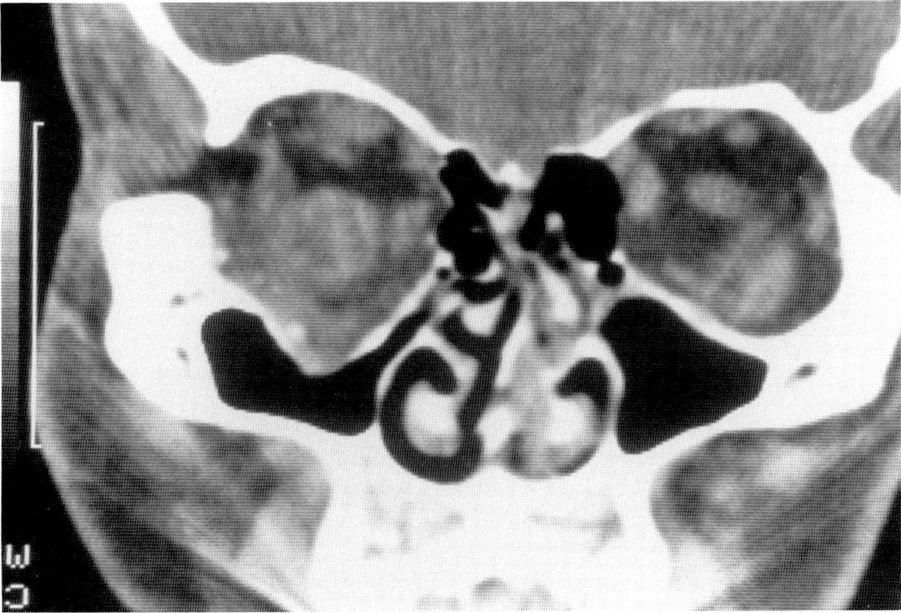

Figure 9. A CT scan six months following the retrobulbar implantation of the autogenous dermis fat graft demonstrated persistence of the graft and augmented orbital soft-tissue.

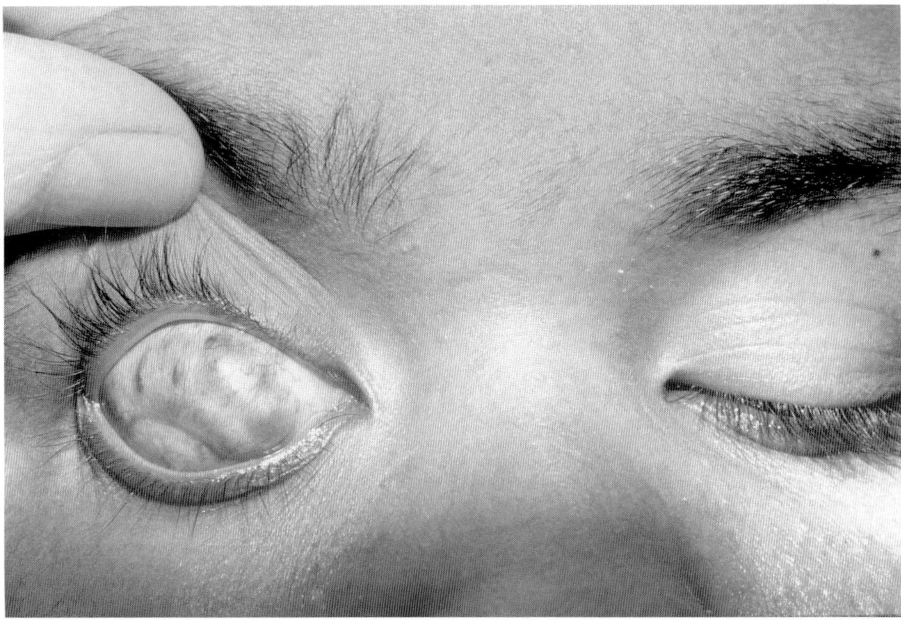

Figure 10. A 17-year-old man developed a prominent anterior staphyloma and a blind right eye following blunt trauma.

productive as it aggravates the orbital volume deficiency. Apparently retention of phthisical globes does not compromise the stability of these autogenous grafts [3] (Figs. 5, 6).

TRAUMATIC CRYPTOPHTHALMOS

In one case of apparent posttraumatic anophthalmos, a phthisical globe was found in a markedly atrophic socket with an extreme superior sulcus defect. The phthisical globe was advanced anteriorly in the socket and supported by a dermis-fat graft inserted behind the globe through a window in the lateral orbital wall. At a second stage a second dermis-fat graft was implanted anteriorly supported by the phthisical globe (Figs. 7, 8, 9).

DERMIS-FAT ORBITAL IMPLANTS AND SOCKET GROWTH

I have long suspected that autogenous dermis-fat grafts may hold some promise when implanted into sockets of pediatric patients who have undergone enucleation or who suffered congenital microophthalmos. I had hoped that the grafts would perhaps grow with the patient and stimulate growth of the orbital cavity. Katowitz's observations in Philadelphia, although preliminary, give reason for optimistic expectation:

"While we currently have many patients in which dermis fat grafting was performed in order to rebuild an anophthalmic or microphthalmic socket, many of these patients did not have preoperative radiologic evaluation to determine orbital volume size or bony hypoplastic defects. The observations that the dermis fat graft grew as the patient advanced in age with

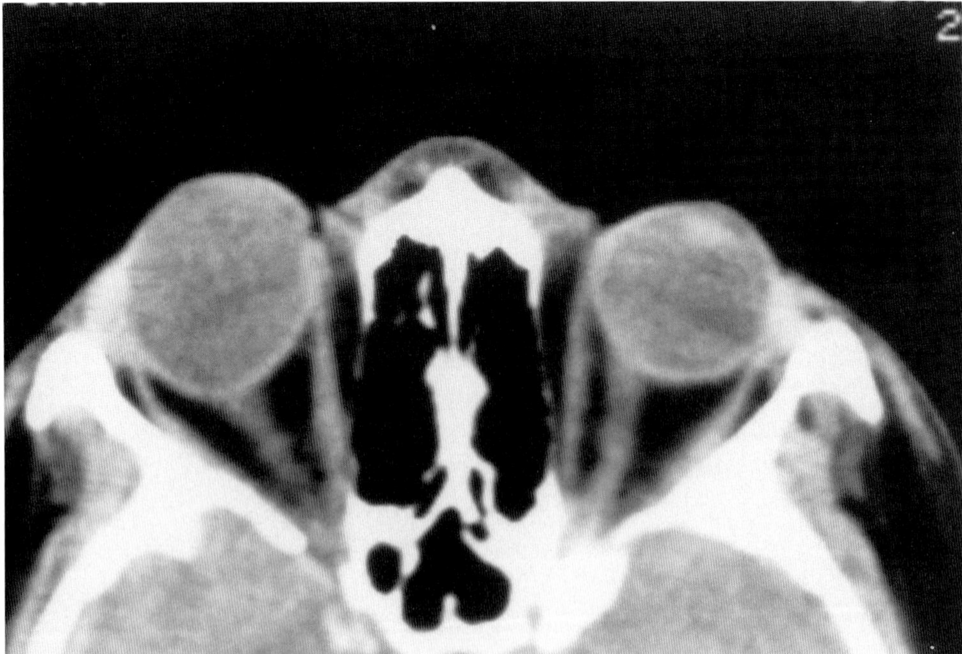

Figure 11. The enlarged globe and attenuated sclera were demonstrated by an orbital CT scan.

subsequent mild or moderate skeletal abnormalities, and that bony orbital volume also increased in relation to the dermis fat graft growth was a delightful, unexpected outcome. We have only recently started prospectively gathering data both radiologically and clinically on our most recent congenital and traumatic enophthalmic sockets implanted with dermis fat grafts in order to stimulate bony growth. Follow-up is short in these patients and currently not adequate for publication at this time" (J. Katowitz, MD, written communication).

INTRASCLERAL IMPLANTATION FOLLOWING EVISCERATION

Dermis-fat grafts have been successfully used in augmenting orbital volume following evisceration [3,4]. As long as adequate avenues for vascular ingrowth have been provided by filleting the sclera posteriorly, the graft will maintain an adequate volume with little resorption. In cases where evisceration with keratectomy has been performed, the only alternative implant would be a small synthetic sphere or hydroxyapatite. When a dermis-fat implant is used, its de-epithelialized dermal surface will be placed anteriorly in the position formerly occupied by the cornea. Conjunctiva will migrate over its anterior surface. An illustrative case follows.

A 17-year-old young man suffered blunt trauma to his right eye, subsequently lost all sight and gradually developed progressive scleral ectasia with prolapsing choroid covered only by conjunctiva (Fig. 10). A CT scan showed a markedly enlarged globe with attenuated sclera (Fig. 11). Because of the possibility of imminent perforation and the chance of even minimal ocular trauma causing a ruptured globe, an evisceration was recommended.

The conjunctiva was dissected off of the anterior staphyloma. An evisceration was per-

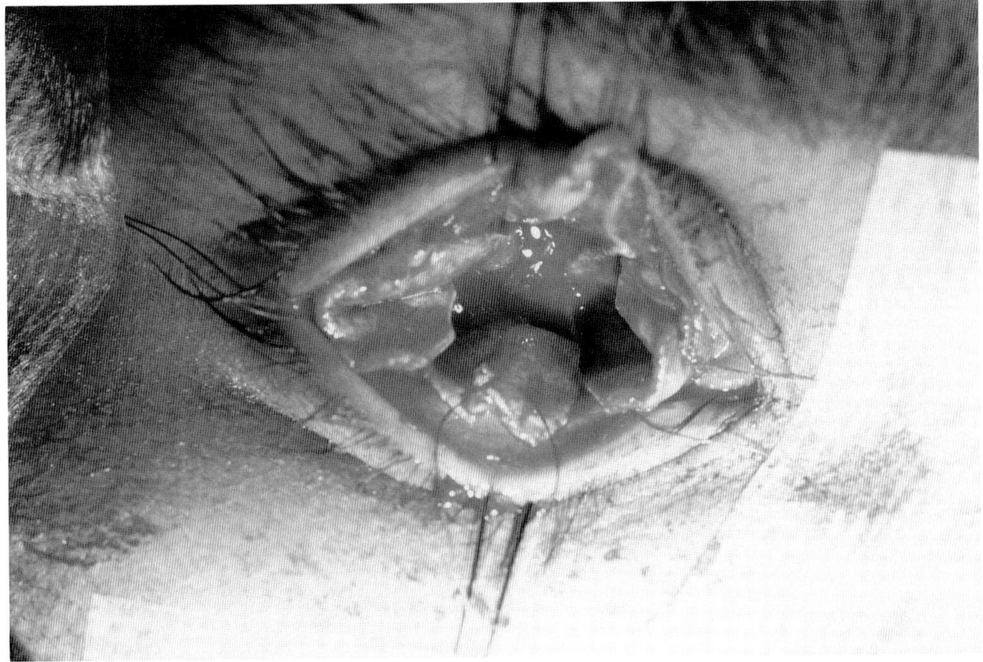

Figure 12. Following evisceration the sclera was filleted posteriorly between the rectus muscles.

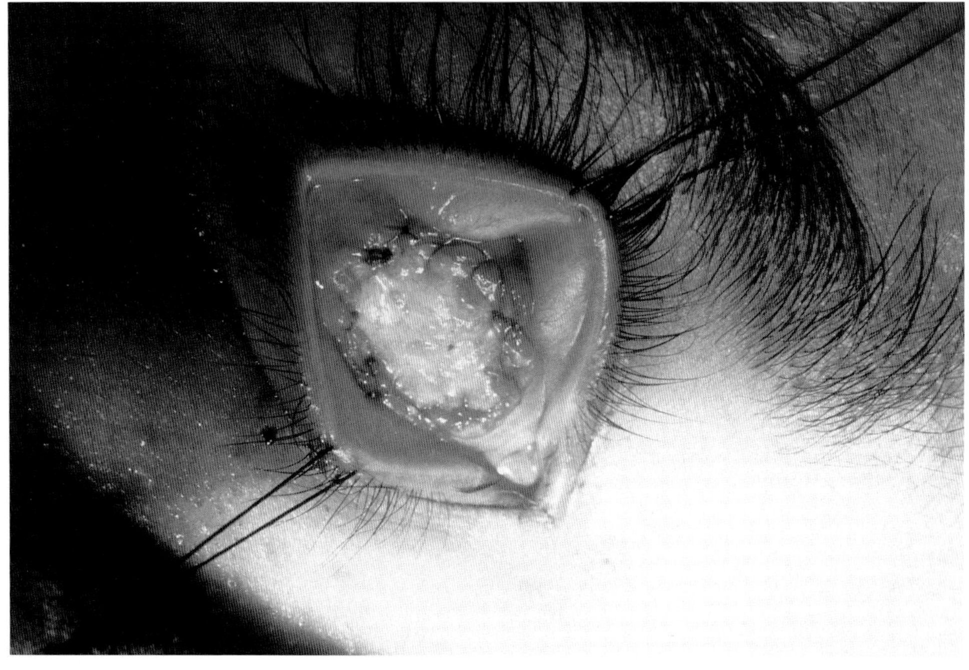

A

B

Figure 13. A de-epithelialized dermis-fat graft was implanted within the scleral shell.

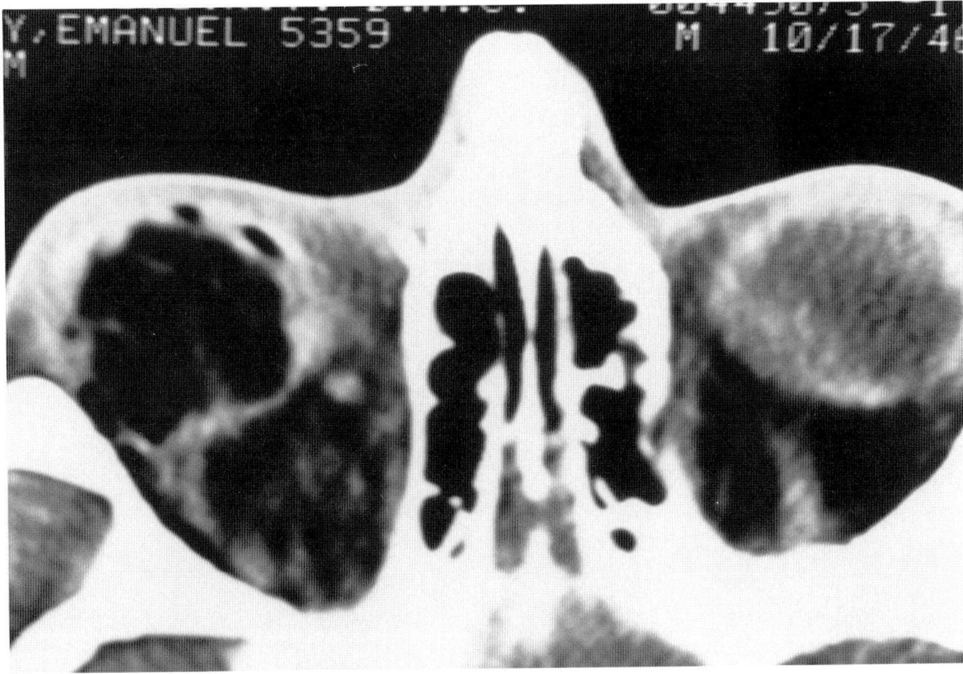

Figure 14. Follow-up eight months following implantation indicated that the graft had maintained its volume.

formed. The sclera was incised posteriorly between the rectus muscle insertions (Fig. 12). A de-epithelialized dermis-fat graft was implanted within the scleral shell (Fig. 13). During the eight months following surgery the graft has maintained its volume well (Fig. 14).

SUMMARY

Although the degree of graft absorption may be accelerated in fibrotic, relatively avascular sockets, autogenous dermis-fat orbital implants may be a useful adjunct in supplementing orbital volume in complex socket deformities if appropriate modifications in surgical technique are implemented.

REFERENCES

1. Naguin HA: Orbital reconstruction utilizing temporalis muscle. *Am J Ophthalmol* 1956; 41:579–621.
2. Bosniak S, Sachs M, Smith B: Temporalis muscle transfer: A vascular bed for autogenous dermis-fat orbital implantation. *Ophthalmology* 1985; 92:292–296.
3. Bosniak SL: Dermis-fat grafts and evisceration. *Ophthalmology* 1989; 96:1276–1277.
4. Archer K, Hurwitz J: Dermis-fat grafts and evisceration. *Ophthalmology* 1989; 96:170–174.

The Role of Flaps in the Management of Contracted Eye Sockets

Bahman Guyuron, M.D.

ABSTRACT

Based on the pathology of the eye socket and periorbital deficiencies, three distinct classes of patients can be recognized:

I. Those who solely have eye socket deficiency with normal orbital and periorbital tissue. The suggested surgical treatment for this class of patient would be a skin or mucosa graft.

II. Patients who have inadequate lining, as well as orbital volume deficiency. The preferred reconstructive approach includes cartilage (rib or ear) with or without fat graft, and skin or mucosa grafts for eye socket expansion.

III. For failed reconstructions of classes I and II or for patients with severe orbital and periorbital deficiencies, the choice is one of three flaps: If the superficial temporal vessels and the postauricular skin is intact, the ideal flap is postauricular fasciocutaneous. If the postauricular skin has previously been used yet the superficial vasculature is intact, a secondary flap is the better choice. In cases where both postauricular skin and superficial temporal vessels have been sacrificed the recommended flap is a free flap with microvascular anastomosis.

INTRODUCTION

Reconstructing a contracted or missing eye socket to provide or restore aesthetically pleasing eye and orbital symmetry is a difficult and often frustrating process. Many techniques have been developed and refined over the years [1,2,3], but the achievement of predictable results remains a challenge. To decrease the failure rate and achieve more consistently successful results, it is crucial to detect and take into consideration all the causal and determining factors. In so doing, the surgical procedure can be planned and custom-designed to suit the needs of each particular patient. The following is a detail of the author's philosophy and technique for the care of these patients.

CLASSIFICATION

The classification of the deformity is important in defining the pathology and properly designing the operation [4].

Class I.   These are the patients that only have insufficient lining of the eye socket, no enophthalmos, no soft tissue or bony deficiency of the orbit or periorbital area.

Class II. These patients have insufficient eye socket lining as well as deficiency in the soft tissue of the orbital content, so that even after the eye socket is successfully reconstructed the prosthetic eye will look enophthalmic.

Class III. These patients not only have deficiencies of the eye socket and orbital soft tissue, but are also deficient in growth of the periorbital tissues and bones.

Classes II and III are more commonly seen in patients who have had enucleation at a younger age and subsequent radiation which resulted in inadequate growth of the orbital and periorbital soft tissue and bone.

MANAGEMENT OF PATIENTS WITH CLASS I DEFORMITY

On these patients who only have contracted eye socket with normal soft tissue volume, shape, and periorbital tissue, the solution lies in expansion of the eye socket with the use of mucosa or skin graft. In general, skin grafts do better and have less chance of contracture in sockets which are missing the majority of the lining. However, when the deficiency is minimal and most of the eye socket is lined with conjunctiva, a small skin graft is then exposed to a large amount of moisture from the surrounding conjunctiva resulting in increased desquamation and epithelial cell accumulation along with fetid odor. Therefore, under these conditions, a mucosa graft might be more suitable. Conversely, moisture is minimal in sockets with practically none or very little conjunctiva and a full-thickness skin graft results in very minimal drainage with a slight amount of unpleasant odor.

Technique. The amount of full-thickness skin or mucosa necessary for the reconstruction is estimated. On an older patient with redundant upper eyelid skin the ideal choice for skin graft is the ipsilateral or contralateral upper eyelid, or both. The skin graft to be harvested is designed, infiltrated with xylocaine with epinephrine, harvested, and the donor defect is closed using 6-0 plain catgut or 6-0 prolene running subcuticular suture. If bilateral upper eyelid skin is needed, the harvested skin sections are sewn together to provide sufficient tissue. The eye socket is then expanded in the appropriate direction by a careful dissection. It is important to take the spacial relation of the eye socket into consideration while dissecting so that expansion is made only where it is necessary and the socket is created only in the area that is missing. The harvested skin graft is then tailored and sewn in position using 5-0 or 6-0 chromic. The area is irrigated copiously with antibiotic solution and an impression of the reconstructed eye socket is taken using Tru-Soft (Harry J. Bosworth Co., Skokie, IL). This material provides the ideal stent for a reconstructed eye socket. It fills the sulcus properly, is flexible enough to be easily removed if necessary, yet firm enough to retain its shape. The Tru-Soft will be a temporary stent until the graft takes, which is approximately two to three weeks. After the two-to-three week waiting period, a permanent or intermediate prosthesis of firm material is created by a prosthetist. The eye socket is checked periodically to ensure proper graft take and lack of infection. During the healing period, Tobramycin eye drops are routinely used and the external incisions are covered with polysporin ophthalmic ointment. I have discovered that early placement of the eye prosthesis eliminates the need to sew the eye socket shut for three to six months. A functional eye socket can be fairly easily achieved in a shortened time period (Fig. 1).

The next best skin-graft choice is the unilateral or bilateral postauricular skin which has minimal donor-site visibility. In general, it should be possible to repair the postauricular skin-

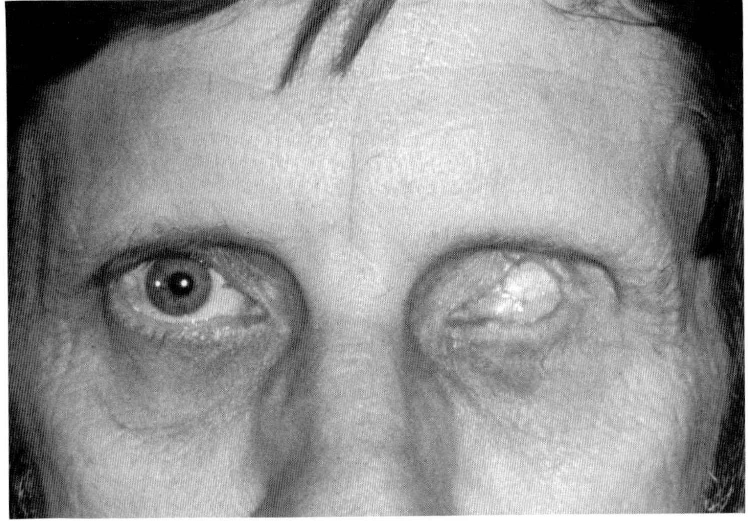

A

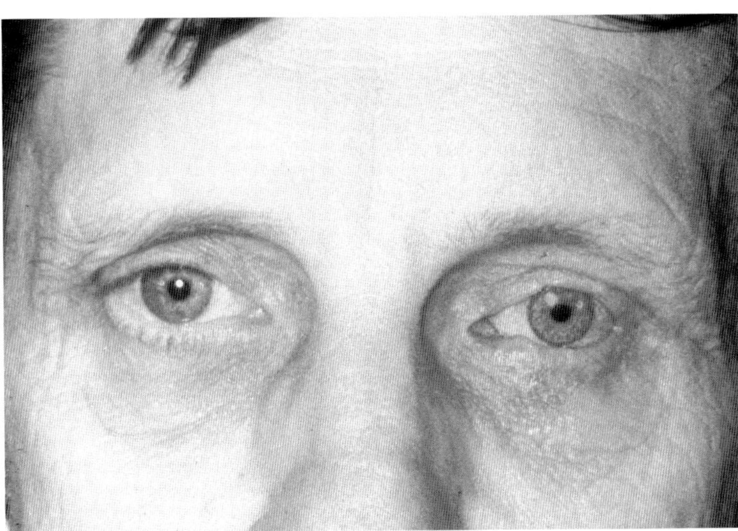

B

Figure 1. A Class I patient with contracted eye socket before (A) and two years following (B) eye socket reconstruction using contralateral upper eyelid skin.

graft donor site with a linear primary closure. When postauricular skin from one side is not adequate, the alternative site is inguinal skin, which similarly has minimal scar visibility. However, if the amount of lining necessary is only minimal, the ideal choice would be a mucosa graft. The steps are much the same regardless of the graft-donor site. The mucosa graft can be obtained either from the oral cavity or from the nasal septum. The donor defect is left to heal with secondary intention.

MANAGEMENT OF CLASS II PATIENTS

These patients not only have an inadequate eye socket, but also deficient orbital content. They require combination skin or mucosa graft for the eye socket (chosen by using the afore-mentioned criteria), as well as augmentation of the intraorbital content (Fig. 2). The material for increasing orbital content can be either synthetic or autogenic. The obviously superior graft choice is the autogenous material. However, in every case all the advantages and disadvantages of the selected material have to be taken into consideration. Synthetic materials used for augmentation of orbital content include: proplast, silicone, methyl-methacrylate, and hydroxyapatite. Synthetic material is seldom used in a previously radiated area because of the high degree of infection and extrusion. Autogenous material includes: rib cartilage, rib bone, cranial bone, illiac bone, ear cartilage, fat or fascia grafts. Illiac bone, because of its significant donor-site morbidity, and fascia grafts, because of their high degree of resorption, are not preferred choices. Rib bone also has a high degree of resorption. Cranial bone has the highest degree of graft take, yet because of the potential dangers and complexity of the harvesting procedure, particularly for an inexperienced surgeon, it is not an ideal graft for this site. Rib or ear cartilage grafts [5] because of their 100% volume retention, and fat grafts be-

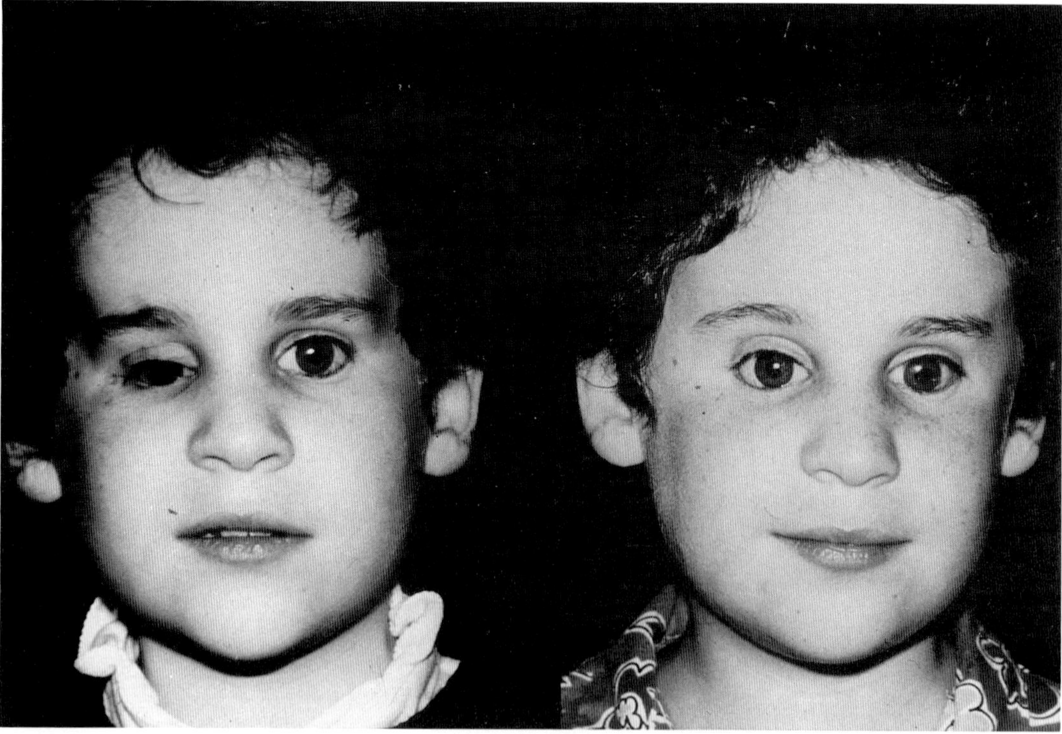

Figure 2. Patient before (left) and one year following left eye socket expansion and acrylic implant to the orbit and temple to correct a radiation induced "hour glass" deformity (right). Photograph used with permission from Guyuron B: The hourglass facial deformity. *J Cranio-Maxillo-Facial Surg* 1990; 18:187–191.

cause of their resemblance to the missing soft tissue from the orbits are more suitable choices. However, each graft choice must be made on an individual basis.

The orbital graft can either be placed through an incision in the existing eye socket or supratarsal fold. In general, to fill in a deep supratarsal fold or to transpose the socket and prosthesis caudally, a fat graft is placed in the cephalad portion of the orbit through a supratarsal incision. Yet in dealing with enophthalmos or caudally dislocated eye sockets, the optimum graft includes thin slices of rib cartilage placed through an incision in the inferior fornix. Occasionally, it is necessary to use a combination of both fat and cartilage grafts. In this case, a submammary incision on a female and a lower chest wall incision on a male allows for harvesting of the rib cartilage graft along with removal of a section of fat. The combination of these two, applied simultaneously, may give more volume retention and also more flexibility. Although the primary choice for eye socket reconstruction for these Class II patients is a skin or mucosa graft, if the recipient bed is significantly scarred or radiated, the graft will most likely fail. This might be true for Class I patients as well. In these grossly suboptimal conditions, the ideal choice is one of the other three flaps discussed in the management of Class III patients.

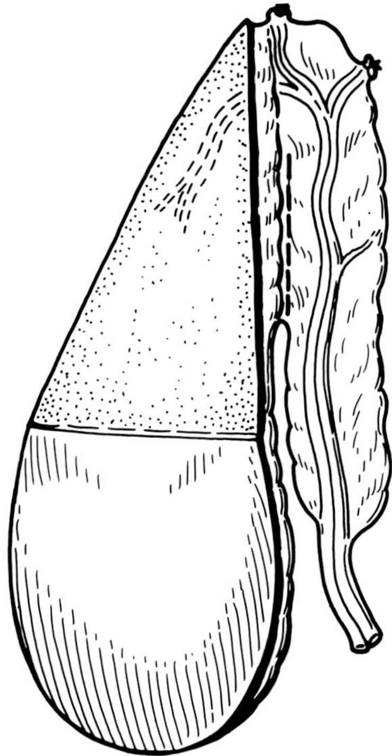

Figure 3. Artistic rendering of the three distinct components of the fasciocutaneous flap including postauricular skin (lower left), triangular de-epithelialized scalp encompassing the posterior branches of the superficial temporal vessels (upper left) and the third portion, temporalis fascia together with the superficial temporal vessels (right, upper and lower sections). (Reprinted with permission from Guyuron B: Retroauricular island flap for eye socket reconstruction. *Plast Reconstr Surg* 1985; 76:527–530.)

MANAGEMENT OF CLASS III PATIENTS

This category of patients suffers not only from enophthalmos, but also from deficiency of the orbital and periorbital soft tissue. With this degree of tissue abnormality, graft failure is almost inevitable. To avoid repeated surgeries and unsuccessful results, it is necessary to take drastic steps and reconstruct the missing or severely contracted eye socket with a combination of the flap and skin graft. In determining what type of reconstruction is suitable for each particular patient, the following anatomical factors must be taken into consideration: presence or absence of superficial temporal vessels and indications of previous surgery in the postauricular area. If the patient has palpable superficial temporal vessels and intact postauricular skin, the choice for reconstructive technique will be fasciocutaneous island flap [6,7] (described later). This flap can be used with or without additional cartilage or bone graft, if deemed necessary. If the postauricular skin has been previously used, which is a common finding, then the choices will be either a temporalis fascia and muscle flap with a skin graft, or even a better choice, a two-staged secondary skin flap (also described later) [8]. However, if neither temporal vessels nor postauricular skin are suitable for eye socket reconstruction, then the reconstructive choice will clearly be a free-flap with microvascular anastomosis [9]. Again, with these flaps further cartilage or bone grafts can be used if necessary.

POSTAURICULAR FASCIOCUTANEOUS ISLAND FLAP

In my experience, this has been the most successful type of reconstruction for Class III patients [6,7].

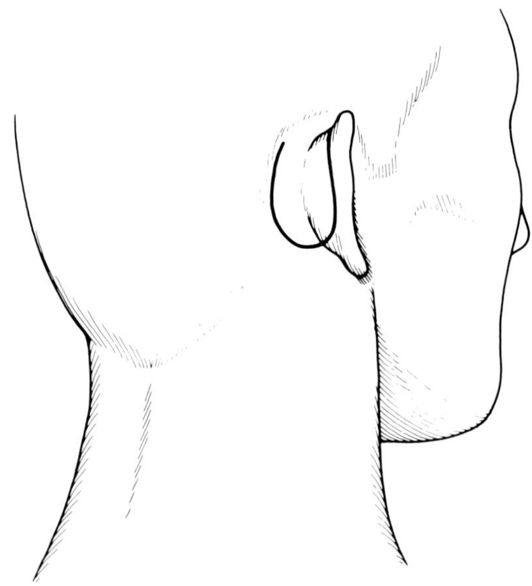

Figure 4. Design of the postauricular (cutaneous) portion of the flap. (Reprinted with permission from Guyuron B: Retroauricular island flap for eye socket reconstruction. *Plast Reconstr Surg* 1985; 76:527–530.)

Anatomy. This flap has three distinct and separate anatomical components: skin, dermis, and fascial portion (Fig. 3). Each of the latter two components has a role in the vascularity of the terminal cutaneous portion, which is the portion used for the eye socket reconstruction. The cutaneous portion of the flap is the hairless skin in the postauricular region. A flap as large as 5 × 6 cm can be harvested from this area. The dermis portion, however, is the triangular-shaped scalp area located just cephalad to the upper portion of the skin flap and helix. The base of the triangle is positioned caudally. This portion of the flap, which is approximately 6 cm long and will be de-epithelialized, encompasses the posterior branch of the superficial temporal vessels — the main blood supply to the flap. The third portion of the flap is the temporalis fascia. The anterior boundary of the fascia is about a centimeter anterior to the superficial temporal vessels to ensure that the vessels are included in the flap. The fascia to be raised with the flap is almost rectangular in shape, about 6 to 7 cm long and about $1\frac{1}{2}$ to 2 cm wide and it will be attached to the remainder of the flap throughout the anterior portion of the triangular segment. If necessary, a cutback is made at the most caudal portion of the triangle between the fascia that contains the superficial temporal vessels, and the triangular portion (dermis and fascia), to augment the reach of the flap through unfolding. This cutback should not be more than 2 or $2\frac{1}{2}$ cm to avoid an injury to the posterior branch of the superficial temporal vessels. The arterial blood to the flap, therefore, will circulate through the superficial temporal vessels and the posterior branch into the triangular-shaped flap. Up to this point the circulation is in an axial pattern; however, the cutaneous portion of the flap that will be used in the eye socket has primarily a random pattern circulation.

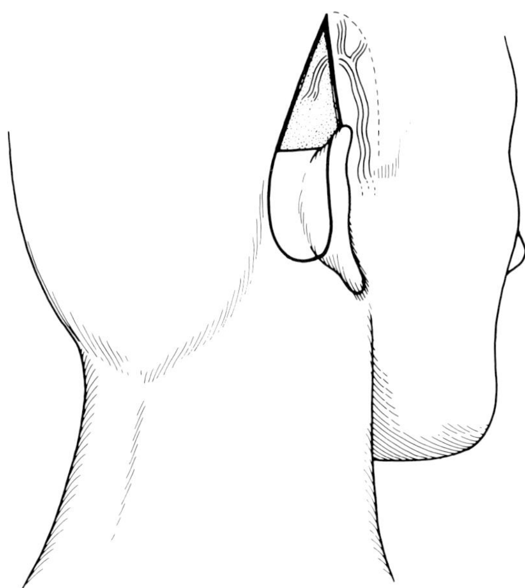

Figure 5. Design of the triangular scalp skin to be de-epithelialized containing the posterior branches of the superficial temporal vessels (dotted areas). The outline of the temporal fascia to be included in the flap is marked with a broken line. (Reprinted with permission from Guyuron B: Retroauricular island flap for eye socket reconstruction. *Plast Reconstr Surg* 1985; 76:527–530.)

Technique of Raising the Flap. Following induction of anesthesia and shaving the scalp above the ear, a postauricular skin flap is designed as large as needed, leaving enough skin along the helix and avoiding hair-bearing skin. Next, the triangular flap is designed (Fig. 4). To mark the posterior rim of the triangular flap a line is drawn 6 cm cephalad to the upper pole of the ear to the most cephalad and posterior portion of the postauricular skin flap (Fig. 5). The base of the triangular skin flap will be the superior edge of the cutaneous flap and the anterior limit is just posterior to the palpable superficial temple vessels. The base of the triangular flap, usually about 3 cm wide, allows for primary closure of the temple defect avoiding any baldness or hair loss in this area.

The incision is started from the posterior boundary of the postauricular flap and is taken down to the subcutaneous tissue, and the flap is raised at the subfascial level. This dissection will be continued cephalad. Next, the skin flap is raised off the ear, with extreme care taken to avoid injury to the perichondrium, so that a vascular bed is provided should a skin graft to the flap donor site become necessary. Next, the posterior border of the triangular flap is incised down and through the fascia. The anterior portion of the triangular flap is incised with extreme care to avoid any injury to the superficial temporal vessels. The incision is taken through the skin only, avoiding the superficial temporal fascia. This incision is then gradually curved back, towards the preauricular area, hugging the anterior border of the helix outline and the tragus. With careful dissection, the superficial temporal vessels are located at the preauricular region and left attached to the fascia, and the dissection is continued cephalad about 6 cm. The postauricular incision is next connected to the preauricular one. If necessary, a cutback incision is made between the vascular pedicle and the flap to augment the reach of

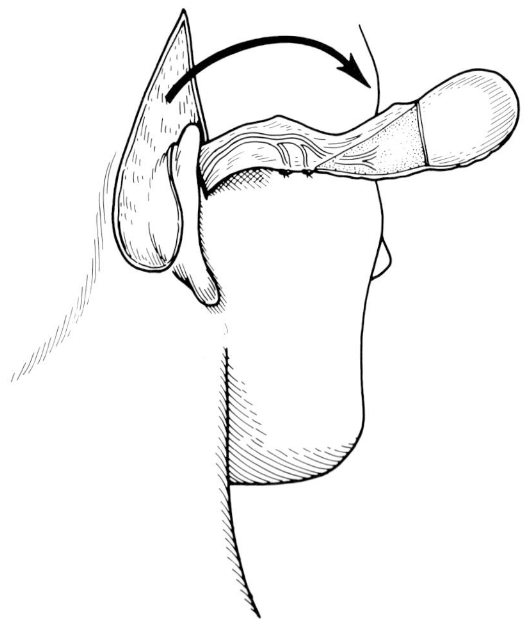

Figure 6. Artist's conception of the flap following dissection of all three parts and having a cutback incision made to augment the reach of the flap. (Reprinted with permission from Guyuron B: Retroauricular island flap for eye socket reconstruction. *Plast Reconstr Surg* 1985; 76:527–530.)

the flap. This incision can be up to $2\frac{1}{2}$ cm and when unfolded can increase the length of the flap up to 5 cm (Fig. 6). Often the posterior branches of the superficial temporal vessels are visible, which makes the cutback safer.

A subcutaneous tunnel is then created between the preauricular area and the orbital region following infiltration with xylocaine containing 1/200,000 epinephrine to minimize bleeding. The upper and lower eyelids and existing eye socket are separated from the orbital content. If there is an adequate amount of mucosa to reconstruct the lid portion of the socket (posterior aspect of the eyelid), it will be done by transferring the appropriate tissue into position. In dealing with an eye socket that is totally missing conjunctiva, an additional thin skin graft is harvested either from the eyelids or from the opposite postauricular region, tailored, and then sewn to the free borders of the flap using 5-0 plain catgut. This is done before the flap is delivered through the tunnel to avoid technical difficulties. The flap is then delivered in position (Fig. 7) and the free caudal margin of the skin graft in the superior fornix is sewn to the caudal margin of the upper eyelid, and the cephalad margin of the skin graft in the lower fornix is sewn to the cephalad portion of the upper eyelid to complete the fixation of the skin graft. The flap is then attached to the medial canthus using through-and-through stitch of 4-0 prolene on a Keith needle and it is tied over a dental roll. The stitches are removed in five to seven days. The donor-site defect is then closed using 5-0 plain catgut over a suction drain. For large donor-site defects that cannot be closed primarily, a skin graft is harvested from the groin, de-fatted, and sewn in position using 5-0 plain catgut. This flap requires very tedious dissection with careful attention to preservation of the vascular pedicle. Occasional congestion of the tip of the flap is noted postoperatively, but usually recovers without significance.

The reconstructed socket is then filled with Tru-Soft, which is replaced with a prosthesis in two to three weeks (Fig. 8).

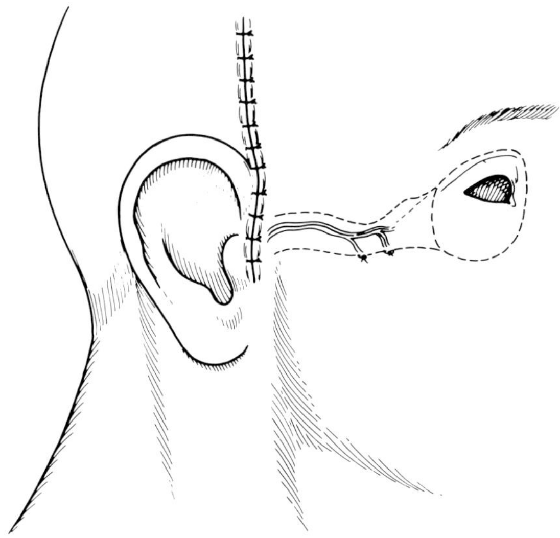

Figure 7. Artistic rendering of the flap having been delivered to the orbit through a subcutaneous tunnel, and showing the donor site repaired primarily. (Reprinted with permission from Guyuron B: Retroauricular island flap for eye socket reconstruction. *Plast Reconstr Surg* 1985; 76:527–530.)

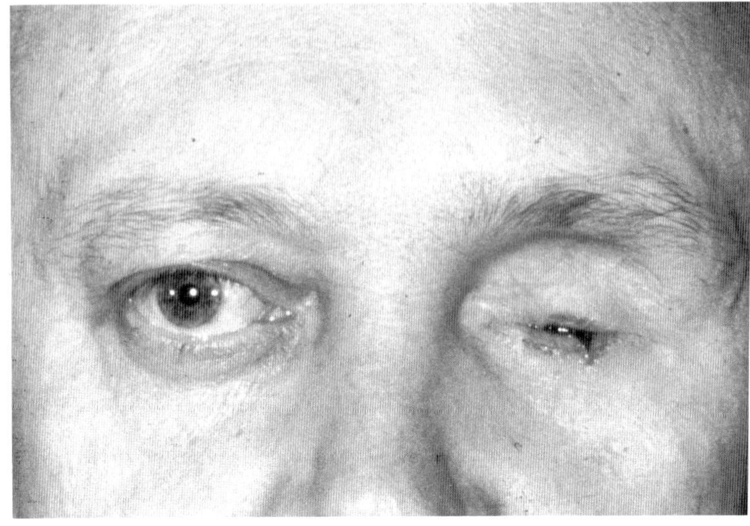

A

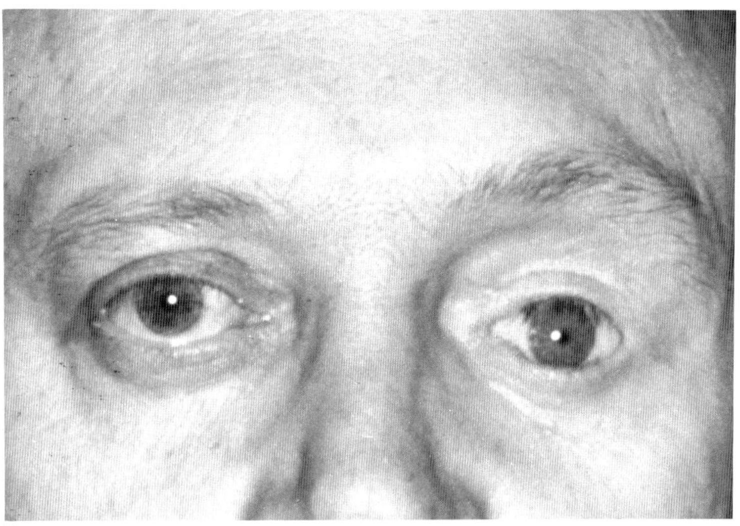

B

Figure 8. An example of a patient with severely contracted eye socket (A), and two years following reconstruction with fasciocutaneous flap (B).

SECONDARY FLAP

If the superficial temporal vessels are present, but the postauricular skin has previously been sacrificed, then a flap of superficial temporal fascia can be raised and buried under the skin of the postauricular region for about two to three weeks, and an island flap is then created for reconstruction of the eye socket [8].

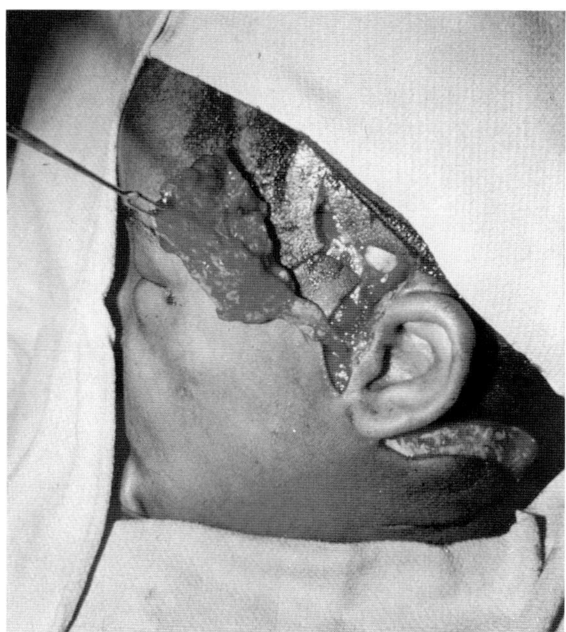

Figure 9. A temporalis fascia flap is elevated.

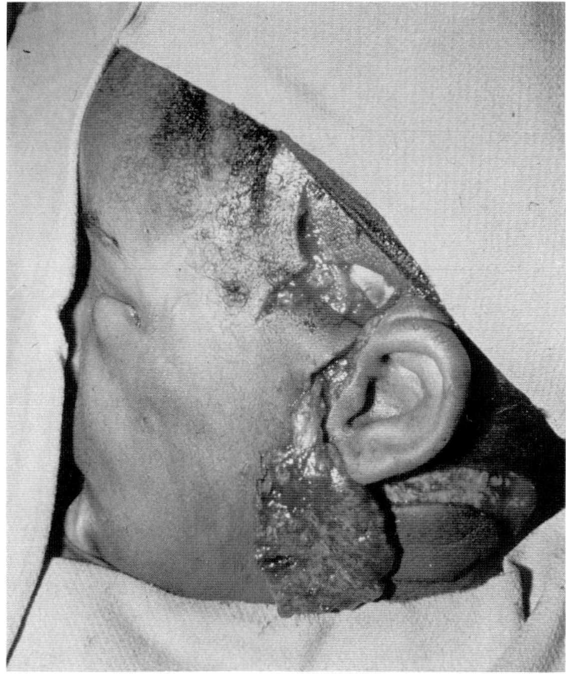

Figure 10. The flap is buried under the skin of the postauricular area and upper cervical region.

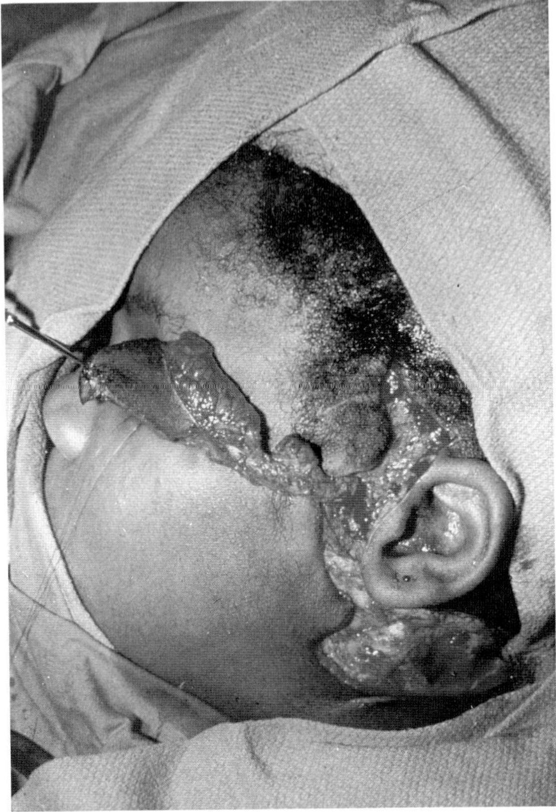

Figure 11. Three weeks later the flap is elevated and transferred to the orbit through a subcutaneous tunnel. If necessary, the eyelids are lined with the full-thickness skin graft. Reproduced with permission from Labandter HP, Guyuron B: Secondary superficial temporal artery–neck flap for orbital reconstruction. In: Strauch B, Vasconez LO, Hall-Findlay EJ (eds): *Grabbe's Encyclopedia of Flaps*. Boston, Little Brown, 1990.

Technique. An incision is started from the preauricular area and is extended cephalad to approximately 8 cm. Extreme care is practiced to avoid injury to the superficial temporal vessels that are left attached to the underlying temporalis fascia. A flap of temporalis fascia is then elevated as depicted in Figure 9, which extends almost to the skull midline. This flap is converted to an island flap and the area is chosen in the postauricular region as illustrated in Figure 10. The skin flap is elevated and the temporalis fascia is smoothly draped under the flap and the skin flap is placed on top of it and sewn in position. Three weeks later, the flap is elevated as a composite tissue containing the previously transposed temporalis fascia and superficial temporal vessels, as well as overlying skin (Fig. 11). By now the skin overlying the fascia will have adequate vascular connection with the fascia and its encompassing superficial temporal vessels so that it can be detached from the surrounding skin safely. This flap is raised and transferred to the orbit through a subcutaneous tunnel as described previously. Again, if necessary, the opposite postauricular skin is used to line the posterior portion of the eyelids (Fig. 12). The donor site is closed primarily, or it is reconstructed with a smaller size skin graft, which gradually contracts and becomes even smaller.

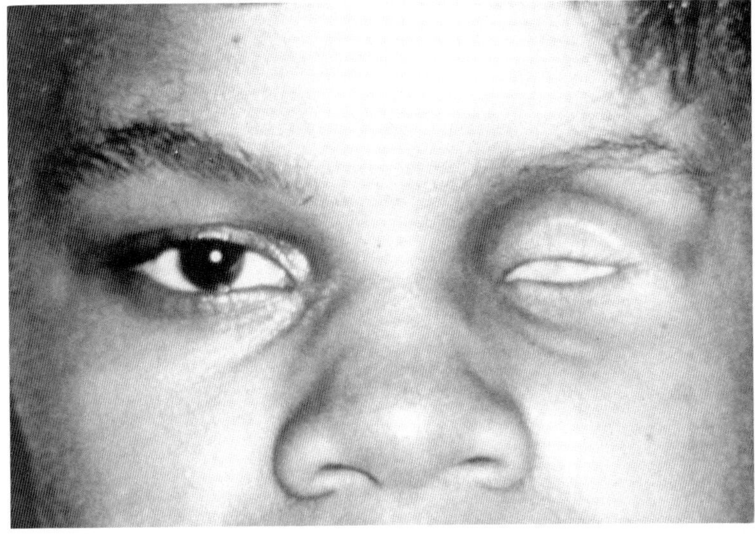

A

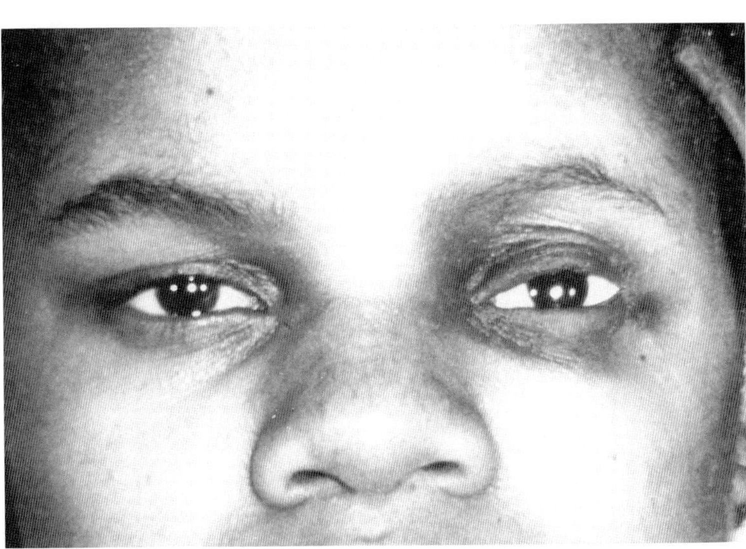

B

Figure 12. A patient with severely contracted eye socket following enucleation and radiation as an infant (A), and following reconstruction using a secondary flap (B).

This type of reconstruction can be accomplished by transferring the temporalis fascia to the orbit initially. The full-thickness skin graft is then applied on the fascia and fixed in position. This one stage operation, however, increases the potential for contraction and loss of eye socket in comparison to the aforementioned secondary skin flap.

FREE VASCULARIZED FLAPS

On patients who have neither suitable superficial temporal vessels, nor available postauricular skin, the choice for reconstruction remains a vascularized free flap using microvascular technology [9]. There are a multitude of available donor sites for use in eye socket reconstruc-

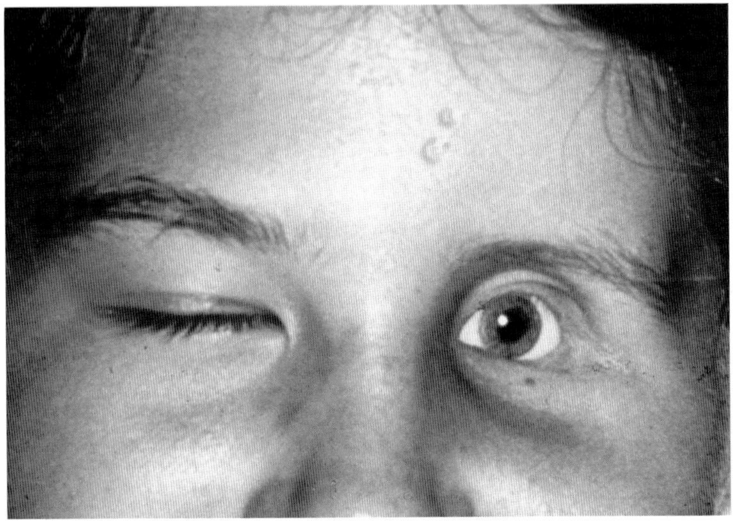

A

B

Figure 13. A patient who had enucleation and radiation resulting in contracture of the eye socket and orbital and periorbital deficiency (A). After reconstruction using dorsalis pedis free-vascularized flap with microvascular anastomosis and rib cartilage graft (B).

tion; however, free-radial forearm flap or dorsalis pedis flap remain the best choices (Fig. 13). The free dorsalis pedis flap is preferred over the free radial forearm flap because the forearm flap leaves a visible scar which is disturbing, particularly for a female patient. The free-flap technique requires microvascular experience and a team approach. The facial artery and external jugular vein are used for microanastomosis. These vessels are identified through a preauricular and cervical incision, and the skin is harvested from the dorsum of the foot and transferred to the face. The microanastomosis is accomplished in an end-to-end fashion between these vessels and dorsalis pedis or anterior tibial vessels under six to 10 magnification and the flap is delivered through a subcutaneous tunnel to the orbit. The eye socket and periorbital deficiencies are reconstructed using this flap. Furthermore, a full-thickness skin graft obtained from the de-epithelialized portion of the flap can be applied to the posterior portion of the eyelid if necessary (Fig. 13). The donor defect is repaired using a skin graft, or primary closure if possible.

REFERENCES

1. Wexler M, Pedled I, Kaplan H: Socket reconstruction using crossarm flaps. *Plast Reconstr Surg* 1981; 68:18.
2. McGraw JB, Furlow LT: The dorsalis pedis arterialized flap. *Plast Reconstr Surg* 1975; 55:177.
3. Erol O, Spira M: Utilization of a composite island flap employing omentum in organ reconstruction: an experimental investigation. *Plast Reconstr Surg* 1981; 68:681.
4. Guyuron B, Labandter HP, Berlin AJ: Fasciocutaneous flap—secondary axial pattern flap and microvascular free flap in eye socket reconstruction. *Ophthalmology* 1984; 91:04–101.
5. Guyuron B: Simplified harvesting of ear cartilage graft. *Aesthetic Plast Surg* 1986; 10:37–39.
6. Guyuron B: Retroauricular island flap for eye socket reconstruction. *Plast Reconstr Surg* 1985; 76:527–530.
7. Guyuron B, Labandter HP: Postauricular delayed fasciocutaneous island flap. In: Strauch B, Vasconez LO, Hall-Findlay EJ (eds): *Grabb's Encyclopedia of Flaps*. Boston, Little Brown, 1990.
8. Labandter HP, Guyuron B: Secondary superficial temporal artery-neck flap for orbital reconstruction. In: Strauch B, Vasconez LO, Hall-Findlay EJ (eds): *Grabb's Encyclopedia of Flaps*. Boston, Little Brown, 1990.
9. Guyuron B, Labandter HP: Doralis pedis free flap for eye socket reconstruction. In: Strauch B, Vasconez LO, Hall-Findlay EJ (eds): *Grabb's Encyclopedia of Flaps*. Boston, Little Brown, 1990.

An Operation for the Removal of the Eye-Ball, Together with the Entire Conjunctival Sac and Lid Margins

John Green, M.D.

Three of the cases now reported were mentioned in a verbal communication made to the American Ophthalmological Society at the meeting of 1882. With the exception of a short abstract which appeared in the following number of Knapp's Archives, no report of them has been published.

In several cases of granulation of the eye-ball, and of partial or total evisceration of the orbit, involving extensive loss of conjunctiva, it has appeared to me judicious to excise the whole conjunctiva, together with the tarsal tissue and the cilia-bearing lid margins, thus preserving large flaps from the very extensible skin and muscle layers of the lids to cover in the cavity, left by the operation and avoiding the subsequent annoyance resulting from the preservation of a useless amount of the conjunctival sac.

The first of these cases was that of a young farmer who had suffered for several years from a malignant ulcer of the inner canthus, which had largely destroyed the conjunctiva on the nasal side of the cornea, together with nearly one-third of the tarsal tissue of both lids. The function of the internal rectus muscle was abolished, and there was a deep cavity extending backward nearly to the equator of the still intact eyeball.

Judging that it was impracticable to save the eye-ball, or a sufficient amount of lid tissue and conjunctiva to admit of the wearing of an artificial eye, I decided to perform enucleation and to combine with it the removal of the lid-margins, the tarsal tissue and the entire conjunctival sac. I was assisted in the operation by Dr. H. H. Mudd.

The diseased tissue at the inner canthus was cut freely away within a curved incision carried down to the bone, and the two ends of this incision were extended through the skin and muscle layers of the upper and lower lid along the ciliary margin. The skin and muscle were then dissected from the tarsal tissue as far as the upper and lower borders of the orbit, and the tendon of the levator palpebrae superioris was lifted on a strabismus hook and divided. The tarsal tissue was then seized with hooked forceps and drawn forwards, and the whole

Dr. John Green's communication is the first American report of a modified exenteration with conservation of the eyelid skin and orbicularis muscle. Although it appeared 300 years after Georg Bartisch's description of an ancient technique (Ophthalmodouleia, Dresden, M. Stökel, 1583, chapter 3, page 208), its publication followed Arlt's description of the modern technique by only 10 years (Operationslehre, in von Graefe A, Saemisch ET: *Handbuch der gesamten Augenheilkunote*, ed 1, Leipzig, Wilhelm Engelmann, 1874, volume 1, page 434). Green's article (*Am J Ophthalmol* 1884; 1:6–9) has been published with permission from The American Journal of Ophthalmology. Copyright by The Ophthalmic Publishing Company.

conjunctival sac was dissected out with scissors so as to expose the tendons of the superior, external and inferior rectus muscles. These were successively taken up on a strabismus hook and divided, the optic nerve was cut through from the temporal side, and the tissues at the nasal side of the orbit were carefully cleaned from the bone from behind forwards. The tumor was thus thoroughly dissected out, leaving the wall of the orbit denuded at the inner side to the extent of perhaps two centimeters in diameter. The flaps formed by the lid integument and orbicularis muscle were easily brought together by means of three or four sutures, so as to cover in the temporal half of the wound, leaving a pretty large opening at the nasal end to heal by granulation. Union along the line of suture occurred without suppuration; the remaining opening, healed rapidly by granulation, and covered itself by drawing in the loose integument of the lids, so that at the end of a month a horizontal linear cicatrix alone remained to mark the site of the incisions. The skin was drawn smoothly over the concave surface of a shallow depression not deeper than that presented, after an enucleation by the sunken eye-lids when unsupported by an artificial eye.

In this case the lachrymal gland was left in situ; no inconvenience resulted from its non-removal. The second case was that of Mrs. J. S., 50 years of age, whom I first saw Oct. 4, 1880. She had lost the left eye twelve years before, from an inflammatory attack accompanied by perforating ulcer of the cornea. The globe was shrunken to about three-fourths of its normal diameter. There was considerable destruction of tissue at the inner canthus resulting from the free use of caustics four months before for the purpose of destroying what had been considered a malignant growth. The lachrymal sac lay widely open and was discharging freely; the adjacent tissues of the lid were slightly ulcerated, but without induration.

The obstructed nasal duct was dilated by repeated probing, canthotomy, with free division of the external tendon of the orbicularis, was performed for the purpose of relaxing the tissue near the inner canthus, and a group of inverted cilia near the nasal end of the upper lid was excised. The patient went home Nov. 22, with seemingly perfect cicatrization of the ulcerated tissues at the inner canthus, with the lids well relaxed, and relieved from the irritation which had been caused by the inverted eye-lashes. In view of the uncertainty regarding the nature of the original affections for which the cauterization had been practised she was cautioned to return promptly in case of any reappearance of trouble. She returned March 27, 1882, with an epithelioma which extended upon the side of the nose to within five millimeters of the median line and involved about one-third of the tarsal tissue of both lids.

Excision of the diseased tissues with enucleation of the globe was performed exactly as in the former case but with the result of leaving a larger gap at the side of the nose to heal by granulation. The inner wall of the orbit in the region of the lachrymal bone was thoroughly scraped and several small portions of the bone were cut away. The wound healed within six weeks, in part by the union of the flaps preserved from the lid integument and orbicularis muscle, and in part by granulation growth from the edges of the surrounding skin. The remnant of the open lachrymal sac filled with granulations and healed smoothly over with the rest of the granulating wound. Two weeks later the patient was discharged with a smooth, firm cicatrix at the side of the nose, and a linear scar extending from it to the external canthus. In this case also the lachrymal gland was left in situ without resulting inconvenience.

A third operation of the same character was performed about two years ago by Dr. A. Alt at the St. Louis City Hospital, upon a patient whom we saw together in consultation. In this case the whole margin of the lower lid together with the lower half of the conjunctival sack had been destroyed by an epithelioma. The skin and muscle of the upper lid gave a flap of sufficient size easily to come into the cavity left by the enucleation and the excision of the remnants of the lower lid.

The fourth and last case is that of H. D., a farmer 55 years of age, who fifteen years ago was struck by a stick of wood upon the right eye. Two months later the eye "ran out." During the past year the orbit began to fill up, and for two months before he consulted me the new growth had increased rapidly until it had considerably distended the eyelids and had become pretty firmly impacted, although still slightly movable by the recti muscles. The tumor was covered in front by the swollen conjunctiva bulbi, in which a small depression seemed to mark the former position of the cornea.

The operation, which was performed May 1, 1884, consisted in the clearing out of the entire contents of the orbit, through the palpebral opening enlarged at the temporal side by scissors. The lid margins were then clipped away, and the tarsal tissue of the upper and lower lids grasped by toothed forceps and dissected out. The thickened bulbar conjunctiva was removed with the tumor. The wound was left without sutures. May 18.—The patient went home. The orbital cavity was already much reduced in size and presented a uniformly granulating surface. The palpebral opening was rapidly closing at both ends, but more at the temperal end, and was about three-quarters of an inch long. There was every prospect of the speedy covering in of the whole granulating surfaces by the integument of the lids leaving a linear scar crossing a rather deep depression.

The advantage which may fairly be claimed for this operation is, that it permits the free excision of very extensively diseased tissues and leaves a firm, smooth, and nearly linear cicatrix, with a minimum quantity of scar tissue.

Indications and Surgical Techniques for Orbital Exenteration

Robert E. Kennedy, M.D.

ABSTRACT

Indications for the mutilating operation of exenteration are enumerated. They usually involve a malignant neoplasm of the orbital contents, primary, direct extension, or adnexal tissue that cannot be controlled by simple excision or irradiation.

Surgically, subtotal exenteration with partial preservation of lids and even conjunctiva may be achieved occasionally. However, total exenteration may be lifesaving. Techniques and precautions are discussed. Advantages and disadvantages of skin grafting that influence the postoperative care are noted.

Exenteration of the orbit is a necessity when malignant neoplasms involving the lids, or the orbital contents, cannot be controlled by irradiation or simple excision. It is successful only when complete eradication of the tumor is accomplished.

For patient acceptance of this mutilating surgical procedure, it is essential that the physician explain in detail the need for it, the type planned, the skin graft areas, and the postoperative rehabilitation, including care, availability and limitations of cosmetic devices.

Indications for exenteration [1] include: (a) malignancies originating in the paranasal sinuses, eyelids, and adnexal tissues; (b) primary orbital neoplasms of adults, excepting lymphosarcomas; (c) orbital sarcomas of children (it is now used much less frequently with rhabdomyosarcomas); (d) secondary malignant melanomas of the orbit, although the value is questioned; (e) advancing meningiomas, plexiform neurofibromas, pseudotumors or granulomas that, in the clinical course, simulate a local malignant disease; and (f) as a palliative procedure in the presence of metastatic disease.

SURGICAL TECHNIQUES

Variations in technique depend on preoperative considerations. Various subtotal procedures in an attempt to preserve some type of socket or lid structure are less disfiguring. However, cosmetic welfare should not be considered if there is a risk of recurrence and if survival is threatened by a less radical procedure than total exenteration.

Presented in combination with the American Society of Ophthalmic Plastic and Reconstructive Surgery at the 1978 Annual Meeting of the American Academy of Ophthalmology. Oct. 22–26, 1978. Published courtesy of *Transactions of Ophthalmology and Otolaryngology* (1979;86:967–973).

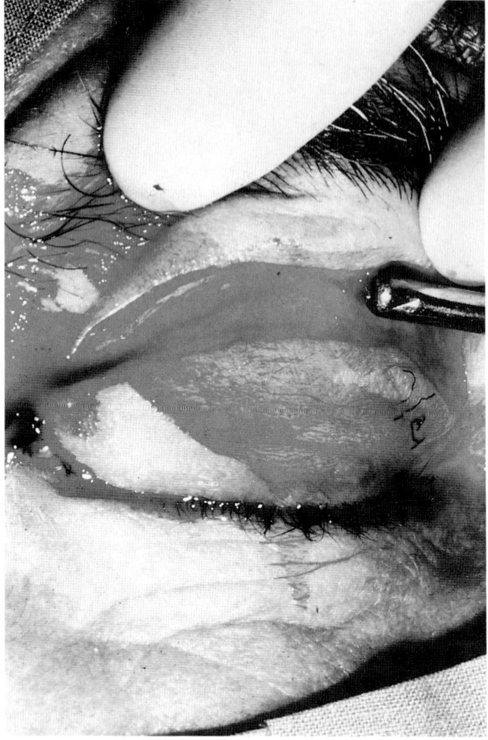

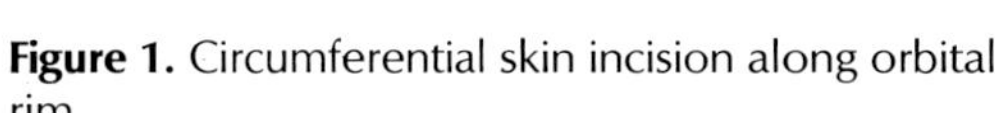

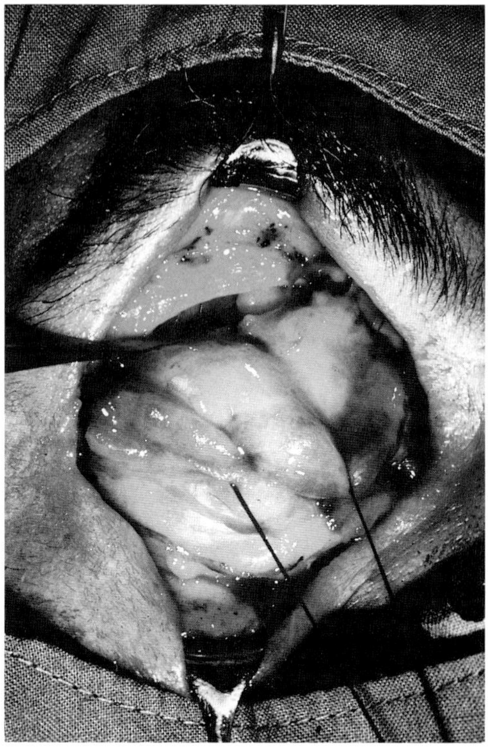

Figure 1. Circumferential skin incision along orbital rim.

Figure 2. Periosteum incised at rim of orbit and periorbita reflected by periosteal elevator.

General anesthesia is required. The patient should be blood grouped and matched. The field is cleansed, as is the donor site of the thigh or abdomen if a skin graft is to be taken.

Skin sutures or a large Allis clamp are applied to the lid margins for traction and guidance of the orbital contents (Fig. 1). A circumferential skin incision overlying the bony rim of the orbit is outlined. There will be less bleeding if a cold knife incision is carried through the skin and then a surgical cutting electrode, such as the Bovie unit, is used to produce a combined cutting and coagulation effect down to the periosteum. Carrying the incision from the less vascular quadrants temporally around nasally allows better visibility before reaching the more vascular upper nasal quadrant. The junction of the periosteum and periorbita at the bony rim is incised, and the peripheral orbital space is entered temporally with a periosteal elevator (Fig. 2). The periorbita separates easily temporally, above, and medially except for the firm attachment of the medial and lateral canthal ligaments and the trochlea, which is best severed with a Bard-Parker knife (No. 15 blade). The thinness of the orbital roof should be realized so that one does not inadvertently penetrate the anterior cranial cavity. Because of the thinness of the nasal orbital wall over the ethmoid air cells, great care must be taken in elevating the periorbita to prevent a future troublesome opening into the nasal cavity (Figs. 3 and 4). The lacrimal sac is removed.

In separating the periorbita along the rim or the orbital wall, the neoplasm may be encoun-

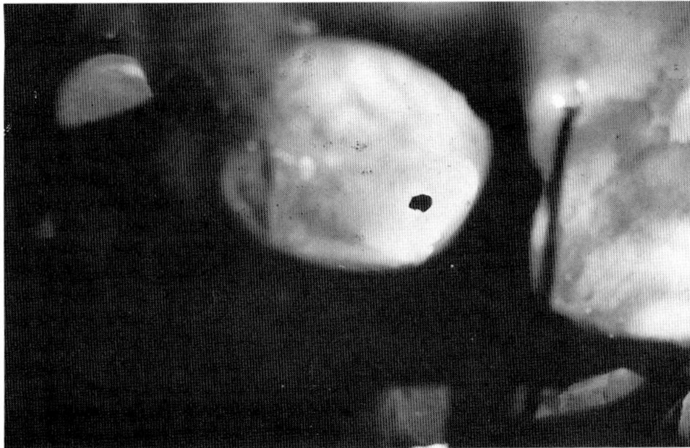

Figure 3. Transilluminated skull showing thinness of nasal wall and roof of the orbit that one must be careful not to penetrate.

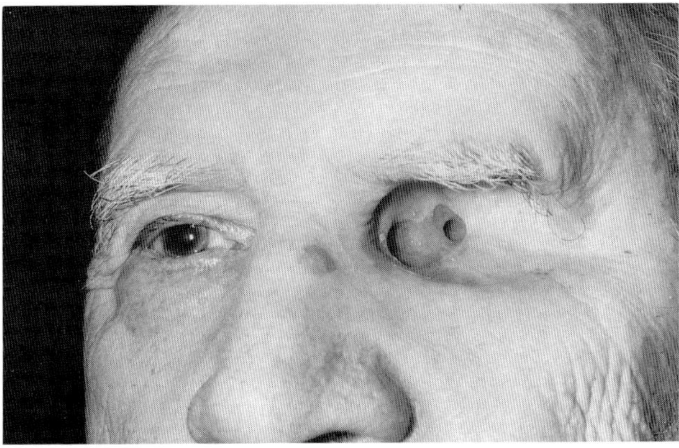

Figure 4. Healed orbit eight years after lacrimal gland carcinoma. Two residual nasal wall openings into nasal cavity are shown.

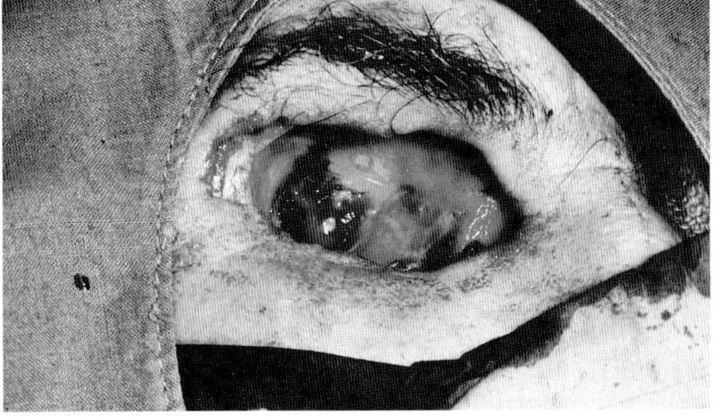

Figure 5. Denuded bone of orbit with contents removed, bleeding controlled.

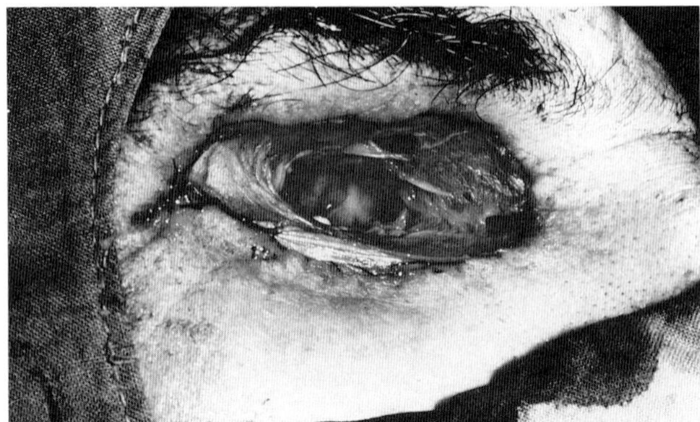

Figure 6. Skin graft in place, sutured to skin margins, with drainage incisions and apex open.

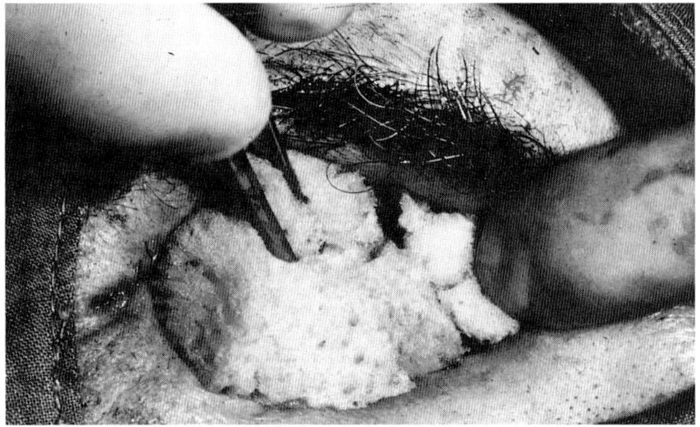

Figure 7. Orbit packed with sea sponge.

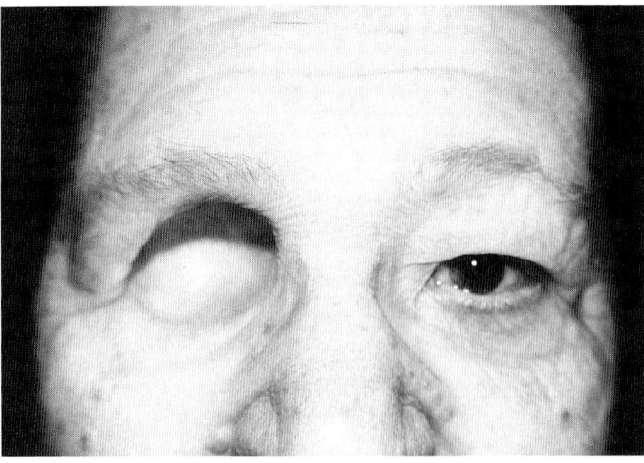

Figure 8. Healed skin-grafted orbit.

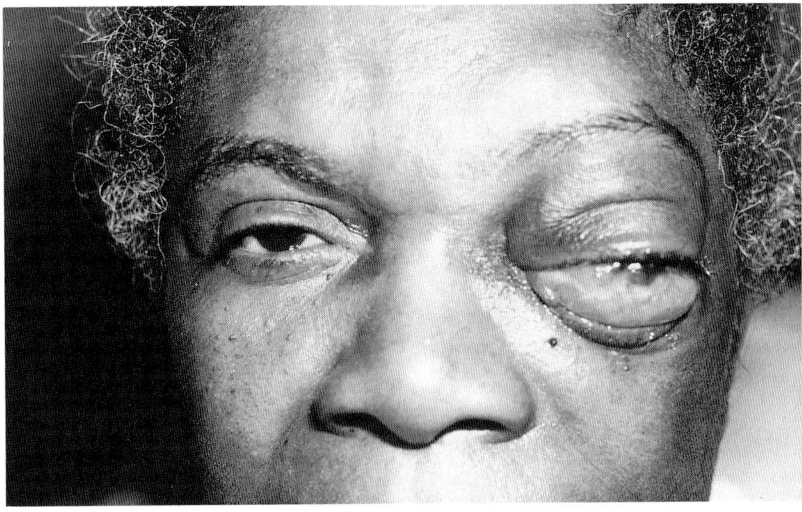

Figure 9. Patient with blind left eye with progressive proptosis, previously operated on neurosurgically for meningioma.

tered invading into or from other areas. This may result in cutting across the malignancy knowingly without full removal, if bone is involved. The periorbita can be freed as far back as the apical stump and along the superior and inferior fissures. These can be clamped and the surgical cutting coagulation electrode applied. The apical stump can be cut with curved neurectomy scissors applied from the nasal side. The stump invariably needs additional clamping and vigorous cautery for the control of bleeding (Fig. 5). The orbit is then packed with

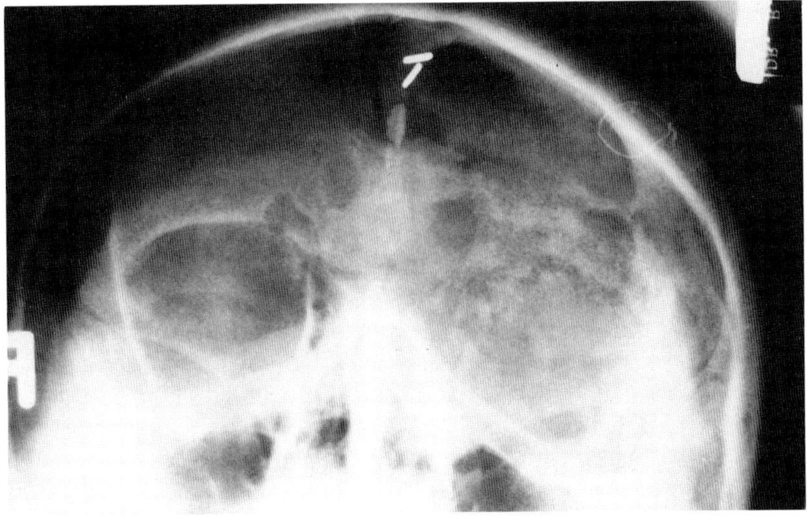

Figure 10. Roentgenogram of patient in Figure 9 with meningioma.

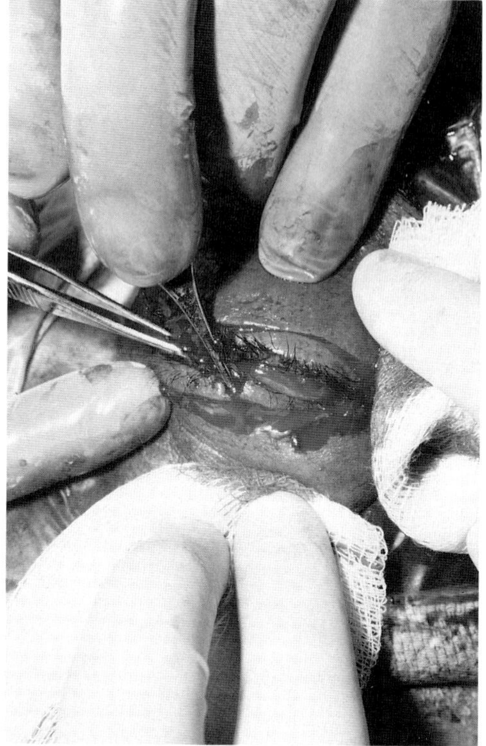

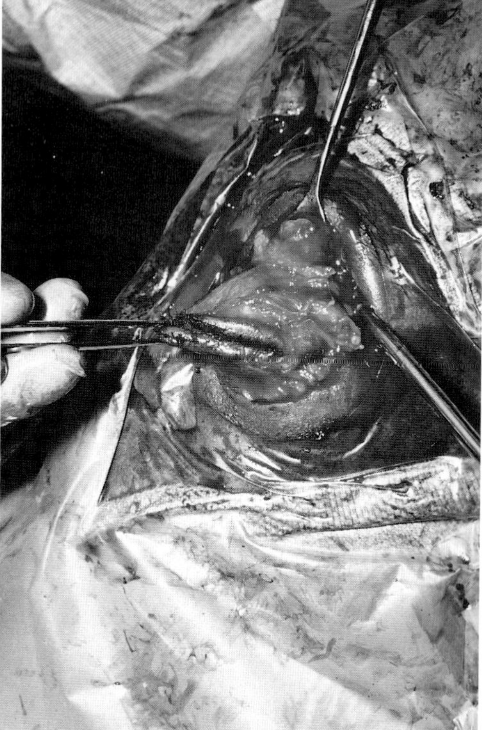

Figure 11. Exenteration in patient in Figure 9, started with incisions near lid margin to save skin.

Figure 12. Orbital tissue about to be removed from patient in Figure 9.

dry gauze. Bone is removed by rongeur where involved with malignancy, even if the sinuses must be entered. Bone removal with lacrimal gland malignancies is particularly important [2]. Bone wax is used as needed to control bleeding. Surgical time can be reduced by 50% or more by liberal use of a surgical cutting coagulation electrode.

Exposed bone can be managed by a variety of methods. Skin grafting to the bare bone can heal the orbit more rapidly than when allowing the orbit to granulate. Any accepted dermatome, such as the Stryker dermatome with oscillating blade, is used to cut a skin graft 1/64 in (0.015 cm) and 2 × 4 in long from the shaven inner surface of the thigh or abdomen. When using clear plastic adhesive tape, as advocated by Iliff [3], the dermatome setting compensates for the thickness of the tape, and the thin graft on the plastic sheet is placed in the orbit in the shape of a cone after the gauze pack has been removed and the orbital bleeding controlled.

The graft is sutured to the skin edges at the rim with many interrupted catgut sutures. The apex of the cone is left open and several stab incisions are placed in the graft to provide drainage (Fig. 6). Strips of petrolatum gauze 1 in wide are used as a thin layer over the graft. Sterile sea sponge is used to line the graft site, and the center is packed with small pieces of sea sponge to provide firm lateral pressure against the bone (Fig. 7). The outer layer is covered with gauze and an elastoplast type of dressing. The donor site is dressed with petrolatum gauze and a firm dressing. The orbital dressing is removed in 10 to 12 days and cleansed with benz-

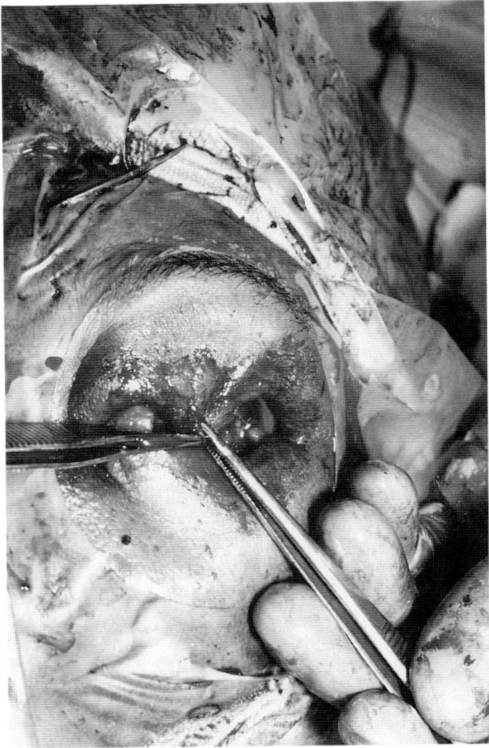

Figure 13. Approximation of skin edges after removal of orbital contents from patient in Figure 9.

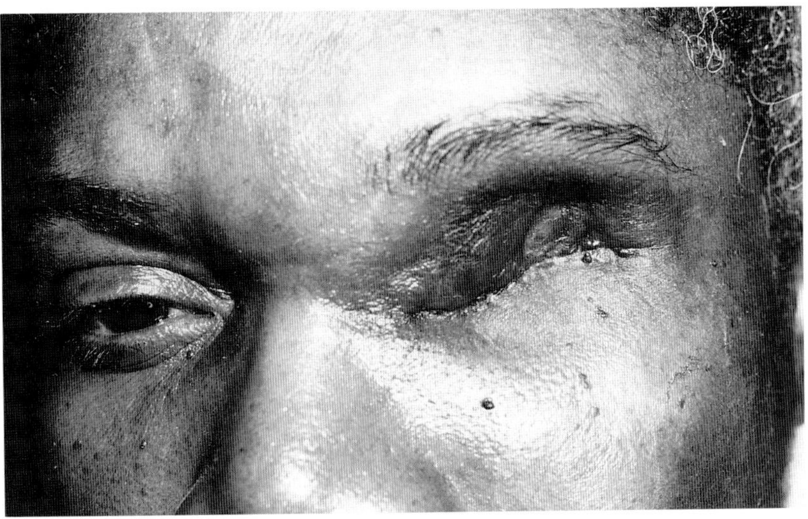

Figure 14. Patient in Figure 9 three weeks postoperatively.

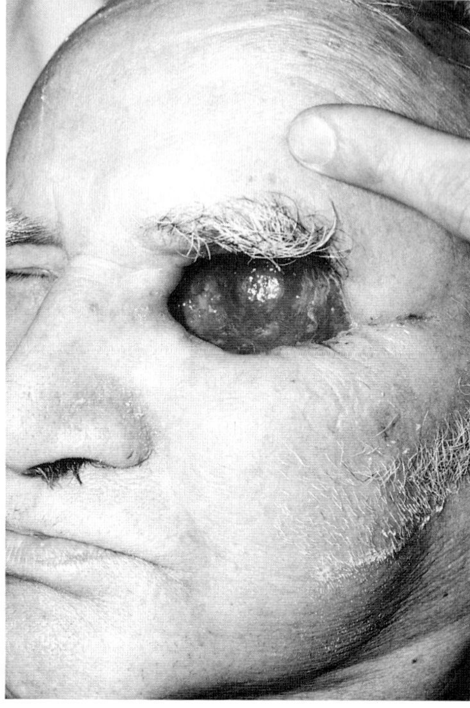

Figure 15. Patient, ungrafted, with orbit granulating, one month postexenteration. Patient had carcinoma of lacrimal gland.

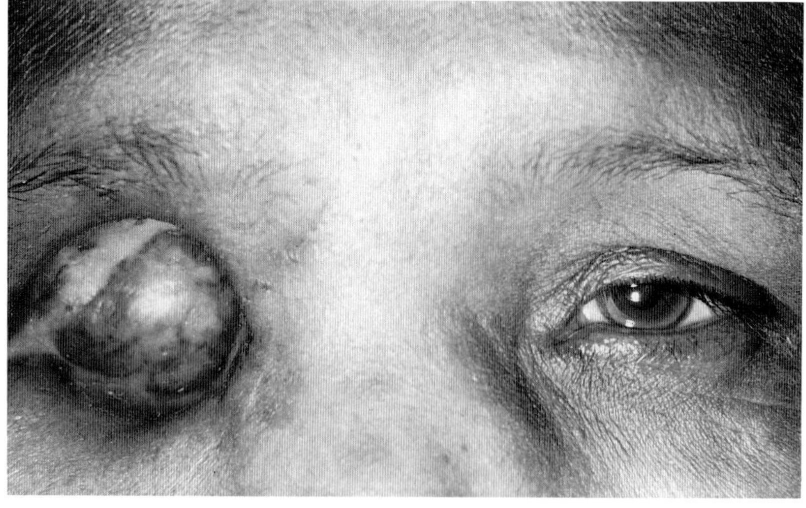

Figure 16. Patient healed by later office pinch grafting to granulating bed.

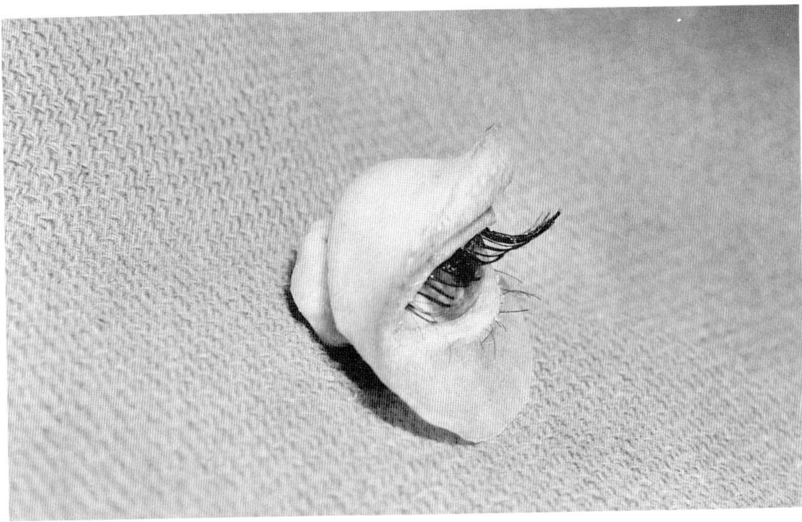

Figure 17. Fabricated, anatomically accurate prosthesis.

alkonium chloride solution (Zephiran), and an antibiotic ointment is applied to prevent crusting. The socket is healed in approximately six weeks with the advantage of the skin-lined socket allowing early detection of recurrences [4] (Fig. 8). Systemic antibiotics are used at least until the dressing is initially removed.

With preservation of the eyelid skin, after bleeding has been controlled, it may be possible to close in a primary manner; this greatly shortens both the operative and postoperative

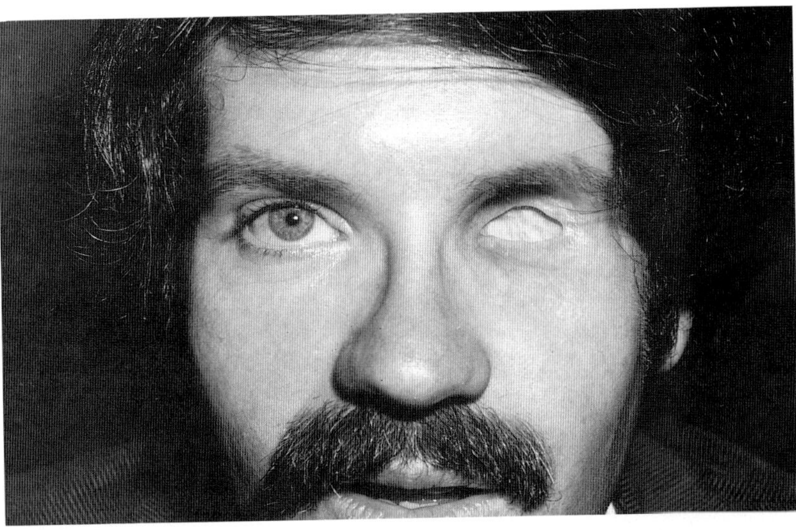

Figure 18. Patient with contracted socket, unable to wear prosthesis, postenucleation for retinoblastoma and irradiation.

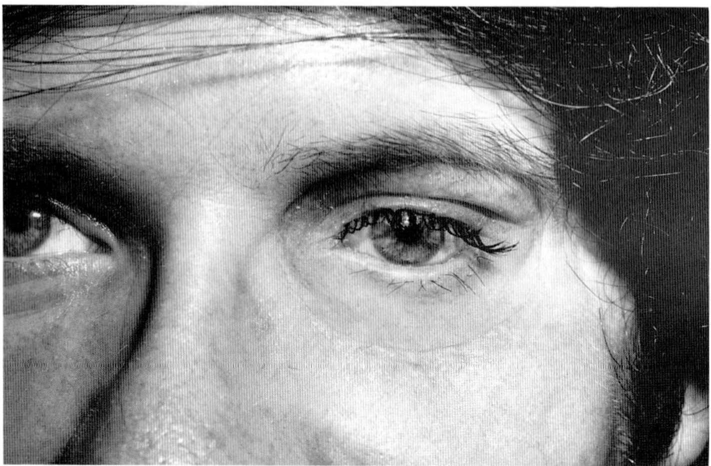

Figure 19. Patient in Figure 18 with prosthesis in place.

course, and hospitalization may be only a few days. Gelfoam and plastics under the skin are readily extruded, however (Figs. 9–14).

Skin grafting may not be performed if the shortest possible anesthetic time is desired or if bleeding persists. Petrolatum gauze can be applied on the skin edges and the walls of the orbit to the apex and packed with sterile sea sponge, gauze, and pressure dressing. This can be allowed to granulate (Fig. 15) and slowly epithelialize over approximately three months or can be skin grafted or pinch grafted later (Fig. 16).

Postoperative patient adjustment is usually surprisingly good, with relief that the tumor has

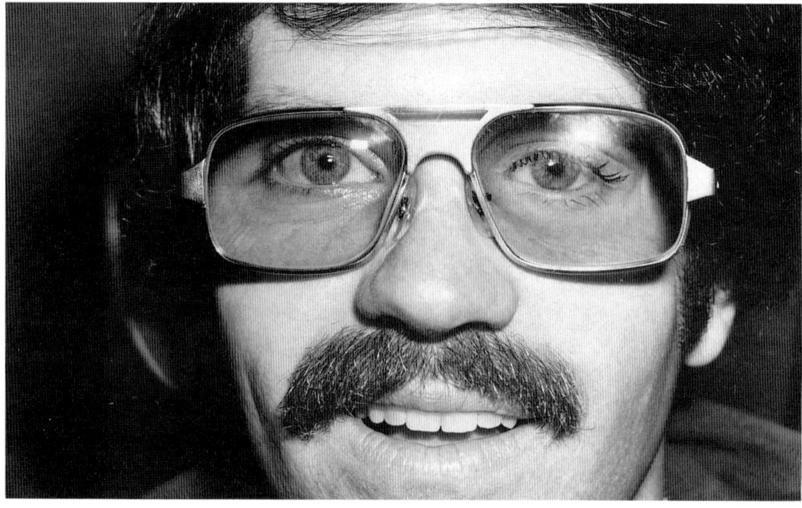

Figure 20. Patient in Figure 18 wearing glasses.

been eradicated. Occasionally, prosthetic devices may be worn satisfactorily (Figs. 17–20), but they are limited in the very young and very old and also by their availability. Most patients prefer simple patch occlusion of the Hathaway Shirt type.

Acknowledgment—Figures 1, 2, 5, 6, and 7 are reproduced with permission from Charles E. Iliff, MD.

REFERENCES

1. Henderson JW: *Orbital Tumors.* Philadelphia, PA, W.B. Saunders Co., 1973:659–673.
2. Reese AB, Jones IS: Bone resection in the excision of epithelial tumors of the lacrimal gland. *Arch Ophthalmol* 1964; 71:382–385.
3. Iliff CE: Results of orbital exenteration with use of cone-shaped skin graft. In Tessier P, Callahan A, Mustarde JC, et al. (eds): *Symposium on Plastic Surgery in the Orbit Region.* St. Louis, MO, C.V. Mosby Co., 1976:371–376.
4. Rathbun JE, Beard C, Quickert MH: Evaluation of 48 cases of orbital exenteration. *Am J Ophthalmol* 1971; 72:191–199.

Radical Orbital Resections

*Renato Frezzotti, M.D., Raffaele Bonanni, M.D.,
Alessandro Nuti, M.D., and Ennio Polito, M.D.*

ABSTRACT

The authors describe the techniques for subtotal, total and radical orbital exenteration. The aspects of primary and late reconstructive surgery are also discussed, with special reference to Frezzotti's personal technique for temporalis muscle transplantation after subtotal exenteration.

INTRODUCTION

Radical orbital resections are one of the most dramatic measures in ophthalmic surgery. This surgery may be indicated for aggressive intraocular tumors, undifferentiated orbital tumors, or secondary orbital tumors (metastatic or contiguous) (Fig. 1).

This procedure may also be required in cases of invasive fungal infiltration of the orbit or severe facial trauma with destruction of the orbital contents.

For the ophthalmologist these surgical indications constitute an unusual event that requires a different mentality using extensive knowledge of the surgical technical difficulties and of the postoperative course. For a long time exenteration had been performed by general surgeons or by other specialists; now it may be considered part of ophthalmic surgery, as are reconstructive aspects of the surgery.

Exenteration is not mentioned in the literature until 1767, when Gooch, in his handbook on surgery, reported an orbit *emptying* in a 16-year-old girl with excellent outcome. Since then, the indications became more numerous and more specific. The entire surgical technique is described by Langenbeck in 1821 and Dupuytren in 1833*, both of them describing the use of different types of cutaneous incisions. Acrel and Derault* describe external canthotomies.

Another important and well-documented description of exenteration was noted in 1833 by J. H. Wishart [2], in which he mentioned an operation for the extirpation of the orbital contents. Subsequently, a subconjunctival variation was described [3–6, also Jamescu, 1899*]. In 1890, Küster was the first to attempt an exenteration sparing the eyelids and the eye. Even then the need to repair the large aesthetic facial mutilation was noted. The first surgical reconstructive attempts consisted of filling the cavity itself and covering it. It was only at the end of the 1800s that the variations of the exenteration technique were classified [3–5,7]. Such a classification remains controversial today because of the great incidence of recurrence in apparently

---

*Cited by Ovio, 1950 [1].

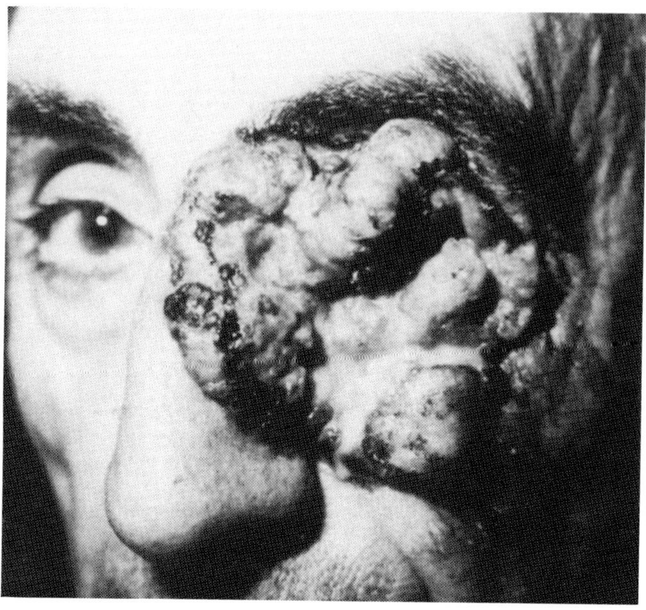

Figure 1. Large basal cell carcinoma of the inferior eyelid (personal observation).

cured cases [8]. Reese [9–11] believes reconstructing the exenterated socket does not mask recurrences any more frequently than granulation within the socket does. We have adopted the following classification based on the amount of tissue to be resected [12] (Fig. 2).

SUBTOTAL EXENTERATION:

Type I: preservation of the eyelids, palpebral and bulbar conjunctiva.
Type II: preservation of the eyelids and palpebral conjunctiva only.
Type III: preservation of the eyelid skin, retaining the underlying muscular layer if possible.

SIMPLE TOTAL EXENTERATION:

Type IV: with complete removal of the eyelids.

RADICAL EXENTERATION:

Type V: with removal of the bony walls (walls of the lacrimal fossa).
Type VI: with extension to the nearby cavities (orbito-sinusal exenteration in collaboration with the maxillofacial surgeon or with the neurosurgeon if beyond the apex of the orbit).

A simple exenteration (Fig. 3) [9] consists of the removal of all the orbital contents, periosteum included. A radical exenteration includes resection of the bony walls and the neigh-

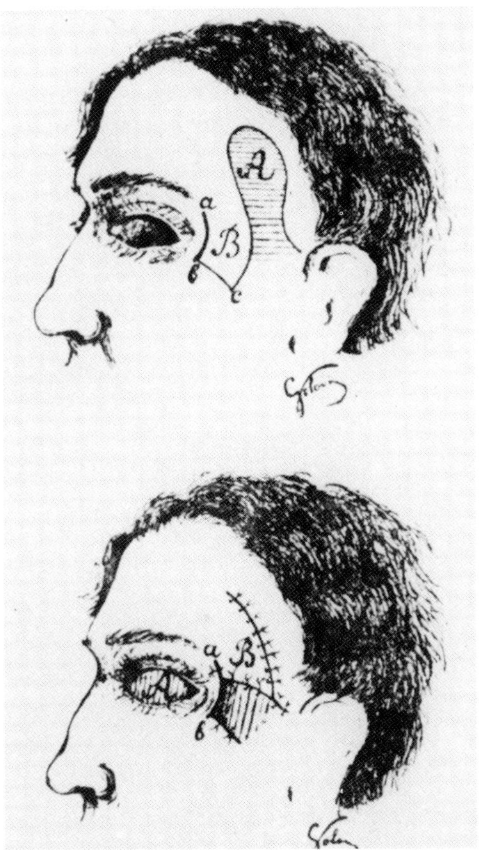

Figure 2. Repair technique after exenteration, proposed by Golovine in 1898, using temporal pedicle flap [6].

boring sinuses when they are involved by the pathological process. Initially, under various names such as *extirpation of the content* (Wishart, 1833 [2]), this surgical technique finally assumed its definitive name of *exenteratio orbitae*. (Previously the latin term *exenteratio* referred to *exenteratio bulbi*). Historically, the various surgical techniques have been divided into four stages (Rollet, 1908 [13]): cutaneous incision; periosteum incision of the orbital margin and its detachment; isolation of the lacrimal fossa and removal of its contents; and incision of the vascular nervous peduncle, and extirpation of the orbital contents. Today these stages still constitute the basis for all of the variations in technique in this procedure.

Modern surgical techniques have offered variations with regard to incisions, hemostasis, and above all, to saving some useful structures for repair and reconstruction.

SUBTOTAL EXENTERATION SURGERY

The surgeon's experience and the specifics of each individual case will dictate the application of this technique.

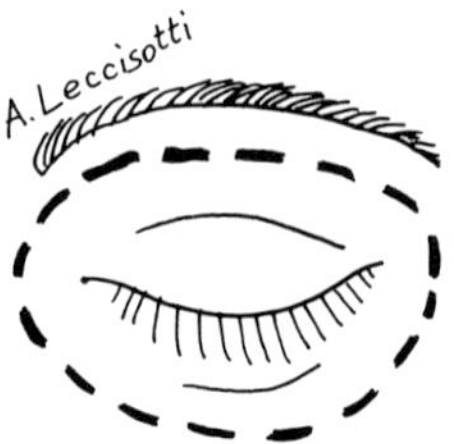

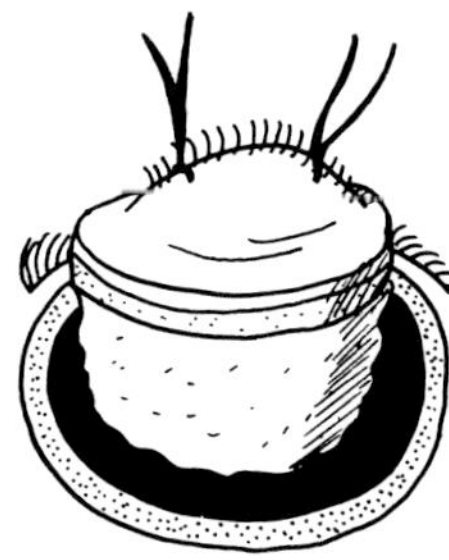

Figure 3. *Exenteratio orbitae* technique as described by Brihaye et al. [25].

The variations include:

Type I: preservation of the eyelids, and conjunctiva; conjunctiva is isolated and conserved as in enucleation.

Type II: preservation of the eyelids and the palpebral conjunctiva; the incision starts in the superior and inferior fornix.

Type III: preservation of only the palpebral skin and muscular layers. A skin muscle flap is separated from the posterior lamella, which is removed (Figs. 4A, B, C). These minor variations are of fundamental importance in establishing the foundation for primary and late reconstructive measures.

Type IV: *Total exenteration.*
This technique is much more dramatic because it includes the complete removal of the eyelids of all the orbital contents, with a circular incision on the bony margins of the orbital cavity (Fig. 5A, B, C, D, E, F).

Type V: *Radical exenteration.*
This is a Type IV exenteration with the addition of a *surgical toilette* (curettage) of the lacrimal fossa bones.

Type VI: This is the most demanding variation that frequently requires interdisciplinary intraoperative collaboration between the orbital, the maxillofacial, and neurosurgeons, because this pathology extends beyond the confines of the orbital cavity (Fig. 6).

No matter what type of exenteration, the interoperative stages include:

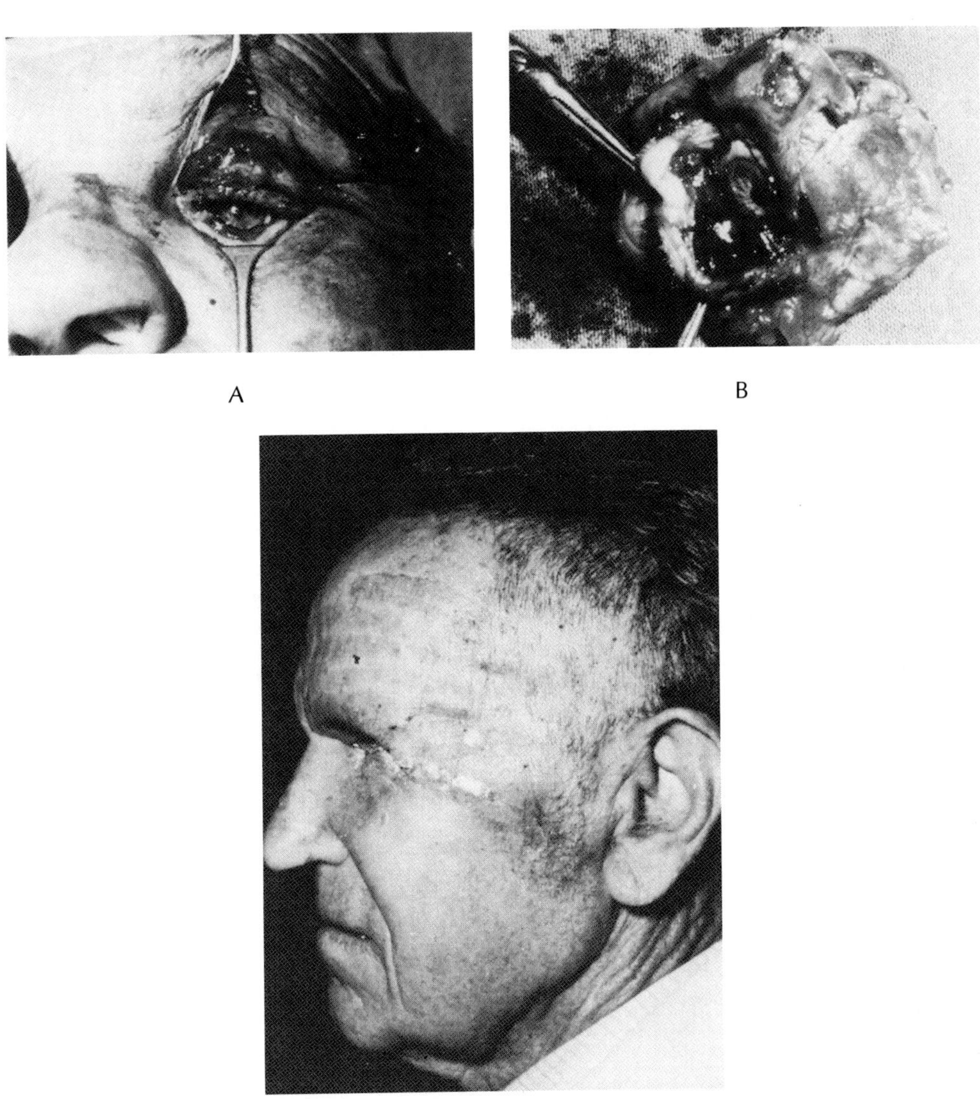

Figure 4. (A) Subtotal exenteration, Type III, with sparing of the lower eyelid cutaneous plane only, in a case of large upper conjunctival fornix melanoma. (B) The "en bloc" excision of orbital contents. (C) Berke incision extending the lateral canthotomy (personal observation).

Cutaneous Incision. The site and extent of the incision depends upon the orbital pathology and the procedure planned. In a simple exenteration, an extended canthotomy is appropriate for better access to the cavity walls. In the subtotal exenteration techniques the enlarged canthotomy is appropriate if the approach is anterior (Fig. 7), although this technique is unnecessary if the approach is hemicoronal [14,15].

On the contrary, an enlarged Berke (1954) [16] type incision is necessary in the Type III

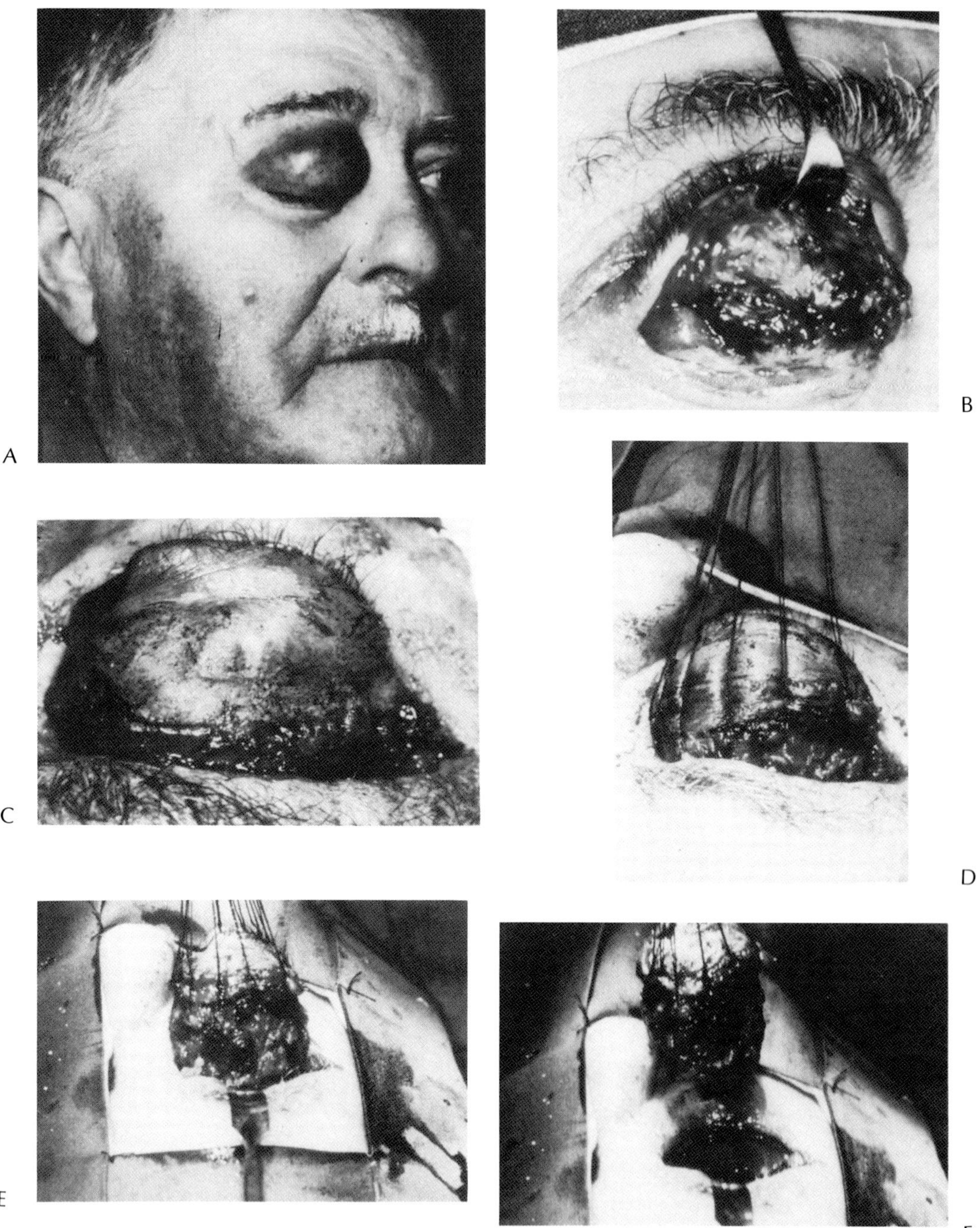

Figure 5. Orbital invasion by choroidal melanoma enucleated a year ago: (A) the patient's appearance upon hospitalization. (B) evident large neoplastic mass everting the eyelids. (C) cutaneous circular incision (exenteration Type IV) at the orbital margins; first stage of exenteration Type IV. (D) the mass including the orbital content and the periosteum, after the elevation from the bony walls of the orbit. (E) after periosteal elevation and resection of the peduncle, the mass can easily be extirpated. (F) exenteration is complete and the orbital floor is clearly seen (observed Nov. 1984).

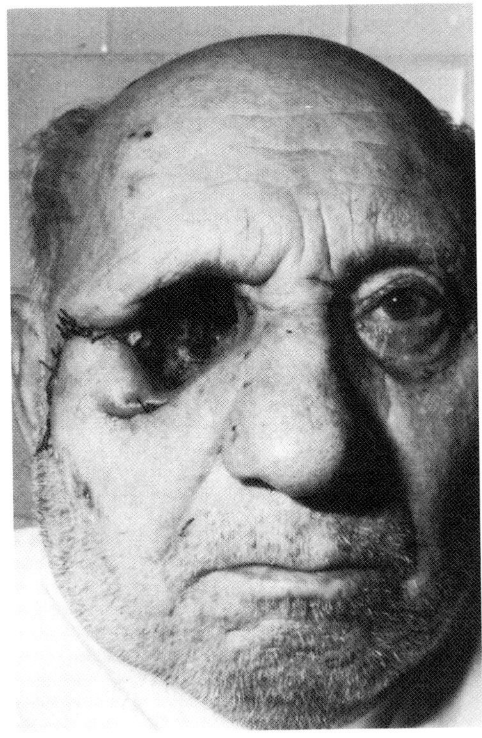

Figure 6. Orbito-sinusoidal exenteration, Type IV, for large squamous-cell carcinoma of the eyelids and conjunctiva infiltrating lids, orbit, ethmoid, and maxillary sinus. Berke's incision is seen, and also the cutaneous incision of the superior portion of the anterior wall of the maxillary sinus (personal observation, Nov. 1982).

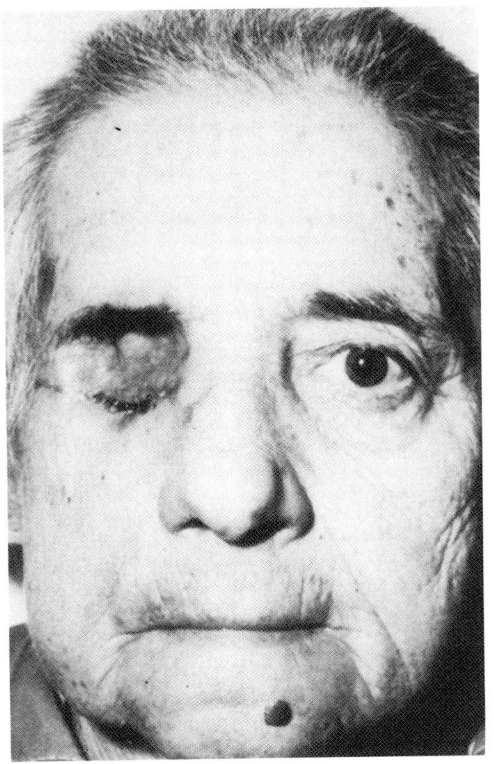

Figure 7. Type III exenteration sparing the superior eyelid, in a case of inferior lid basal cell carcinoma with invasion of the orbit (personal observation, Apr. 1975).

operations (Fig. 8) when the temporal muscle must be reflected to expose the external surface of the temporal orbital wall before a bony window is created.

We agree with Rougier (1977) [14] that in these cases the hemicoronal approach can include a better aesthetic result. However, the extended Berke [16] incision may provide better exposure than the hemicoronal approach (Fig. 9).

Periosteal Incision and Elevation. An electric scalpel or cutting cautery is used to open the periosteum with the least possible bleeding and also to avoid neoplastic dissemination. The periosteum should be incised at the bony margin at a safe distance from possible tumor infiltration.

The elevation of the periosteum must be performed with a smooth instrument or a finger, especially at the apex, to avoid any laceration of the periosteum itself and fracture of the fragile bony areas of the orbital walls (i.e., ethmoid and nasal orbital floor). Such precautions are not necessary in the presence of obvious tumor infiltration for which orbital-sinusoidal exenteration is required. Special attention should be paid to the superior and inferior orbital fissure areas where there is tenacious adherence of the periosteum to the neovascular bundle which must be lysed with scissors or electric scalpel.

Excellent hemostasis can be achieved with a Frazier suction cannula connected to a unipolar coagulator or bipolar forceps.

Emptying of the Lacrimal Fossa. When indicated this is performed with a smooth periosteal elevator. It may be necessary to open and curette the nasolacrimal duct osteum.

Sectioning the Neurovascular Peduncle. The neurovascular peduncle which includes the optic nerve, ophthalmic artery, and neurovascular bundle coming from the superior orbital fissure and orbital apex is sectioned as close as possible to the optic foramen, after placement of metal clips across the peduncle for hemostasis. It is helpful to cauterize the peduncle itself before sectioning. Bleeding may nevertheless sometimes follow which can be stopped by tamponade and unipolar cautery applied to the Frazier suction tip.

Closure. If a Type III exenteration has been performed, a partial or complete blephorrhaphy to retain an exenteration socket implant is appropriate, while awaiting eventual reconstruction (Figs. 7 and 8).

Primary Reconstructive Surgery. Mustardé (1980) [8] rejected primary reconstruction because it could make radiation treatment less effective and conceal recurrence. Radiation therapy may

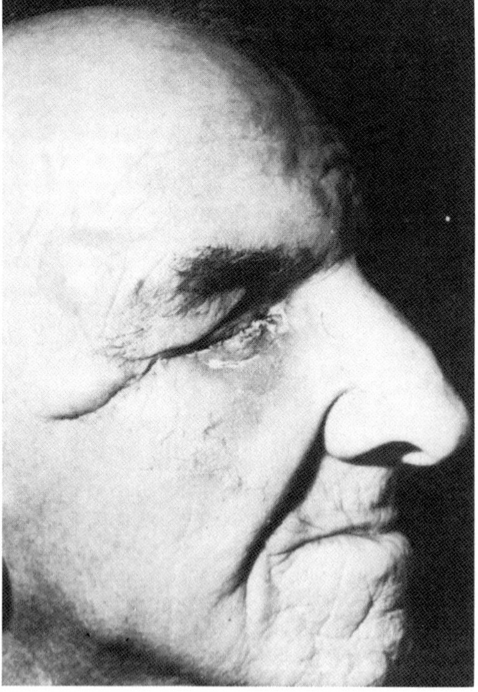

Figure 8. Type III exenteration in a case of orbital extension of malignant melanoma of the choroid (Feb. 1972).

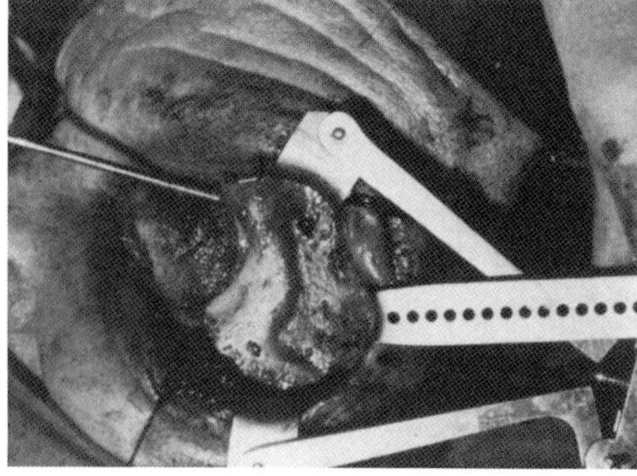

Figure 9. The Reese retractor permits a good view of the whole field.

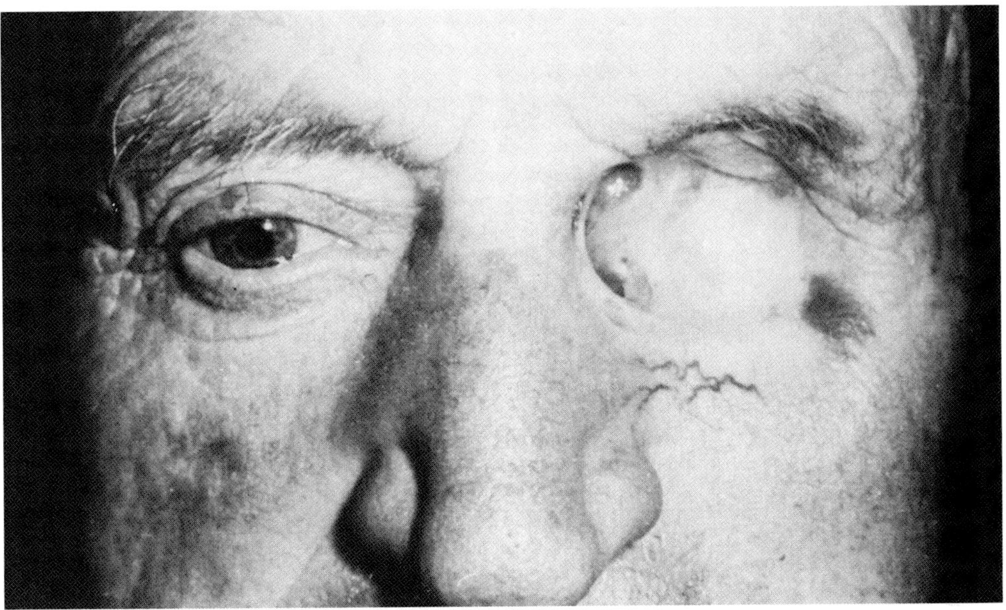

Figure 10. Type IV exenteration; the orbital cavity is filled by granulation tissue.

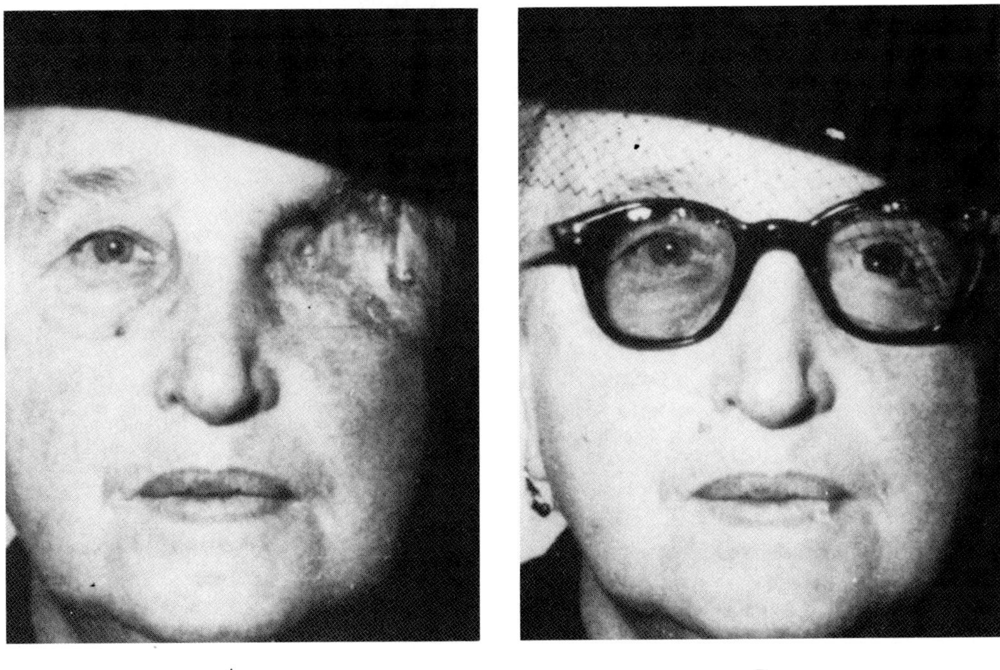

A   B

Figure 11. (A) Repair after orbital exenteration; (B) epiprosthesis covering, Type IV exenteration.

Table 1. Repair Techniques after Orbital Exenteration

A Wheeler technique: epidermal graft.
B Inert material filling technique.
C Temporal muscle transplantation, Naquin 1956 [21]; modified by Frezzotti, 1959 [22].
D Personal technique, Frezzotti, 1964 (from: Frezzotti R, Bonanni R) [28].

also compromise the viability of the free grafts and pedicles used to reconstruct the socket. Late reconstruction can be performed following radiation therapy. Reese advocates primary reconstruction with certain exceptions. Contraindications to primary reconstruction, according to Reese, are: tumors of the lacrimal gland, orbital infiltration of basal cell carcinomas of the eyelids, malignant vascular tumors, malignant lymphomas, and orbital extension of conjunctival and uveal melanomas. Apart from the malignant lymphomas, which are now treated conservatively, we generally agree with Reese (1963). However, primary reconstruction is recommended in those rare cases of uveal melanoma with limited extrascleral extension. Such extension has been observed in only five out of 114 enucleated cases of choroidal melanomas (personal series of cases 1974–84) [17].

It is controversial whether to fill the cavity with granulation tissue or to cover the cavity with a free skin graft as described by Wheeler (1922) [18], particularly following a Type III or a Type IV exenteration (Table 1-A). After a year the appearance of the cavity, healed by granulation tissue alone (Fig. 10) and camouflaged with an epiprosthesis (Fig. 11A and B) is more acceptable.

The advantages of a primary reconstructive procedure are evident. When dealing with this type of surgery an attempt to limit its disfiguring outcome is always made. The first reconstructive measures were by Busachi [4], Romano, Catania [5], and Golovine [6], with free or pedicle skin flaps from the temporal area. These date back to the end of the last century (Fig. 2). The decision to reconstruct primarily, however, is a delicate decision influenced by multiple clinical factors including the histopathology, the intraoperative findings, the patient's quality of life, and the surgeon's personal insight.

The reconstructive measures performed primarily include the following:

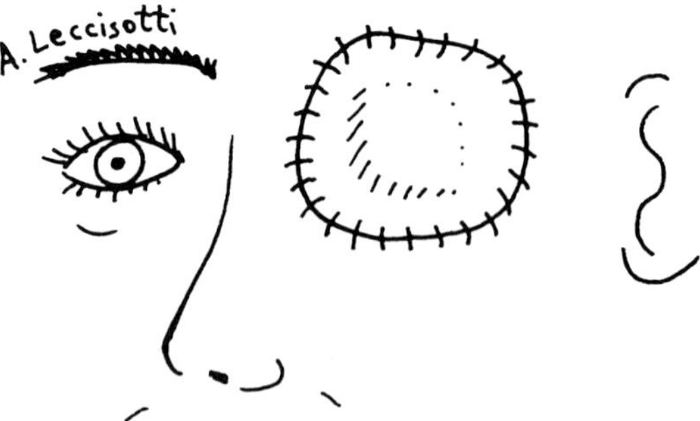

Figure 12. Free skin graft (Wheeler technique).

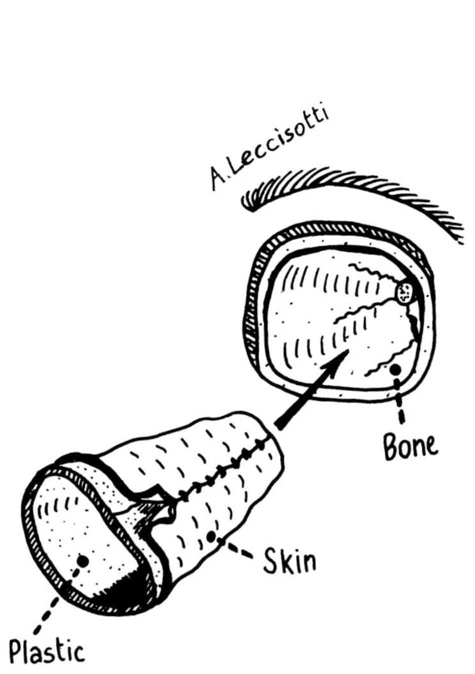

Figure 13. Iliff and Ossofsky technique to repair an orbital exenteration Type IV.

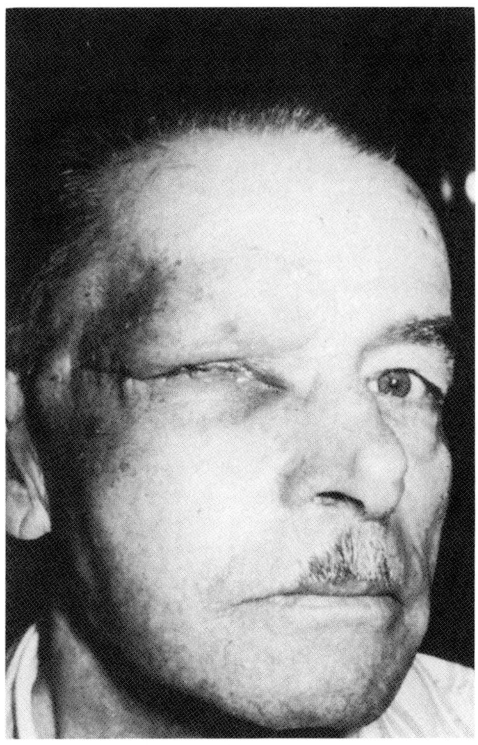

Figure 14. Type III exenteration for orbital exenteration of uveal melanoma. Repair technique by Naquin-Reese, using temporalis muscle (personal observation, Dec. 1960).

1. *Skin lining.* (Type III and Type IV exenterations) Free skin grafts (Wheeler, 1922) of 6 × 12 cm and approximately 0.2 mm thick are removed from the abdomen or from the medial or anterior aspect of the thigh with a dermatome and are used to line the cavity (Fig. 12). In another technique [19] the skin strip is shaped in the form of a truncated cone and is inserted into the cavity (Fig. 13). After about a week the conformer of sterile sponge is removed.

2. *Filling the socket with inert material.* This technique follows a Type III exenteration that saves the eyelids. Gass [20] has used an externally molded acrylic implant. The myocutaneous eyelid remnants are sutured onto the alloplastic material; the result is a filled and sealed cavity, suitable to support an external prosthesis (Table 1-B).

3. *Transplantation of the temporalis muscle.* This technique can be performed after a Type I, II, or III exenteration. Proposed by Naquin in 1954 [21] and modified by Reese [9,10], temporalis transposition provides a viable filling for the cavity (Fig. 14). A second reconstructive procedure allows the creation of a palpebral aperture and the establishment of a socket suitable to support an ocular prosthesis. In a variation proposed by Frezzotti in 1959 [22] (Ta-

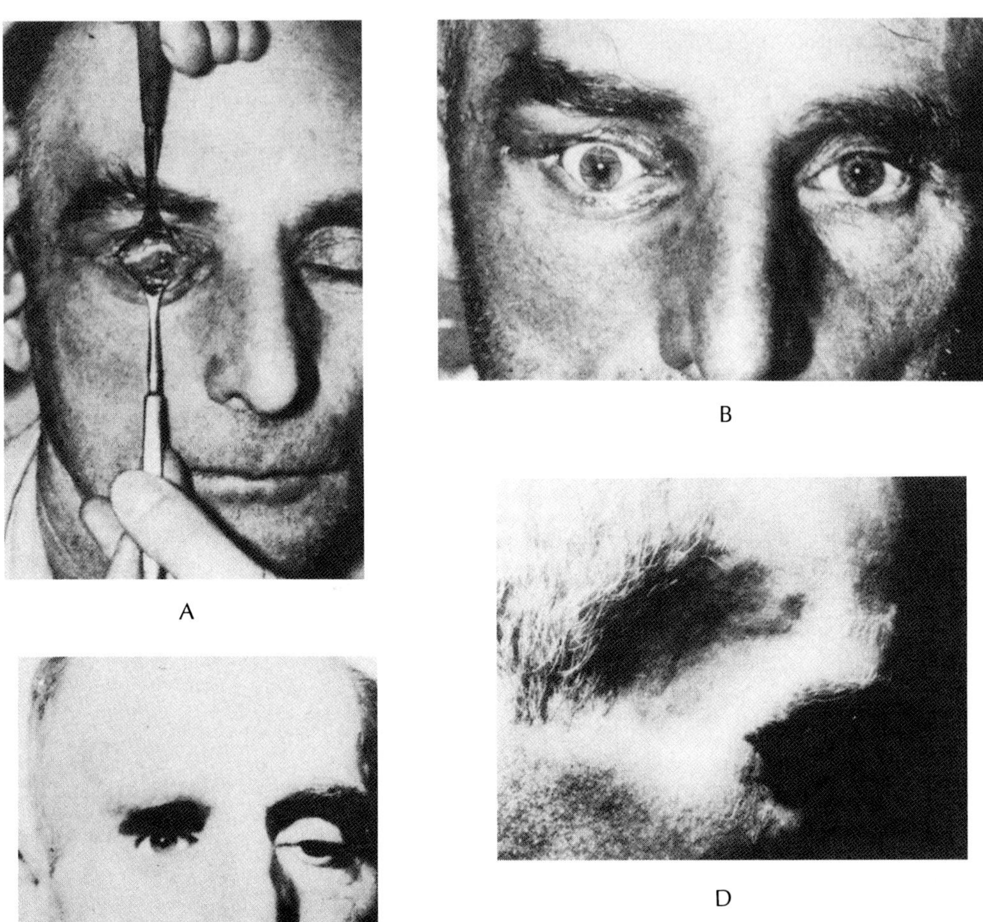

Figure 15. Type I orbit exenteration for orbital extension of malignant melanoma. Temporal muscle implant, Frezzotti's technique (1959): (A) restoration of the socket with preserved conjunctiva. (B) the same patient wearing a common prothesis 15 days later. (C–D) the patient four years later: sinking of the temporal fossa and enophthalmic effect caused by muscular atrophy (personal observation, Jan. 1959).

ble 1-C) after a Type I exenteration, the preserved conjunctival sac which overlies the transposed temporalis muscle can be reconstructed. Therefore, an ocular prosthesis can be applied as early as the tenth postoperative day (Fig. 15A and B).

In 1964 Frezzotti proposed an additional modification [23,24] of temporalis muscle transplantation following a Type I exenteration. Long-term follow-up of the techniques of Naquin, Reese, and Frezzotti, showed atrophy of the transplanted temporalis muscle within the socket, with progressive enophthalmos of the prosthesis and an unaesthetic depression of the tempo-

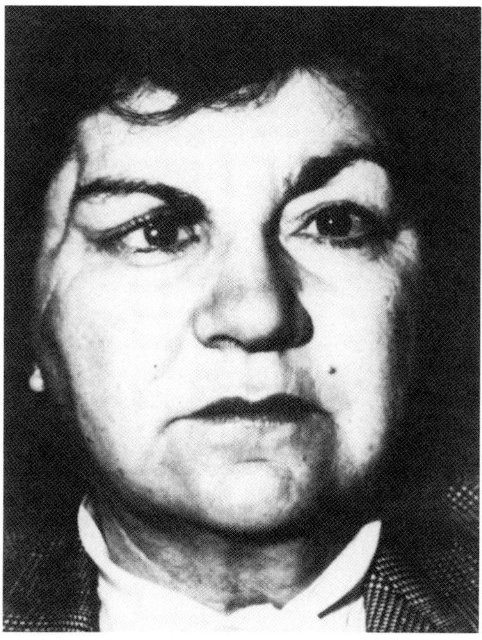

Figure 16. Type I exenteration; temporalis muscle transplant, reconstructed conjunctival sac and insertion of a common prosthesis (personal observation, March 1983).

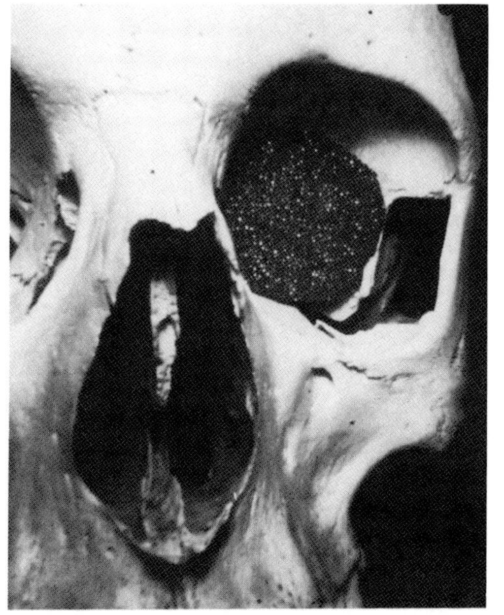

A

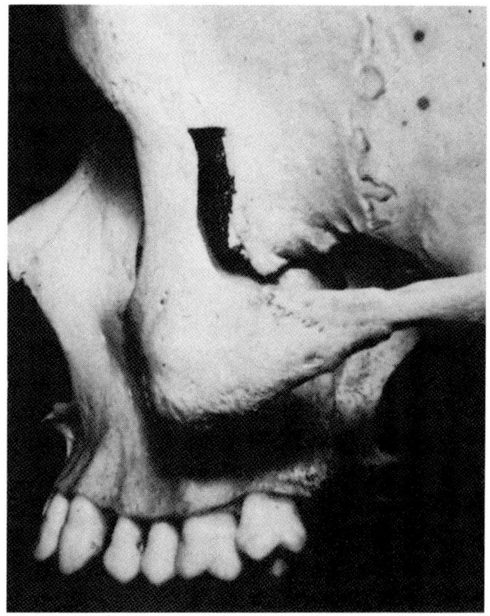

B

Figure 17. (A & B) The Silastic® cone is well-seen through the bone window.

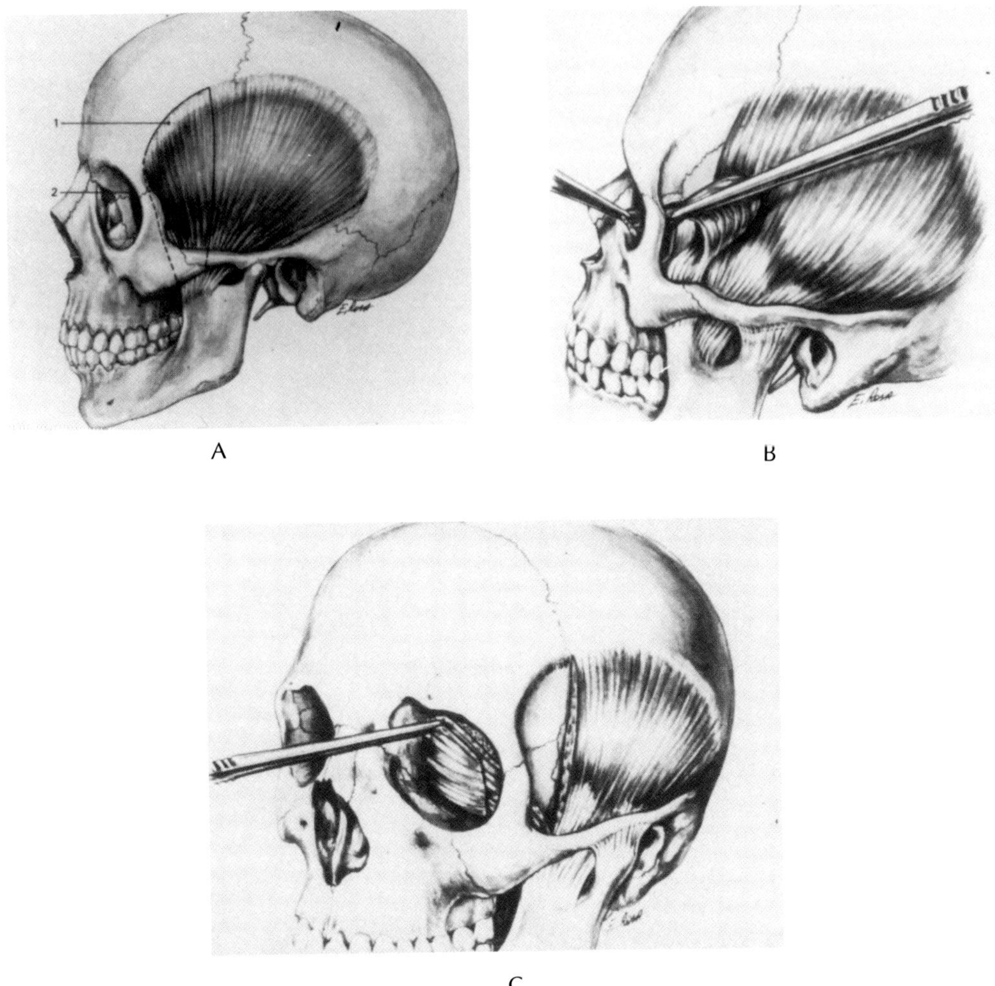

Figure 18. Surgical steps of exenteration in Frezzotti's modified technique. (A) isolation of the anterior third of the temporalis muscle. (B–C) temporalis muscle ceiling over the Silastic® cone (from Frezzotti, 1984) [27].

Table 2. Orbit Exenteration (according to Frezzotti)

A Bone window of approximately 18 × 10 mm to accommodate the temporalis muscle.

B Exenteration is already performed; the temporalis muscle on the right is transposed into the orbital cavity.

C Filling of the posterior two-thirds of the orbital cavity with Silastic® (Dow Corning, Midland, Michigan, USA).

D Silastic® is now covered with a layer of temporalis muscle. The portion of the transposed muscle is sutured to the inferomedial and superomedial orbital margins. The hollow of the temporal fossa is carefully filled with flakes of silicone sponge (from: Frezzotti R., Bonanni R.) [28].

ral region (Fig. 15C, D, and 16) (Table 1-D) [18]. Tessier (1982) [15] who proposed temporalis muscle transposition in 1977, did not mention progressive enophthalmos as a sequela of this procedure. Because of the aforementioned difficulties of temporalis muscle transposition alone, the posterior two-thirds of the cavity can be filled with an appropriately shaped silicone cone (Silastic®, Dow Corning, Midland, Michigan, USA) (Fig. 17A and B). Following the isolation of the conjunctiva and extirpation of the orbital contents, a lateral canthal incision extending 5 to 6 cm inferiorly and posteriorly is made. The superficial temporalis muscle fascia is incised along the posterior margin of the orbital process of the zygomatic bone. Sutures are placed at the wound edges for retraction. The temporalis muscle is exposed and the anterior one-third of the muscle is disinserted (Fig. 18A). Using a smooth periosteal elevator the muscle is separated from the deep temporalis fascial or the periosteum of the temporalis fossa. The adhesions between the temporalis muscle and the zygoma are bluntly dissected as far inferiorly as the coronoid process of the mandible. Only by these means can the anterior third of the temporalis muscle achieve the necessary mobility (Fig. 18B–C) [19]. A 20 × 10 mm bony window in the temporal orbital wall is fashioned with a Stryker or Feldman electric saw (Fig. 17 and Table 1A). The mobilized temporalis muscle is transposed into the orbit through the bony window. The muscle must be placed over the Silastic cone (Table 2A–B) and sutured to the margins of the periosteal incisions and to the medial orbital periosteum (Fig. 18C) (Table 2C–D). The temporal depression is filled with a silicone sponge (Table 2D). With the use of the Silastic orbital implant the amount of muscle needed in the orbital cavity and the resultant temporal fossa defect are reduced. The layered closure of the temporalis fascia and skin conclude the procedure (Fig. 19). A drain can be left in the temporal fossa. Frezzotti's 1964 modification provides a number of advantages: less muscle is needed in the orbital cavity, a smaller bony window is made, there is less late enophthalmos and temporal depression,

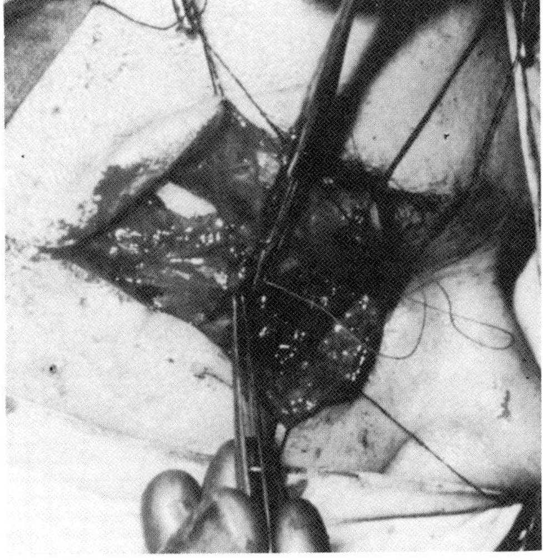

Figure 19. Repair after exenteration surgery by Frezzotti, 1964. The silicone sponge is completely covered by a temporalis muscle flap transposed into the orbital cavity through a bone window.

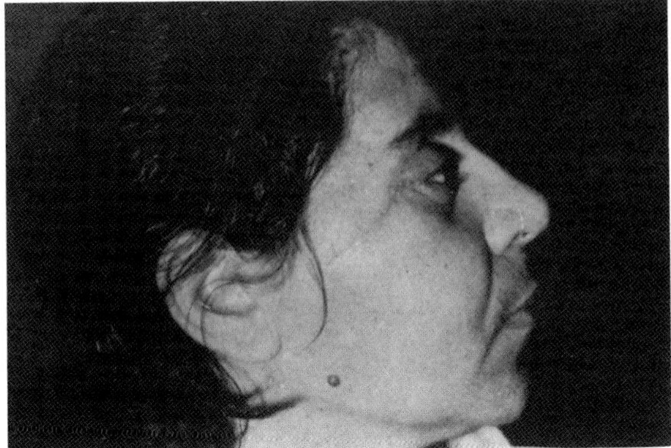

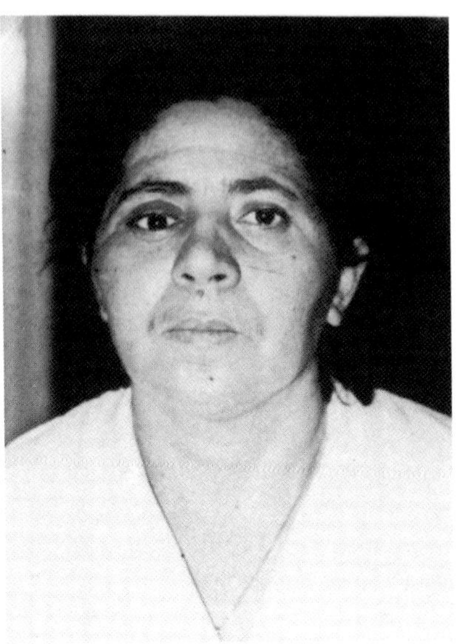

A

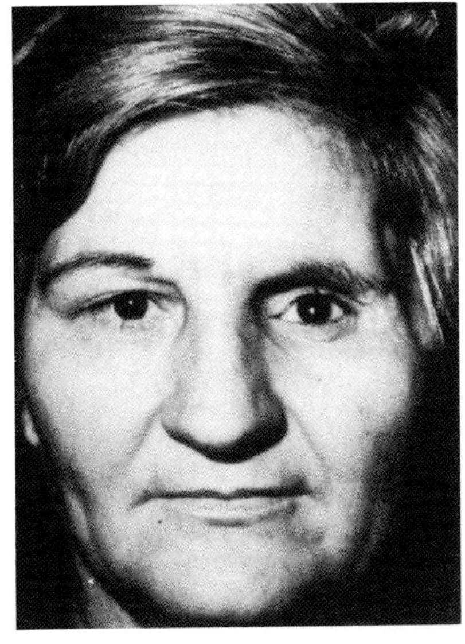

Figure 20. Long-term results of reparative surgery: (A) exenteration for orbital extension of uveal melanoma, two years after surgery. (B) exenteration for orbital extension of uveal melanoma, four years after surgery; slight sinking of the eyelids, not enophthalmos (personal observations, July 1978).

B

and there is better intraorbital support of the prosthesis. The execution is relatively simple, and there is an excellent overall esthetic result (Fig. 20A and B).

Late Reconstruction. Such surgery is generally required for Type IV, V, and VI exenterations for poorly differentiated tumors, and for orbital invasion by contiguity, as well as in exenteration following severe craniofacial trauma. In such cases, cooperation among ear, nose and throat, neurosurgical, and oculoplastic surgeons is essential. In our experience, the need for these operations has diminished. In the decade 1966–75 the ratio of radical to circumscribed exenteration was 4:10, and in the following decade was 3:10.

Using Frezzotti's technique we attempted to reconstruct the orbit as described above. Since 1959, follow-up data are available from nine patients sharing a diagnosis of circumscribed extraocular extension of uveal melanoma. The average age of the patients is 53.8 years (43–70 years). One of them was operated on with the Naquin-Reese technique, two by Frezzotti's original technique, and the remaining six with the modification of that technique [28]. Of the nine patients, four died after seven, five, five, and two years from the date of surgery, all from hepatic metastasis. The remaining five have been followed for two to 14 years, with an average of seven to eight years. The first patient operated on in 1959, then 55-years-old, was alive 14 years later. None of the patients, both the dead and living, demonstrated any local recurrence after an average follow-up of eight years.

In our experience radical exenteration is a necessary procedure which offers the patient a viable solution to a life-threatening problem.

Acknowledgments—We are grateful to Dr. Doris Hadjistilianou and Dr. Jeffrey Schiller for the English version of this chapter. Thank you to Dr. Antonio Leccisotti for drawing Figures 3, 12, and 13.

REFERENCES

1. Ovio G: *Storia dell'oculistica.* Cuneo, Ghibaudo 1950; vol. II:282.
2. Wishart JH: A case of extirpation of the eyeball. *Edinburgh Med and Surg J* 1833; 40:274.
3. Küster: Die Deckung der Augenhoehle nach Ausraehmung derselben. *Zentrlbl f Chir* 1890:25.
4. Busachi: Come si debba coprire la cavita' orbitaria dopo averla svuotata. *La Riforma Medica* 1891; 4:467.
5. Romano Catania A: Un nuovo processo di plastica per la copertura della cavita' orbitaria nella "exenteratio orbitae." *Arch d'Ottalmol* 1904; 1:209.
6. Golovine SS: Procedè' de closture plastique de l'orbite après l'exenteration. *Arch d'Ophthalmol* 1898; 19:679.
7. Lagrange F: Report sur le diagnostic et le traitment des tumeurs de l'orbite. *Soc Franc d'Ophthalmol* Congres de 1903, Paris, Steinheil, 1903.
8. Mustardé JC: *Repair and Reconstruction in the Orbital Region. 2nd ed.* Edinburgh, Livingstone, 1980:239–244.
9. Reese AB: Exenteration of the orbit with transplantation of the temporalis muscle. *Am J Ophthalmol* 1958; 45:386.
10. Reese AB: Exenteration of the orbit and repair by transplantation of the temporalis muscle. *Am J Ophthalmol* 1961; 51:217.
11. Reese AB: *Tumors of the Eye. 2nd ed.* New York, Harper & Row, 1963:570–577.
12. Frezzotti R: The ophthalmologist's approach to orbital surgery. *J Neurosurg Sci* 1982; 26:140.
13. Rollet: Revue gen. de Ophthalmol. 1908.
14. Rougier J, Tessier P, Hervouet F, Woillez M, Lekieffre M, Derome P: Chirurgie plastique orbito-palpebrale. *Soc Franc d'Ophthalmol* Paris, Masson, 1977:33–43.
15. Tessier P, Krastinova D: La transposition du muscle temporal dans l'orbite. *Ann Chir Plast* 1982; 3:213.
16. Berke RN: A modified Kroenlein operation. *Arch Ophthalmol* 1954; 51:609.
17. Tosi P, Frezzotti R, Cintorino M, Sforza V, Nuti A, Polito E, Hadjistilianou T: Quantitative morphological parameters for evaluating the propensity of choroidal melanomas to orbital extension. *Orbit* 1987; 6:139.
18. Wheeler JM: The use of epidermic graft in plastic eye surgery. *Internat Clinics* 1922; 3:292.
19. Iliff CE: The lateral approach for orbital tumors and exenteration. *Trans Am Soc Ophthalmol Otolaryngol* 1966; 70:612.
20. Gass D: Technique of orbital exenteration utilizing methil-metha-crylate implant. *Arch Ophthalmol* 1969; 82:789.
21. Naquin HA: Exenteration of the orbit. *Arch Ophthalmol* 1954; 51:850.
22. Frezzotti R: Trapianto del muscolo temporale nella cavita' orbitaria dopo "exenteratio orbitae." *Boll Oculist* 1959; 38:801.

23. Frezzotti R: Remarks on the exenteration of the orbit with temporalis muscle transplant as a method for the treatment of uveal malignant melanoma. *Ophthalmologica* 1966; 151:819.
24. Frezzotti R, Nuti A: Repair after orbital exenteration: personal technique. *Acta Neurochir* 1982; 60:119.
25. Brihaye J, Hoffmann FR, Francois J, Brihaye M: Les ophthalmie neuro-chirurgicales. *Neurochirurgie* 1968; 14:187.
26. Iliff CE, Ossofsky KJ: *Tumors of the eye and the adnexa in infancy and childhood.* Springfield, IL, Charles Thomas, 1962.
27. Frezzotti R: Chirurgia demolitrice dell'orbita. In: Paletto AE (ed.): *Trattato di Tecnica Chirurgica.* Torino, UTET, vol X, 1984:649–663.
28. Frezzotti R, Bonanni R: *Chirurgia orbitaria e problemi inerenti la ricostruzione delle parti molli dopo exenteratio.* Atti del Simposio di Chirurgia Orbitaria, Bari, 1979.

Dermis-Fat Graft for Orbital Reconstruction after Subtotal Exenteration

John W. Shore, M.D., Randy Burks, M.D., Charles R. Leone, Jr., M.D., and Clinton D. McCord, Jr., M.D.

ABSTRACT

A surgical technique for reconstruction after subtotal orbital exenteration uses an autogenous dermis-fat graft. A musculocutaneous flap is advanced over the graft to provide the anterior vascular supply for the free dermis-fat graft. The periorbita and remaining orbital tissue provide the vascular supply posteriorly. This technique eliminates extensive skin grafting and delayed spontaneous healing. Wound healing is rapid and surgical morbidity is minimized. We have used this procedure in three patients with sebaceous gland adenocarcinoma, two patients with severe posttraumatic contracted sockets, and as a palliative procedure in one patient with a fungating choroidal melanoma and widespread metastasis.

INTRODUCTION

Orbital exenteration is indicated for the treatment of specific ocular or adnexal malignancies, large periorbital tumors when radical craniofacial resection is required, and, occasionally, periorbital fungal infections that require radical but lifesaving treatment [1]. Additionally, exenteration has been proposed as a treatment for orbital deformities associated with neurofibromatosis and for the management of the severely contracted anophthalmic socket when there is little chance for successful reconstructive surgery [2,3]. Our technique of dermis-fat grafting to orbits after subtotal exenteration expedites surgical recovery and minimizes postoperative care.

MATERIAL AND METHODS

The procedure is best performed with the patient under general anesthesia; however, local infiltrative or regional anesthesia may be used if necessary. One hour before surgery, the patient is given 1 g of sodium cephapirin over a 30-minute period to obtain high tissue levels of antibiotics. The patient is placed in a 15° reverse Trendelenberg (head up) position. The

Published previously in *The American Journal of Ophthalmology*, August 1986, Volume 102, pages 228–236. Published with permission from The American Journal of Ophthalmology. Copyright by the Ophthalmic Publishing Company.

The views herein are those of the authors and do not necessarily reflect the view of the U.S. Air Force or the Department of Defense.

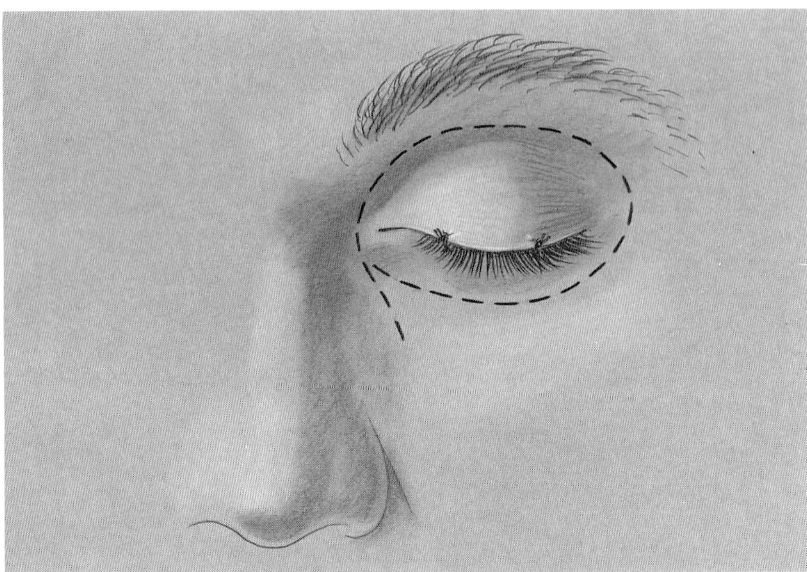

Figure 1. (Shore and associates). The surgical incision should be planned so all involved eyelid and orbital tissue can be excised. A relaxing incision may be outlined in the nasal-jugal fold or out over the zygoma. Actual incisions should not be made until the exenteration has been completed and free surgical margins have been obtained since simple undermining may be sufficient to close the wound.

proposed skin incision is marked with a surgical marking pen (Fig. 1). Sufficient margins should be planned to expedite frozen section evaluation of the surgical margins. The skin and subcutaneous tissue is infiltrated with lidocaine 1% with epinephrine 1:100,000. The donor site for the dermis-fat graft and the entire face are prepared in separate surgical fields.

The subtotal exenteration is performed first. Traction sutures of 4-0 silk are passed through the tendons of the medial and lateral recti muscles. Intermarginal sutures of 4-0 silk are placed, leaving the traction sutures protruding through the palpebral fissure. At the time of skin incision, 4 mg of dexamethasone is administered intravenously to reduce postoperative swelling. The skin incision is made as marked and carried through the orbicularis oculi muscle. The orbital septum is opened and cut free from the arcus marginalis. This dissection begins superiorly and inferiorly and proceeds medially and laterally. The medial and lateral attachments of the canthal tendons are exposed and the cutting unipolar cautery is used to free the tendons from their insertions. A surgical plane is then developed between the orbital fat and the periorbita (Fig. 2). The dissection is bloodless if performed in the proper surgical plane and is easily accomplished with malleable retractors, cotton-tipped applicators, and, if necessary, unipolar cautery. Anterior traction is maintained with the traction sutures to facilitate the dissection.

In the area of the lacrimal sac the dissection proceeds directly next to the periosteum of the medial orbital wall. It is necessary to transect the fundus of the lacrimal sac in most cases. If indicated, the lacrimal sac may be avoided by keeping the dissection more superficial. In this situation, the common canaliculus is transected as it enters the lacrimal sac, avoiding an in-

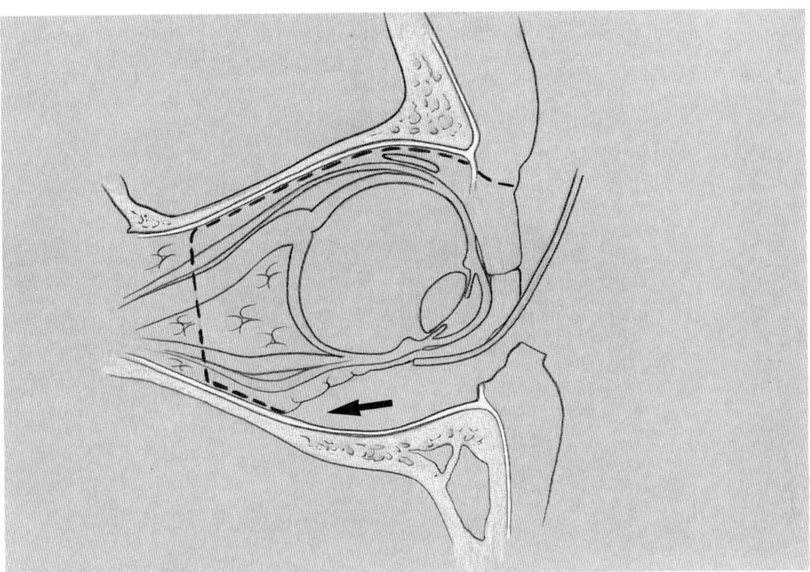

Figure 2. (Shore and associates). Dissection of the orbital tissue proceeds in the plane between the orbital fat and the periorbita. This plane is easily entered at the arcus marginalis and proceeds with minimal bleeding if anterior traction is maintained with malleable retractors and traction sutures (not shown).

cision in the lacrimal sac proper. This is possible because, unlike conventional exenterations, the dissection is not subperiosteal and does not extend to the apex of the orbit.

As the dissection proceeds posteriorly toward the apex of the orbit, the orbital contents prolapse anteriorly. Enucleation scissors are used to cut through the orbital contents posterior to the globe. Some orbital contents remain in the apex of the orbit (Fig. 3). The periorbita and arcus marginalis are left intact. When contracted, anophthalmic sockets are exenterated, all the mucosa must be excised and the orbital implant removed; however, the orbital tissue posteriorly is left in place.

In tumor cases, all surgical margins are sampled for evidence of residual tumor. It is most important to get complete and tumor-free frozen sections on all margins. If the margins are free, reconstruction proceeds; if there is any question of tumor remaining, the wound is left open to heal spontaneously. As a minimum, the margins sampled should include the skin, orbicularis oculi muscle, periorbita, deep orbital tissue, and the lacrimal sac area if there is any question of tumor progressing in that area. Other margins may be sampled as indicated.

Hemostasis is obtained by gently packing the orbit with cellulose sponges and standard surgical packing sponges. Cauterization of deep orbital fat should be avoided. If necessary, bipolar cautery may be used sparingly. Bleeding must be controlled before the dermis-fat graft is placed.

Once tumor-free margins have been obtained and the orbital packing is in place, the dermis-fat graft is harvested from the left lower quadrant of the abdomen just superior to the iliac crest. Grafts of sufficient size cannot be harvested from the buttocks or thigh [4]. We obtain an elliptical graft 4 × 2.5 cm wide with sufficient fat attached to overfill the partially ex-

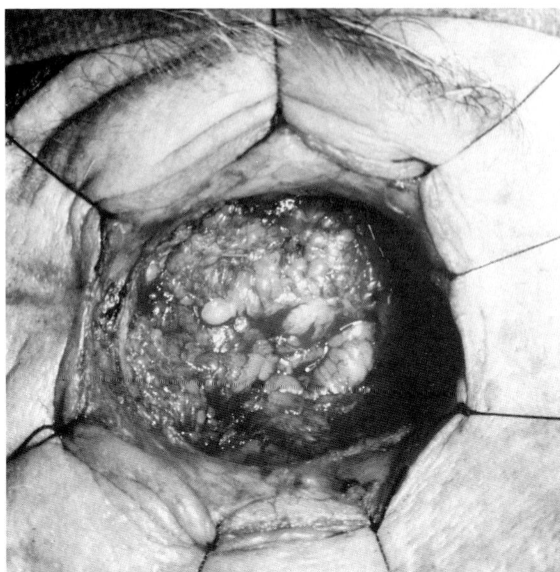

Figure 3. (Shore and associates). Once the subtotal exenteration has been performed, soft tissue remains in the apex of the orbit. All bony surfaces are covered by the periorbita. In tumor cases, all margins must be sampled to assure the tumor has been completely excised.

enterated socket by 20%. The graft must be handled cautiously to prevent excessive trauma. Once harvested, the graft is irrigated with saline and carefully placed in the orbit after the orbital packing is removed. The fat and dermis of the graft are trimmed to fit the surgical defect (Fig. 4). The dermis is sutured to the arcus marginalis with interrupted 5-0 Vicryl (Ethicon,

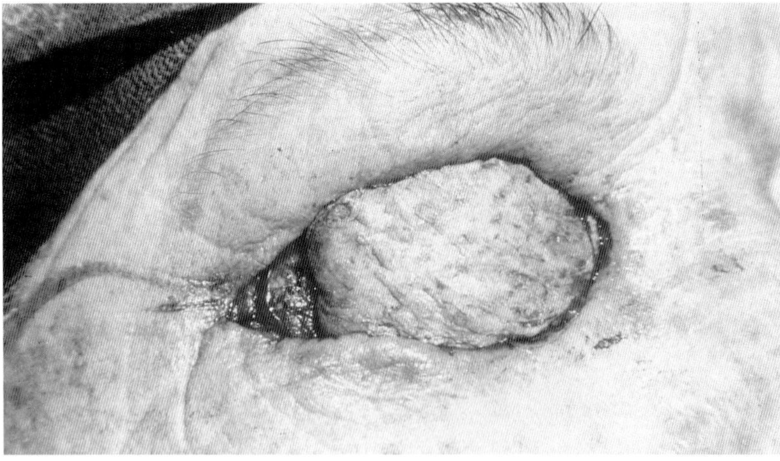

Figure 4. (Shore and associates). The dermis-fat graft is properly shaped and carefully placed in the orbital defect. It should be sized at least 20% larger than the surgical defect to allow for postoperative graft shrinkage and secondary volume loss.

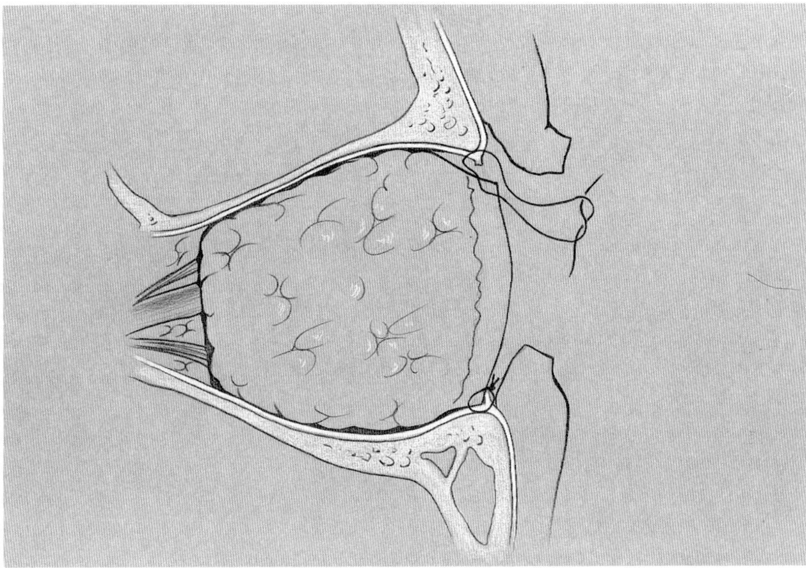

Figure 5. (Shore and associates). The dermis is sutured to the arcus marginalis with interrupted 5-0 Vicryl sutures placed circumferentially around the orbital margin. The deep orbital tissue and fat are not sutured.

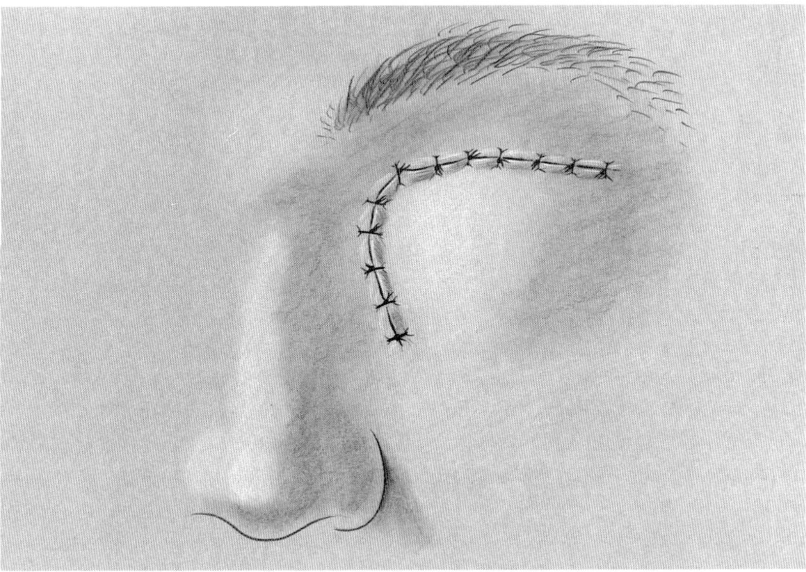

Figure 6. (Shore and associates). A musculocutaneous flap is used to close the defect over the front surface of the graft. Simple undermining of the wound margin may be all that is required. If necessary, a relaxing incision can be made to develop a local advancement or rotational flap to close the wound. A surgical drain may be used (not shown).

Johnson and Johnson) sutures (Fig. 5). Meticulous hemostasis is maintained to prevent hematoma formation under the graft. Once sutured, the dermis portion of the lipodermal implant should protrude 1 cm anterior to the orbital rim.

The remaining skin and orbicularis oculi muscle form musculocutaneous flaps that can be placed anteriorly over the dermis-fat graft (Fig. 6). In elderly patients with redundant skin, the flaps can be developed by undermining and advancing the wound margins. If excessive eyelid skin has been resected to obtain clear surgical margins, or if sufficient skin is not present to close the wound without tension, a rotation or advancement cheek flap such as a Mustarde or Tenzel flap [5] can be mobilized to cover the defect. The musculocutaneous flap should be sutured to the dermal elements of the free graft with interrupted 3-0 Vicryl sutures. In this way, the potential space between the dermis portion of the free graft and the undersurface of the musculocutaneous flap is obliterated. A small penrose drain may be placed subcutaneously and brought out through the wound laterally to reduce the chance of hematoma formation. If used, the drain is removed on the first or second postoperative day. A soft compressive dressing is applied and left in place for five to seven days.

The patient remains in a head-up position for three days. The graft donor site is managed in a standard fashion. Patients undergoing exenteration for cancer should have a baseline orbital computed tomographic scan within three months of surgery and periodically thereafter to search for evidence of recurrent disease.

CASE REPORTS

CASE 1

A 59-year-old woman had a three-year history of unilateral blepharoconjunctivitis unresponsive to all modes of medical therapy. A full-thickness left upper eyelid biopsy performed by her referring ophthalmologist had confirmed his clinical diagnosis of sebaceous adenocarcinoma. The patient was referred to Wilford Hall USAF Medical Center for definitive treatment.

Her visual acuity was 20/20 in the right eye and 20/25 in the left eye. Positive findings were limited to the left orbit. There was extensive erythema and thickening of the margin of the left upper eyelid. The meibomian gland orifices were inspissated and the cilia were distorted and reduced in number. A notch was present centrally in the left upper eyelid in the area of previous biopsy. The conjunctiva over the tarsus was thickened and there was a diffuse papillary conjunctival reaction. The bulbar conjunctiva was erythematous but smooth, without evidence of diffuse thickening or a local nodular reaction. The superior fornix was shortened. A corneal pannus extended circumferentially from the corneoscleral limbus centrally and encroached upon the visual axis. A computed tomographic scan failed to disclose evidence of orbital involvement. There was no regional lymphadenopathy and a metastatic evaluation was negative. Further biopsies showed carcinomatous involvement of the bulbar conjunctiva and superior fornix.

The patient underwent subtotal exenteration. Multiple superficial cutaneous and deep orbital frozen-section biopsy specimens demonstrated clear surgical margins. The periorbita was preserved. An elliptical dermis-fat graft was used to fill the partially exenterated socket. A significant amount of eyelid skin had been sacrificed and therefore a musculocutaneous advancement flap was used to cover the graft. The wound healed in ten days and orbital swelling had subsided within three weeks (Fig. 7A, B, and C).

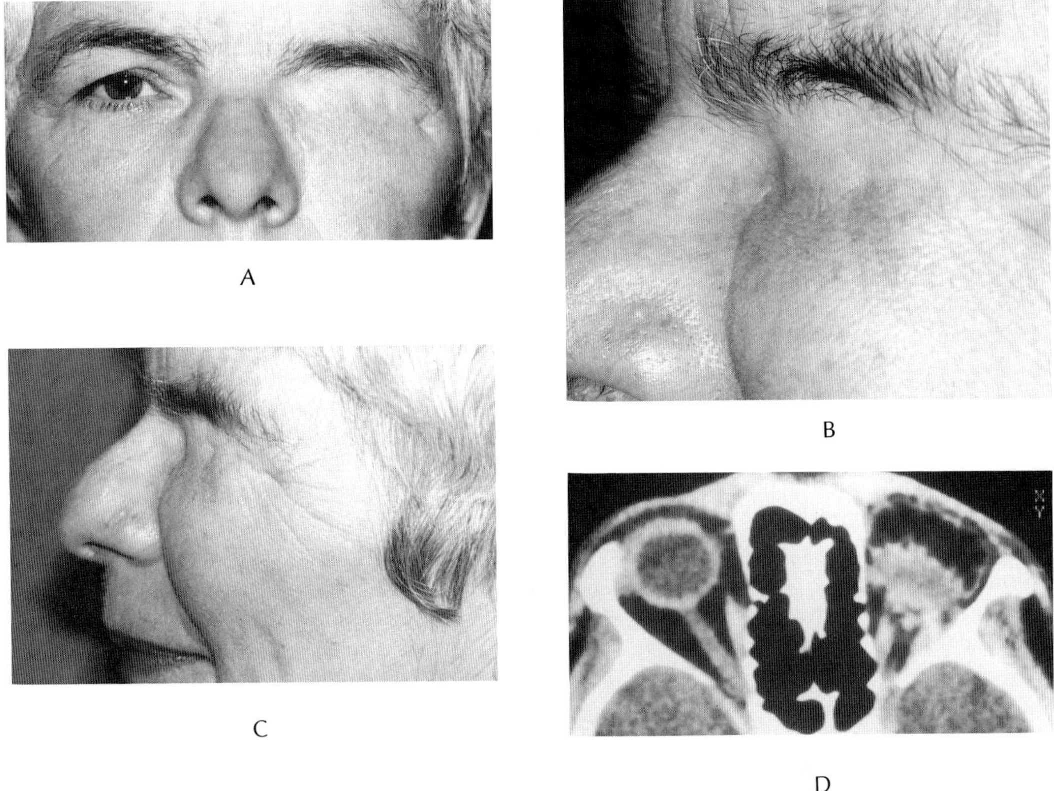

Figure 7. (Shore and associates). Case 1. (A, B, and C) The postoperative appearance of a 59-year-old woman 18 months after subtotal orbital exenteration of the left orbit for sebaceous adenocarcinoma of the left upper eyelid. (D) A computed tomographic scan obtained 29 months after surgery shows no evidence of recurrent tumor. The graft, host-graft interface, and posterior orbital structures are easily identified.

A baseline computed tomographic scan obtained six weeks postoperatively clearly demonstrated the implanted dermal-fat graft, the residual orbital contents, including the extraocular muscles and proximal portion of the optic nerve, and the graft-host interface. Clinically there has been no significant volume loss during three years of follow-up. This was confirmed on a recent computed tomographic scan 29 months following surgery (Fig. 7D). The patient has no problems with socket hygiene and is comfortable appearing in public without a patch.

CASE 2

A 53-year-old man was struck on the left side of the head by a motorboat propeller while water-skiing. There was extensive damage to the facial soft tissue and a corneal-scleral laceration with partial loss of the ocular contents. The upper and lower eyelids on the left side were partially avulsed. The patient underwent extensive facial plastic and ophthalmologic reconstructive surgery over an 18-month period but eventually developed a phthisical left eye and was referred to the Oculoplastic Surgery Service at Wilford Hall USAF Medical Center for enucleation.

Examination showed a phthisical left globe with a dense cyclitic membrane, total retinal detachment, and no light perception. The left upper eyelid was completely blepharoptotic and without measurable levator palpebrae superioris muscle function (Fig. 8A and B). The lateral half of the inferior fornix was absent. There was extensive scarring of the lateral canthus that extended superiorly and inferiorly into the lateral portions of the left upper and left lower eyelids. This cicatrix had resulted in long-standing lymphedema of the left upper eyelid. The upper and lower lacrimal puncta were scarred and the canaliculi were not patent. There was no evidence of sympathetic ophthalmia.

Enucleation followed by a prolonged course of eyelid and socket reconstruction was discussed with the patient; however, the patient was not interested in wearing an ocular prosthesis and stated on several occasions that he only wanted to be free of orbital pain and to return to work as quickly as possible.

The patient underwent subtotal exenteration followed by primary dermis-fat graft reconstruction. The skin was closed so as to accentuate the scar in the palpebral fissure. This was accomplished by partially inverting the skin edges during wound closure and by suturing the skin edges to the dermis portion of the graft. This enhanced the horizontal scar in the midorbital region, simulating a "closed eyelid" appearance (Fig. 8C). A small hematoma formed despite the use of a penrose drain but resolved in seven days and did not require surgical drainage.

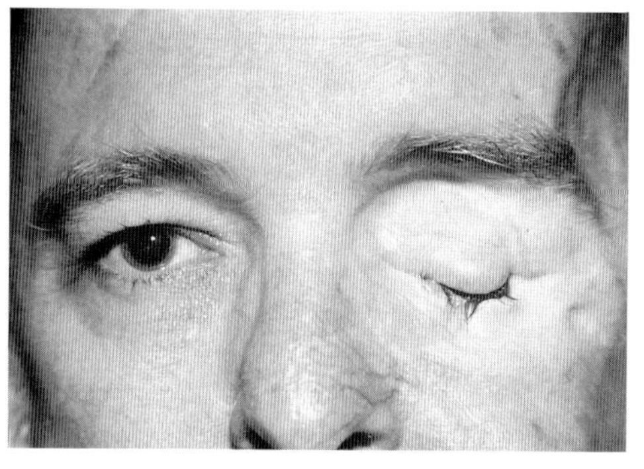

A

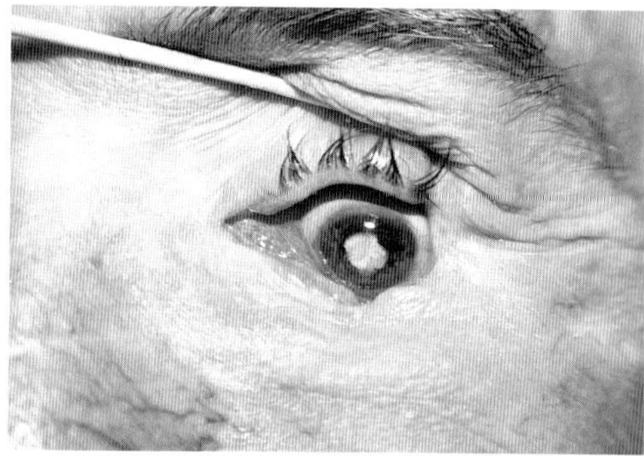

B

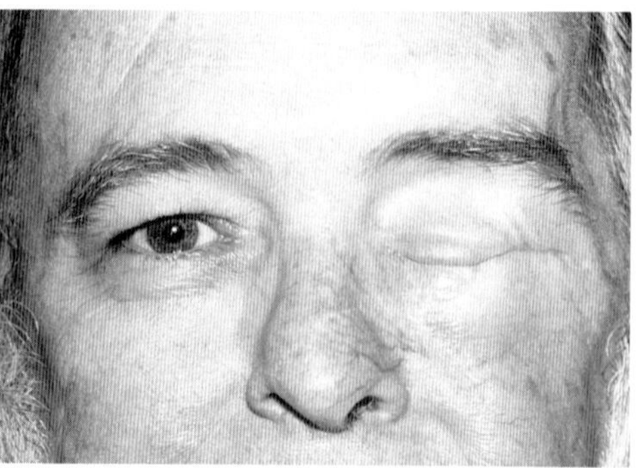

C

Figure 8. (Shore and associates). Case 2. (A) A 53-year-old man with chronic left upper eyelid edema, and complete blepharoptosis, and eyelash ptosis eight years after severe ocular and adnexal trauma. (B) A phthisical left eye and severely deformed lower eyelid and lateral canthus make socket reconstruction difficult. (C) Twelve weeks after subtotal exenteration and dermis-fat graft reconstruction, the orbit is well healed and the patient is comfortable and pleased with the cosmetic result.

Six months postoperatively a small amount of lymphedema was still present in the area of the previous left upper eyelid. The patient is now pain-free and has no socket discharge. Further surgery is not anticipated.

RESULTS

We have used the dermis-fat graft to reconstruct six orbits over a five-year period (Table 1). This includes three patients with sebaceous adenocarcinoma of the eyelid requiring subtotal exenteration. There is no evidence of tumor recurrence in any case after follow-ups ranging from 12 to 32 months. The cosmetic results in two cases were excellent. In the third case, the socket developed a sunken appearance postoperatively. The initial result was excellent but within four months excessive volume loss was evident in the superior aspect of the orbit (Fig. 9). We believe this complication was the result of inadequate volume replacement during the initial procedure. Further volume loss has not occurred. The other five patients who underwent this procedure received larger grafts and did not develop this complication.

One patient with a severely contracted and inoperable anophthalmic socket had chronic socket discharge and underwent excision of the deformed eyelids and socket mucosa. An anterior orbital exenteration was performed. The periorbita, apical orbital contents, and remaining eyelid tissue were used for reconstruction. A large dermis-fat graft was placed with excellent results. Another patient with severe ocular and adnexal deformities after trauma (Case 2) also achieved a satisfactory cosmetic and functional result. Both patients returned to full employment within three weeks of surgery with no postoperative socket care other than to remove the sutures. Neither patient has required further reconstructive surgery.

Another patient underwent resection of a fungating choroidal melanoma with orbital extension. The posterior orbit was uninvolved. The patient had widespread metastasis and a short life expectancy. A palliative subtotal exenteration of the involved orbital tissue was performed followed by immediate dermis-fat graft reconstruction. The wound healed uneventfully and the patient returned home to live the remainder of her life free of the crusting, bleeding, and unsightly tumor.

Wound healing has been rapid and without complication in all cases to date. Generally, patients have returned to work within two or three weeks following surgery. One patient (Case 2) developed a hematoma between the dermis and the overlying musculocutaneous flap. The hematoma resolved without surgical intervention. We recommend placement of a surgical drain to reduce the chance of hematoma or seroma formation. The drain should be removed as soon as possible after surgery to reduce the chance of wound infection. A light compressive dressing allows for good tissue apposition and further reduces the chance of hematoma formation. We give our patients perioperative antibiotics, especially if a surgical drain is used.

We have not had a wound infection to date but this complication should be expected in a larger series of cases.

DISCUSSION

When exenteration is performed, wound healing may be delayed for eight to 14 weeks if the exenterated socket is allowed to heal spontaneously [1,6]. Wound healing will be more rapid if the orbital cavity is skin-grafted but exenteration with skin graft requires cleaning of the desquamated epithelium; this is not the case with wounds allowed to granulate. If the or-

Table 1. Summary of Clinical Data

Patient no. Sex, Age (yrs)	Diagnosis	Follow-up	Eyelids preserved	Closure	Complications	Status
1, F, 59	Sebaceous adenocarcinoma, left upper eyelid	29 mos	No	Flap*	None	Disease-free; wears spectacles
2, M, 53	Phthisis bulbi, left eye, with severe posttraumatic eyelid and adnexal deformities	24 mos	Yes	Direct	Hematoma	Comfortable; wears spectacles
3, F, 73	Sebaceous adenocarcinoma, right upper eyelid	32 mos	No	Direct	None	Disease-free; wears spectacles
4, F, 74	Sebaceous adenocarcinoma, left lower eyelid and medial canthus	12 mos	No	Direct	Inadequate volume replacement	Disease-free; wears spectacles
5, M, 28	Severely contracted anophthalmic right socket with 80% ankyloblepharon	14 mos	No	Flap*	None	Comfortable; wears eyepatch†
6, F, 74	Fungating choroidal malignant melanoma with metastasis, right eye	10 days	Yes	Direct	None	Unknown‡

*Musculocutaneous rotation-advancement flap.
†The patient had extensive posttraumatic facial scarring. He wears a beard and continues to cover the orbit with a patch to mask the facial deformities.
‡The patient had widespread hepatic and bone metastasis. She never returned after suture removal on the tenth postoperative day. At that time the wound was well healed and the patient was comfortable.

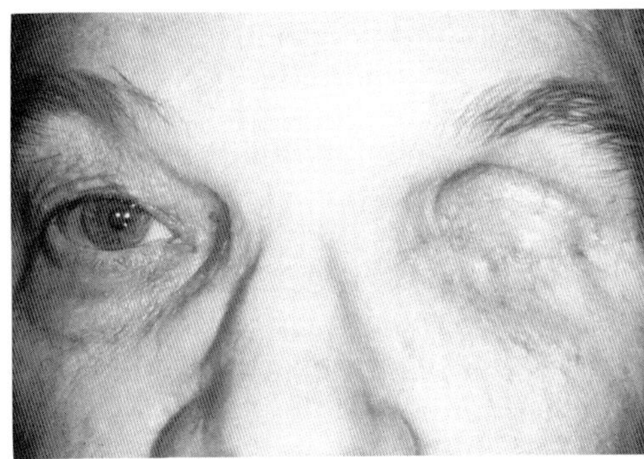

Figure 9. (Shore and associates). Case 4. Hollow appearance in a 74-year-old woman 12 weeks after exenteration and dermis-fat graft reconstruction for sebaceous adenocarcinoma of the left medial canthus. An undersized graft was used for reconstruction. Subsequent graft shrinkage led to the volume undercorrection evident here. The wound is well healed.

bital walls are penetrated at the time of surgery, chronic, nonhealing sino-orbital or nasal-orbital fistulas may form. Such fistulas can be bothersome to patients because of malodorous discharge, crusting, constant wound breakdown, difficulty in blowing the nose, and speech disturbances.

Prosthetic devices that cover large facial deformities are available and lately there has been an improvement in the appearance, comfort, and wearability of exenteration prostheses [7]. Nevertheless, these prosthetic devices require daily cleaning, constant care, are adynamic, and, in our experience, are poorly accepted by some patients.

Although total exenteration may be required to manage certain diseases, the less radical procedure of subtotal orbital exenteration may be possible in properly selected cases [8]. It is most important to get frozen sections of all margins. If they are free, the reconstruction proceeds; if there is any question of tumor remaining, the wound is left open to heal spontaneously. Since 1978 there has been a resurgence of interest in and the use of dermis-fat graft implants for reconstruction of anophthalmic sockets [4,9–15]. Our experience in anophthalmic patients [15] led us to use the procedure for reconstruction after subtotal orbital exenteration.

Patients with inoperable socket contracture and patients with severe ocular and adnexal deformities after trauma are good candidates for this procedure. We use subtotal exenteration rather than complete exenteration in these cases and have found the procedure to be particularly helpful when the deformities are so great that there is little chance for cosmetic or functional improvement even with multiple surgical procedures staged over a period of years. In such cases, excellent results can be achieved by using a dermis-fat graft to reconstruct the partially exenterated orbit. We do not advocate socket exenteration when conventional socket reconstructive surgery is indicated.

Dermis-fat graft reconstruction is useful in cases in which a palliative subtotal exenteration must be performed to achieve local control of a tumor. Wound healing is rapid and postoperative morbidity is minimized. The patient is able to return to normal life more quickly than if total exenteration had been performed.

Other indications for the procedure include eyelid malignancy requiring subtotal exenteration. To be safe in such cases, it is essential that the tumor be restricted to the anterior orbit, that wide surgical margins are attainable, and that all margins are shown to be free of tumor by meticulous frozen-section sampling [16]. Once the tumor has been totally excised, the remaining orbital tissue and a free dermis-fat graft can be used for orbital reconstruction.

Volume loss can be a problem any time a free dermis-fat graft is used for head and neck reconstruction. Reports of volume loss after dermis-fat grafting in anophthalmic sockets range from none to 75% [4,9–11,13–15] of the donor graft size. We experienced excessive volume undercorrection in one patient in whom a graft that was too small was placed. To compensate for expected graft atrophy, we recommend the graft be at least 20% larger than the surgical defect. Also, trauma to the free graft must be minimized during surgery. Guberina and associates [14] emphasized the need to handle the graft expeditiously and with great care. Hemostasis must be achieved but the use of cautery should be minimized. Hemostasis is best achieved with surgical packing sponges which must be removed before the graft is placed in the recipient bed. We have not experienced any donor site wound complications; however, this complication has been reported previously [15].

Hair growth and epidermization of dermis-fat grafts placed in anophthalmic sockets has been reported [11,15]. Because the graft is taken from a relatively hairless area, the lower left abdomen, there is usually little chance for hair growth and discharge. Nevertheless, care must be taken to insure all epithelial elements are removed as the graft is harvested. Otherwise there is a potential for pilosebaceous growth in the buried implant. We have not experienced this complication in any patient to date.

The advantages of subtotal exenteration followed by dermis-fat graft reconstruction are rapid wound healing, enhanced cosmesis, comfort, and freedom from chronic socket problems such as fistula formation, skin desquamation, and continuous wound breakdown. We advocate its use in carefully selected patients in whom subtotal exenteration is performed.

UPDATE

As with any new surgical procedure, time and follow-up allow critical evaluation of long term results. Since publishing this article in 1985, I have operated on an additional six patients. All have achieved excellent results. Complications and volume loss have not occurred. The patients have remained tumor and pain free. Some patients elect to wear a patch, others cover the defect with tinted glasses, and a few leave the surgical site uncovered. Two patients have been fit with a maxillofacial prosthesis without difficulty. Most patients have not been fit because there is no purchase for the prosthesis to rest on. This must be discussed with the patient preoperatively because some patients desire a prosthesis and do not like the smooth appearance of the partially exenterated socket. I usually show patients pictures of both options and ask them to decide how they wish to proceed.

The dermis-fat graft is an excellent technique for reconstruction following subtotal orbital exenteration. Patients must be prepared for the postoperative result and advised of all reconstructive options.

REFERENCES

1. Lindberg JV, Orcutt JC, and Van Dyk HJL: Orbital surgery. In: Duane TJ (ed): *Clinical Ophthalmology*. Hagerstown PA, Harper and Row, 1985: 5:38–43.
2. Small RG, and Lafuente H: Exenteration of the orbit in selected cases of severe orbital contracture. *Ophthalmology* 1983; 90:236.

3. Jackson IT, Laws ER, Jr, and Martin RD: The surgical management of orbital neurofibromatosis. *Plast Reconstr Surg* 1983; 71:751.

4. Smith B, Bosniak SL, and Lisman RD: An autogenous kinetic dermis-fat orbital implant. An updated technique. *Ophthalmology* 1982; 89:1067.

5. McCord CD, Jr, and Nunery WR: Reconstruction of the lower eyelid and outer canthus. In McCord CD, Jr. (ed.): *Oculoplastic Surgery*. New York, Raven Press, 1981:192–201.

6. Putterman AM: Orbital exenteration with spontaneous granulation. *Arch Ophthalmol* 1986; 104:139.

7. Eaton LD, Dryden RM, Popp JC, and Harner D: Functional anatomical reconstruction in an oculofacial prosthesis. *Ophthalmology* 1984; 91:984.

8. Grove AS, Jr: Surgery of the orbit. In Spaeth GL (ed.): *Ophthalmic Surgery. Principles and Practice*. Philadelphia, PA, WB Saunders, 1982:541–544.

9. Smith B, and Petrelli R: Dermis-fat graft as a movable implant within the muscle cone. *Am J Ophthalmol* 1978; 85:62.

10. Smith B, Bosniak SL, Nesi F, and Lisman R: Dermis-fat orbital implantation. 118 cases. *Ophthalmic Surg* 1983; 14:941.

11. Aguilar GL, Shannon GM, and Flanagan JC: Experience with dermis-fat grafting. An analysis of early postoperative complications and methods of prevention. *Ophthalmic Surg* 1982; 13:204.

12. Bullock JD, and Brickman KR: Dermis-fat graft in socket reconstruction. Theoretical and experimental considerations. *Ophthalmology* 1984; 91:204.

13. Nunery WR, and Hetzler KJ: Dermal-fat graft as a primary enucleation technique. *Ophthalmology* 1985; 92:1256.

14. Guberina C, Hornblass A, Meltzer MA, Soarez V, and Smith B: Autogenous dermis-fat orbital implantation. *Arch Ophthalmol* 1983; 101:1586.

15. Shore JW, McCord CD, Jr., Bergin DJ, Dittmar SJ, Maiorca JP, and Burks WR: Management of complications following dermis-fat grafting for anophthalmic socket reconstruction. *Ophthalmology* 1985; 92:1342.

16. Condon GP, Brownstein S, and Codere F: Sebaceous carcinoma of the eyelid masquerading as superior limbic keratoconjunctivitis. *Arch Ophthalmol* 1985; 103:1525.

Orbital Exenteration with Spontaneous Granulation

Allen M. Putterman, M.D.

ABSTRACT

Excision of the orbital contents by orbital exenteration is required in the treatment of some eyelid and orbital carcinomas. Allowing the orbit to heal spontaneously with granulation tissue has several advantages over the popular technique of lining the orbital walls with a split-thickness skin graft. The use of granulation tissue is simpler, since it avoids the need for obtaining a skin graft, and the final result is cosmetically more acceptable, because a shallower cavity occurs compared with the skin graft technique. The main disadvantages are that it takes longer for the orbit to heal and dressing changes are required more frequently. The spontaneous granulation technique has provided excellent results in 12 patients with exenterated orbits.

INTRODUCTION

Orbital exenteration with removal of the eyelids, eye, and orbital contents is necessary at times to treat orbital and eyelid carcinomas [1,2]. Many surgeons reconstruct the exenterated orbit by lining it with a split-thickness skin graft [3]. An alternative technique is to allow the orbit to heal spontaneously without a skin graft [4,5]. It is the purpose of this report to convey the results of spontaneous granulation of the exenterated orbit in 12 patients.

SURGICAL TECHNIQUE

An incision is made with a No. 15 knife blade (Bard-Parker, Rutherford, N.J.), a hot knife, or a cutting cautery through skin, orbicularis muscle, and periosteum for several millimeters peripheral to the orbital rim over 360° of the orbital entrance (Fig. 1A). Bleeding is controlled with electric (Bovie) cautery.

The sharp end of a Tenzel (St. Louis, MO) periosteal elevator is used to dissect periosteum from the orbital rim (Fig. 1B). The blunt end of the same elevator is then used to dissect periosteum from the four walls of the orbit (Fig. 1C). (Care is taken to avoid undue pressure on the medial wall and floor of the orbit because the orbital bones in these areas are thin.)

A large, curved scissors then amputates the posterior portion of the orbital tissues (Fig. 1D). (At times, the posterior one-third of the orbital contents can be spared; at other times, it is

Published previously in *Archives of Ophthalmology*, January 1986, Volume 104, pages 139–140. Copyright 1986, American Medical Association. Reprinted by permission.

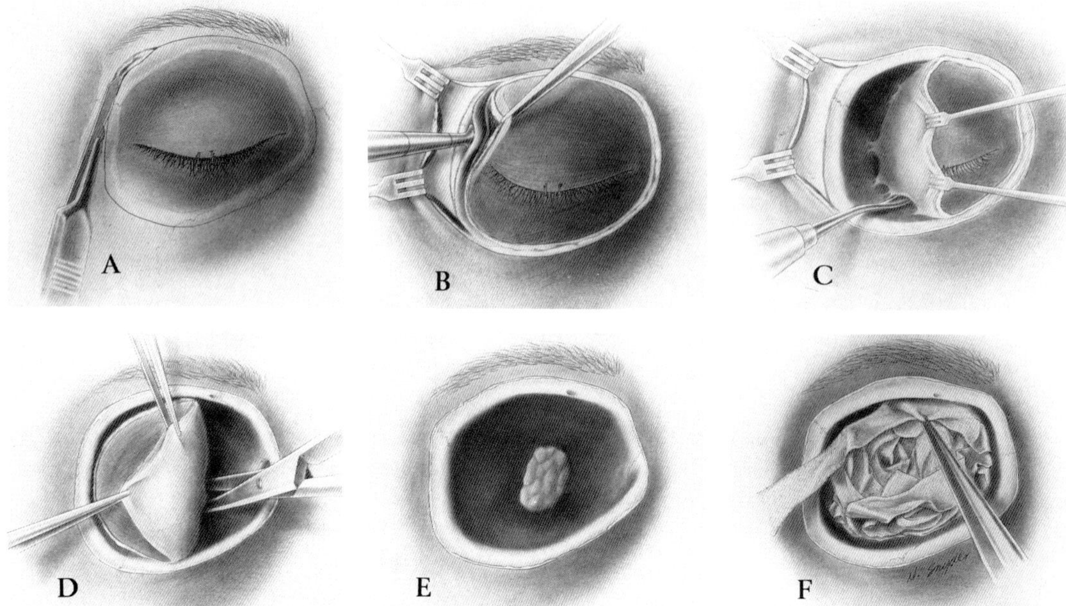

Figure 1. (A) Skin, orbicularis muscle, and periosteum are severed for 360° peripheral to orbital entrance. (B) Sharp edge of Tenzel periosteal elevator dissects periosteum from orbital rim. (C) Blunt edge of Tenzel periosteal elevator dissects periosteum from orbital wall. (D) Scissors is used to sever optic nerve and apical orbital tissues. (E) Variable amount of orbital tissue may remain at orbital apex following exenteration. (F) Orbit is packed with petrolatum gauze.

necessary to sever the tissues exactly at the apex (Fig. 1E), depending on the depth of invasion of tumor.) Bleeding, is controlled with electric (Bovie, Largo, Florida) cautery, pressure, and gauze saturated with a 1:100,000 solution of epinephrine injection.

Strips of petrolatum gauze, 2.5 × 150 cm, are lubricated with bacitracin or gentamicin sulfate ointment. The strips are used to line and pack the orbital cavity until the gauze is slightly above the anterior surface of the orbital entrance (Fig. 1F). (Four to eight strips are usually necessary.) A pressure dressing of 10 × 10-cm gauze fluffs and flexible (Micropore, St. Paul, MN) tape is then applied. The patient is placed on a regimen of ampicillin trihydrate, 250 mg four times a day, and is usually discharged from the hospital one to two days postoperatively.

The external dressing of a 10 × 10-cm gauze pad or eye pad is changed daily, and topical gentamicin or bacitracin ointment is applied to the external surface of the petrolatum gauze dressings. On the third or fourth postoperative day, the gauze is completely removed from the orbit and is replaced with additional petrolatum gauze strips saturated with antibiotic ointment. The orbit is packed slightly looser than at surgery, and fewer strips are necessary. These dressings are changed twice a week for the first two weeks postoperatively and then weekly for one to two months thereafter. (The dressings can be changed by the surgeon, the patient's family, or a visiting nurse.) During this time the orbit will gradually fill with granulation tissue and fewer strips will be necessary to pack the orbit.

Usually two to three months postoperatively, the orbit will heal sufficiently for the patient to be fit with a prosthesis. (Some patients are content to wear an eye pad or black patch.)

COMMENT

Lining the orbital walls with a split-thickness skin graft after orbital exenteration is advocated by many surgeons [3]. This procedure leads to rapid healing of the exenteration site and avoids the necessity for frequent dressing changes. It requires the surgeon to be skilled in the technique of obtaining a split-thickness skin graft, however; it also frequently leads to a deep, wide, and disfiguring orbital cavity.

Allowing the orbital cavity to heal with granulation tissue is a relatively simple technique and avoids the need to obtain and apply a split-thickness skin graft. It leads to a shallower orbital cavity, as the orbit fills with granulation tissue, which is cosmetically more acceptable. Also, many ocularists find the shallow orbital cavity easier to fit with a prosthesis (W. Cox, BCO, R. Scott, BCO, oral communication, 3 September 1985). The main disadvantages of the granulation technique over the skin graft procedure are that healing takes longer and dressing changes are required more frequently. Also, the eyebrow is sometimes drawn downward.

The described technique of orbital exenteration with granulation healing has been used in 12 patients, with healing completed in eight to 14 weeks postoperatively (Fig. 2A–D). Patients have been followed up for four to 30 months after surgery. No postoperative infections or other complications have been noted. Patient acceptance of the healed orbit has been good.

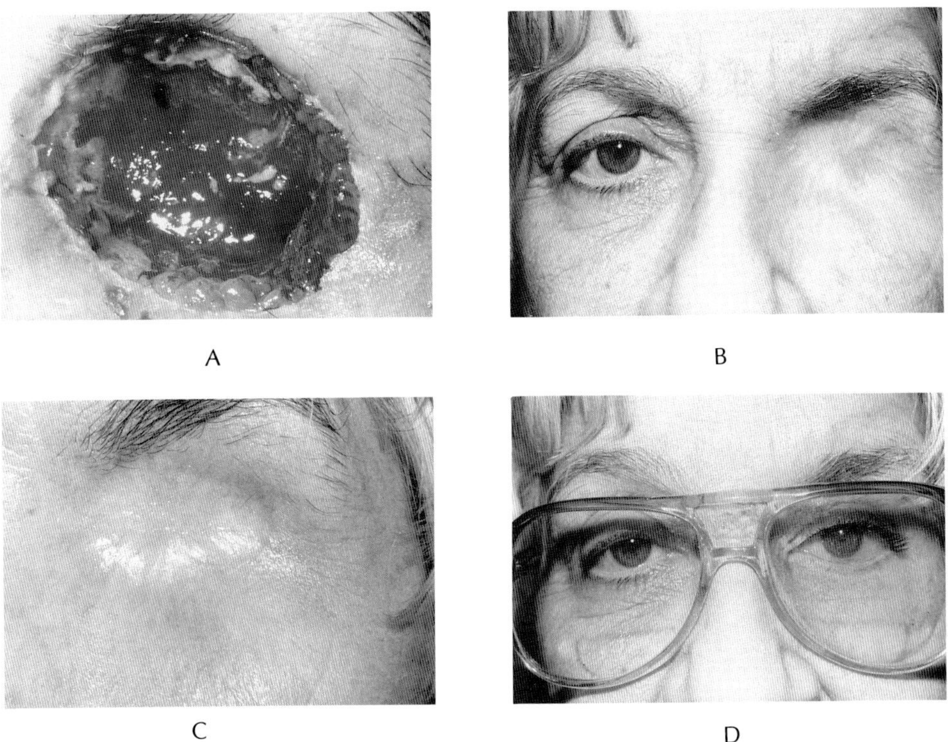

A

B

C

D

Figure 2. (A) Orbit one week after exenteration for sebceous gland adenocarcinoma with spontaneous granulation. (B and C) Same eye shown at top left, three months postoperatively. (D) Patient wears orbital prosthesis to camouflage exenteration site.

Acknowledgments— This investigation was supported in part by core grant EY 1792 from the National Eye Institute, Bethesda, Md.
    I thank Nancy Snyder for the illustrations.

REFERENCES

1. Kennedy RE: Indications and surgical techniques for orbital exenteration. *Ophthalmology* 1979;96:867–873.
2. Schlernitzaver DA, Font RL: Sebaceous gland carcinoma of the eyelid. *Arch Ophthalmol* 1976;94:1523–1525.
3. Quickert MH: Exenteration in problems and treatment of contracted sockets, exenterated orbits and alkali burns. In Guibor P, Gougelmann H (eds): *Problems and Treatment of Enucleation, Evisceration, and Exposure.* New York, Grune & Stratton Intercontinental Medical Book Corp, 1973:119–126.
4. Silva D: A typical orbital exenteration. In Guibor P, Gougelmann H (eds): *Techniques of Anophthalmic Cosmesis.* New York, Grune & Stratton Intercontinental Medical Book Corp, 1976:89–96.
5. Tenzel R, in discussion, Anderson RL, Blodi FC, Boniuk M, Callahan A, Guibor B, Jakobiec, F, Stassion O, Tenzel R, Wilkins R. and Wobig J (eds): *Symposium on Diseases and Surgery of the Lids, Lacrimal Apparatus, and Orbit: Transactions of the New Orleans Academy of Ophthalmology.* St. Louis, MO, CV Mosby Co. 1982:459.

Orbital Exenteration with Spontaneous Granulation: Editorial Comment

Stephen L. Bosniak, M.D.

In January, 1986, Allen Putterman described a technique of orbital exenteration with spontaneous granulation in the *Archives of Ophthalmology*. It provided excellent cosmetic results without skin grafting, but it took much longer to heal.

Spontaneous granulation following orbital exenteration can yield results that are quite satisfying. However the patient and the surgeon must be prepared for the gaping, raw orbital socket, which may not be completely healed for years.

The following case illustrates the postoperative course when using this technique.

A 66-year-old male with basal cell carcinoma that eroded the left side of his face and his left eye (Fig. 1) underwent wide resection and exenteration (Figs. 2 and 3) in November 1986.

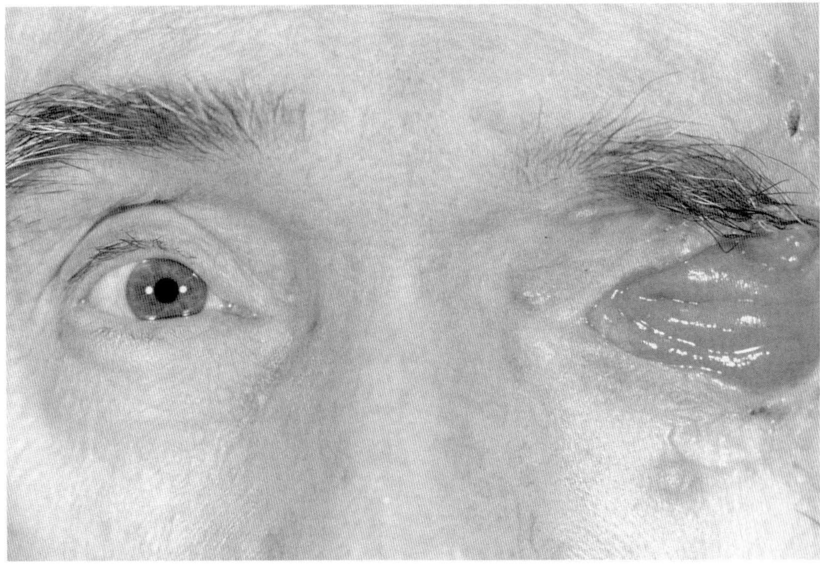

Figure 1. A 66-year-old man with a basal cell carcinoma that infiltrated the left side of his face and his left eye.

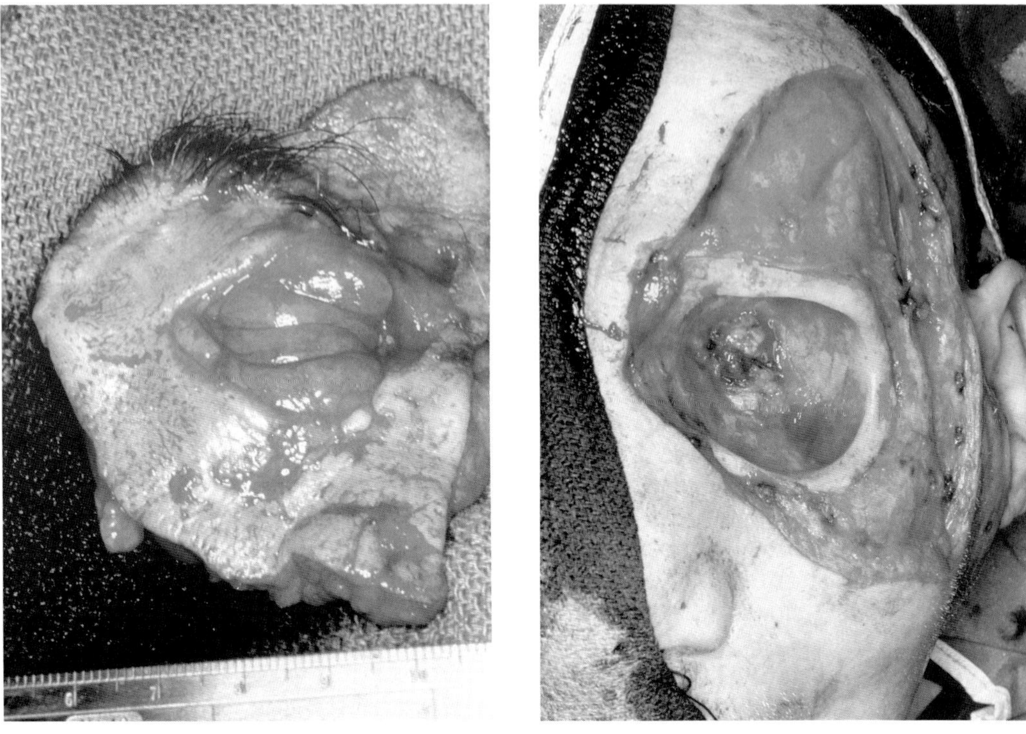

Figures 2 and 3. Wide resection of the tumor and an exenteration were performed.

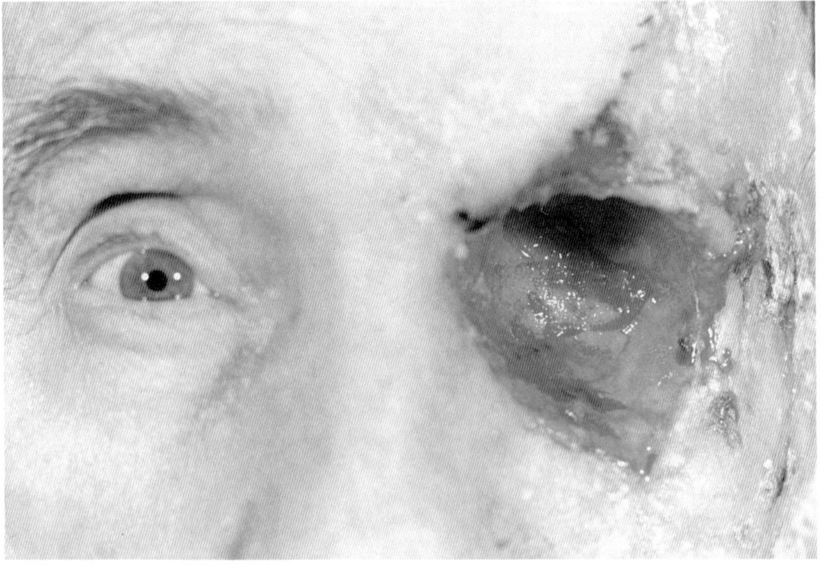

Figure 4. Granulation tissue filled the socket within three months of the initial surgery.

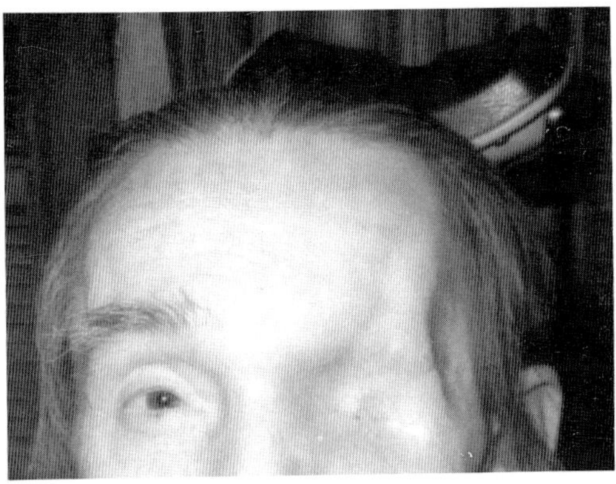

Figures 5 and 6. By the ninth postoperative month only a small epithelial defect persisted in the socket.

His postoperative course proceeded smoothly and granulation tissue began to fill in the socket by the end of January 1987 (Fig. 4). Epithelialization of the granulation tissue bed followed. By mid-June only a small epithelial defect of the socket persisted (Figs. 5 and 6). However, the socket was not completely healed until February 1988 (Fig. 7).

The patient was quite pleased with the ultimate result of his surgery, but refused to be fitted for a prosthetic device, and continues to wear his black patch.

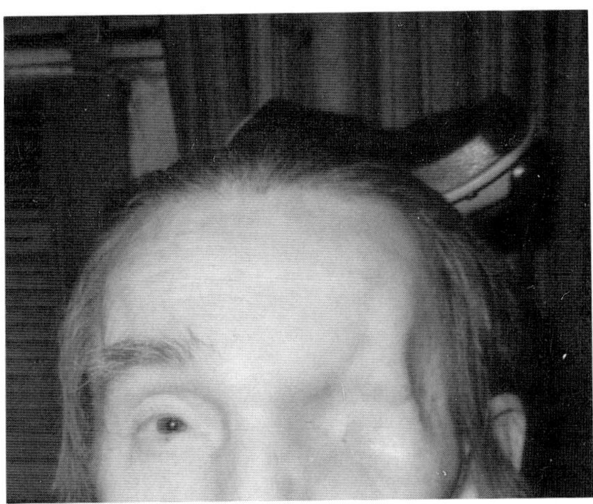

Figure 7. Complete epithelialization did not occur until the 15th postoperative month.

Operation for Retention of an Artificial Eye after Exenteration of the Orbit

Isadore Goldstein, M.D.

It was Bartisch [1] who introduced the medieval and Arlt [2] the modern method of exenteration of the orbit. To overcome this dreadful deformity, Axenfeld [3] suggested the operation in which the conjunctiva, lids and hair lines are preserved. Later the conjunctiva and lids are

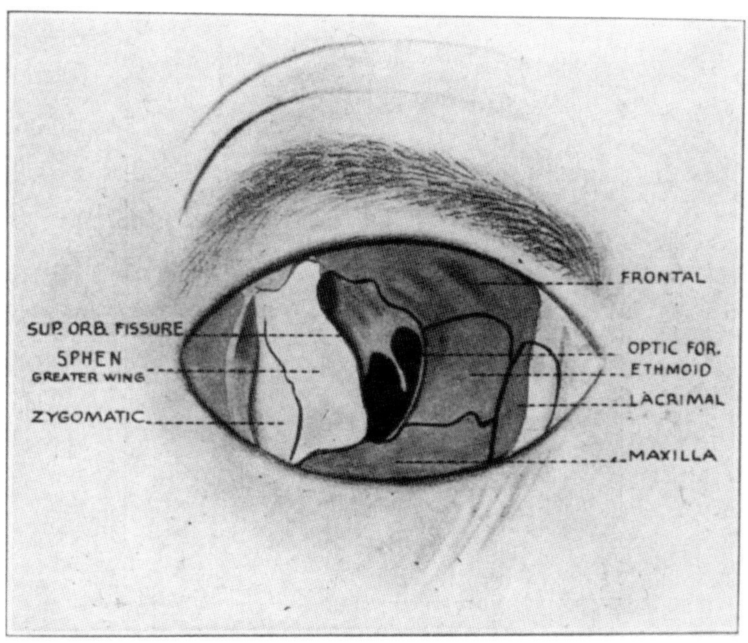

Figure 1. Appearance of the orbital cavity after exenteration.

This article was read before the Section on Ophthalmology of the New York Academy of Medicine on Dec. 16, 1935.

I. GOLDSTEIN

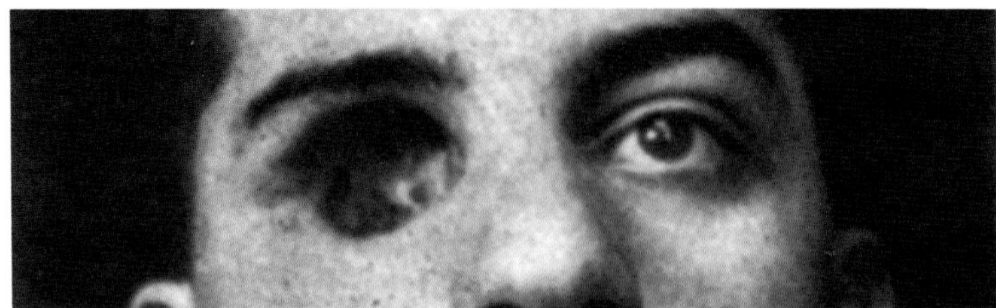

Figure 2. Aspect of the orbital cavity after exenteration when covered with a Thiersch graft.

sutured. Other surgeons, Küster [4], Busache [5], Rollet [6], G. Worms [7], and Romano-Catania [8], used mucous membrane grafts, skin flaps, Thiersch grafts, and sliding skin flaps to obviate the deformity without the introduction of a prosthesis. Few surgeons, however, have attempted to correct this deformity so that an artificial eye could be worn. Pólya [9] conceived the idea of introducing artificial bone into the orbital cavity and suturing the lids over it. In this manner a support is obtained for a prosthesis. Probably the best known procedure is the operation devised by Golovine [10] in which a temporal pedicle flap is taken, passed through a vertical opening at the outer canthus, carried into the orbit and sutured in place to the surrounding structures.

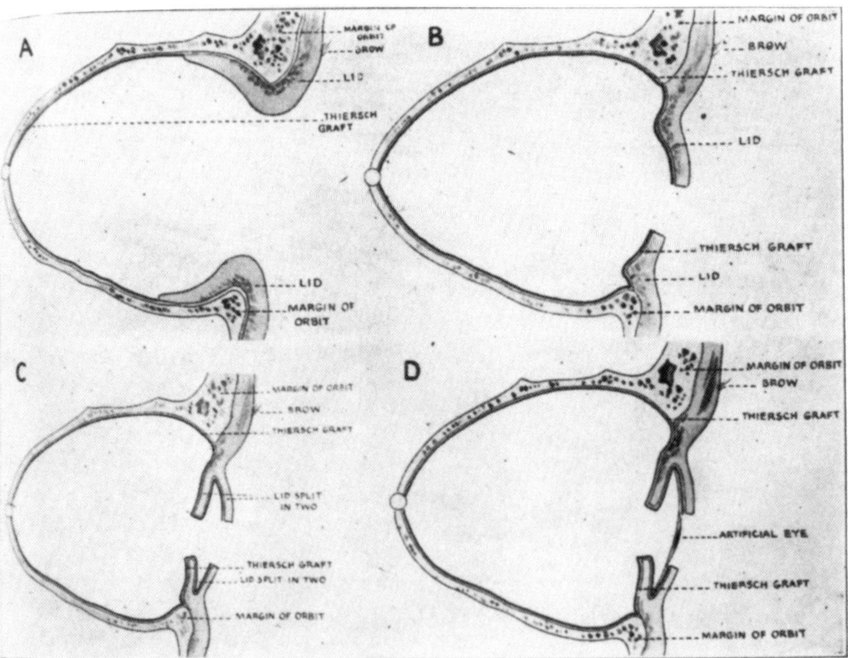

Figure 3. Sagittal sections of the orbit: (A) The orbit lined with a Thiersch graft and the lids adherent to the bone; (B) the orbit and the back of the lids covered by Thiersch grafts; (C) Thiersch grafts covering the orbit, the posterior surface of the lids and the sulcus formed by splitting the lids; (D) the Thiersch-lined sulcus formed by splitting the lids retaining the artificial eye.

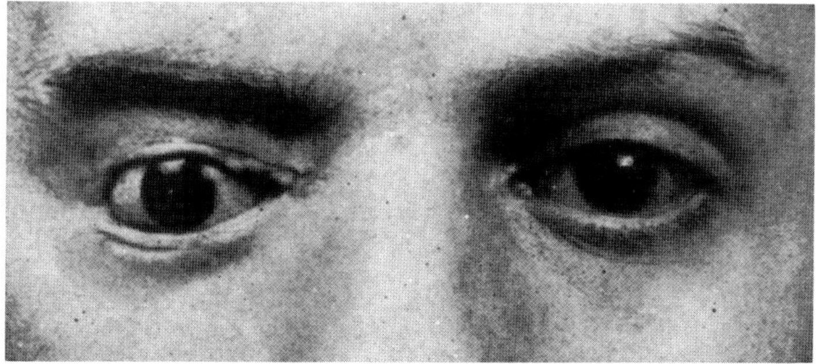

Figure 4. Patient wearing the artificial eye.

I employed the following technique after exenteration of the orbit for a spindle cell sarcoma: The bony cavity (Fig. 1) was previously lined by Thiersch grafts (Fig. 2), and the remaining portions of the lids were placed within the orbit, where they became adherent to the bone. Six weeks later the adherent lids (Fig. 3A) were freed. This was readily done. Thiersch grafts were placed (Fig. 3B) on the denuded areas on the bone and on the back of the lids. The grafts were held in place by gauze packings. In this manner the upper and lower lids were partially restored. Three weeks later the lids were divided on their margins from the inner to the outer canthus, and the dissection was carried almost to the margins of the orbit. The horizontal division of the lids for their entire length gave the effect of four lids, two upper and two lower ones (Fig. 3C). Into the sulcus formed by separating the upper lid into two parts was placed a thin mold of Kerr's dental modeling compound. The mold was 1 mm in thickness, 15 mm in its vertical diameter and 50 mm in its transverse diameter. The mold was covered by a Thiersch graft placed in the sulcus and kept in position by temporary sutures holding the two parts of the divided lid together. A similar mold covered by a Thiersch graft and placed in the sulcus of the divided lower lid was held in place by suturing the split lid. By placing a packing in the orbit and on the lids immobilization was obtained.

The plastic procedures described permit the formation of accessory lids which act as a diaphragm and in turn give support to the artificial eye (Fig. 3D). The hair lines were reconstructed following the method of Wheeler [11]. Destruction of the lashes is not advisable; they should be retained if this is feasible (Fig. 4).

REFERENCES

1. Bartisch G: *Ophthalmodouleia*, Dresden, M. Stökel, 1583:208.
2. Arlt: Operationslehre. In von Graefe, A, and Saemisch, ET; Handbuch der Gesamten Augenheilkunde, ed. 1, Leipzig, Wilhelm Engelmann, 1874:111:434.
3. Axenfeld: Ueber plastischen Verschluss der Orbita, Verhandl. d. Gesellsch. *Deutsch. Naturf. u. Aerzte* 1904; 2:301.
4. Küster: Die Deckung der Augenhöhle nach Ausräumung derselben, *Centralbl. f. Chir.* 1890; 17:25.
5. Busache: Come si debba coprire la cavità orbitaria dopo averla suturata, *Riforma med* 1894; 4:467.
6. Rollet: Occlusion de l'orbite et suppression des paupières, *Rev gén d'opht* 1908; (July) 27:289.
7. Worms, G: Bull. Soc. d'opht. de Paris, Jun 1932, p. 358.
8. Romano-Catania, A: Un nuovo processo di plastica per la copertura della cavità orbitaria nella exenteration orbitae, *Arch di ottal* 1893; 1: 209.
9. Pólya, SJ: Szemeszet, no. 4, 1904; abstr., Michel's Jahresb., 1904, p. 367.
10. Golovine: Procédé de clôture plastique de l'orbite après l'exentération, *Arch d'opht* 1898; (Nov.) 18:679.
11. Wheeler: Restoration of the margin and neighboring portion of the eyelid by free graft from lower part of eyebrow and skin directly below it. *JAMA* 1920; (Oct. 16) 75:1055.

Exenteration of the Orbit and Repair by Transplantation of the Temporalis Muscle

Algernon B. Reese, M.D. and Ira S. Jones, M.D.

INTRODUCTION

In a previous paper one of us (A.B.R.) reported a technique for repair of the exenterated orbit by utilization of the temporalis muscle (Fig. 1) [1]. Since that time the technique has proved its worth, and has now been used in a total of 20 cases.

The operation gives a cosmetic result much more acceptable to the patient than the previously practiced simple exenteration with a split-skin graft. Furthermore, after we have thought tumor recurrence unlikely, we have been able to reconstruct the socket for a prosthesis in two cases. An additional advantage has been that no postoperative dressings are necessary after a week to 10 days.

More experience with the operation has led to some improvements in technique and likewise in our results. The present technique employed follows.

TECHNIQUE OF TEMPORALIS MUSCLE TRANSPLANT

The upper and lower lids are halved by an incision with a scalpel through the gray line from one end of the lid to the other (Fig. 2). At the extremities of the lids this incision may be completed with scissors. This halving of the lids leaves, anteriorly, the cilia and skin, and, posteriorly, the tarsus, orbicularis, conjunctiva, palpebral muscle, and fascial planes. This division of the upper and lower lids is carried out to the orbital margin above and below.

A skin incision is made from the external canthus horizontally for from two to three centimeters (Fig. 3). The dissection of this skin is continuous with that of the skin of the upper and lower lids and is carried out above and below to expose the entire region over the temporalis muscle. When these upper and lower flaps, including the skin of the upper and lower lids and the skin of the temporal region, are now reflected, the entire orbital cavity is exposed together with a wide area in the temporal region.

The next step is to incise the periosteum around the entire orbital circumference and to perform an exenteration, including the periosteum (Fig. 4).

Next, an incision is made in the deep fascia along the origin of the temporalis muscle. The deep fascia with its underlying temporalis muscle is reflected from the temporal fossa (Fig. 5). The fascia is incised from the upper margin of the zygomatic process where it is adherent (Fig. 6).

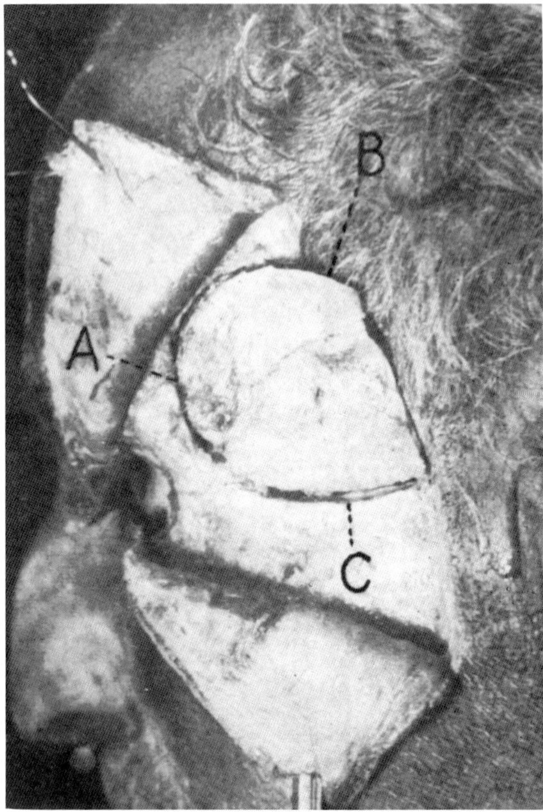

Figure 1. Cadaver dissection to show area of temporalis to be transplanted. The skin flaps have been reflected in the fascial plane overlying the temporalis muscle and the portion of the muscle to be utilized is outlined. (A) Beginning of the muscle dissection. (B) Extension of incision around thin edge of muscle. (C) Separation of thick fascia from zygoma.

The muscle is dissected down under the zygomatic process to its insertion into the coronoid process of the mandible. The muscle and fascia are freed until they are sufficiently mobile to reach the orbit easily.

With the Stryker saw, a round opening is made in the lateral wall of the orbit. This is enlarged with ronguers, particularly below, but the anterior orbital margin is left (Fig. 7). A 20-mm gold sphere is placed in the apex of the orbit (Fig. 8). When the opening in the lateral wall of the orbit has been made sufficiently large, the temporalis muscle and its fascia are passed through the opening into the orbit and sutured to the remaining periosteum in such a way that the muscle and fascia are fanned out to fill uniformly as much of the orbit as possible. The lid margins are approximated with two double-arm catgut sutures. A pressure dressing is applied (Fig. 9).

The differences in the technique just described and in that used earlier are as follows: The orbital periosteum is not preserved. This was originally used for a suture anchor, but the cut edges of periosteum at the orbital rims are sufficient. About two-thirds of the temporalis mus-

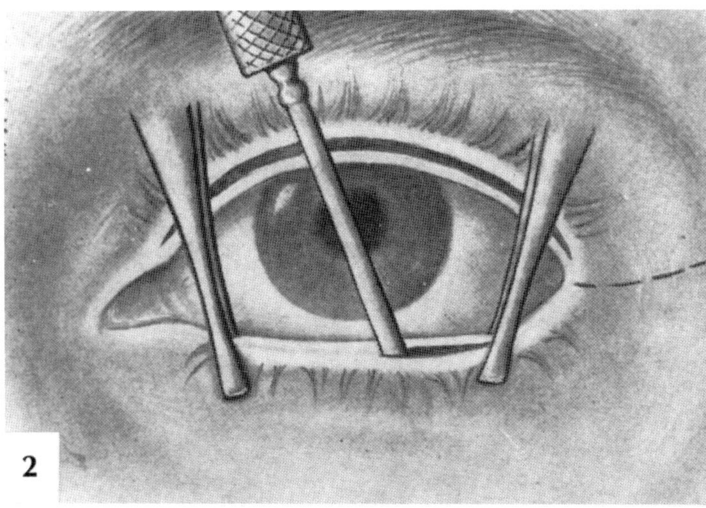

Figure 2. Modified exenteration procedure which is used when temporalis muscle transplantation is to be done. The upper and lower lids have been halved, leaving, anteriorly, the cilia and skin, and, posteriorly, the tarsus, orbicularis, conjunctiva, palpebral muscle, and fascial planes.

cle was formerly used to obtain enough tissue to fill the orbital defect. The present technique utilizes about half of the muscle. Part of the difference is in the use of a larger gold sphere, but most of the difference is due to obtaining more of the heavy muscle fascia from its attachment to the zygoma and to a freer mobilization of the muscle.

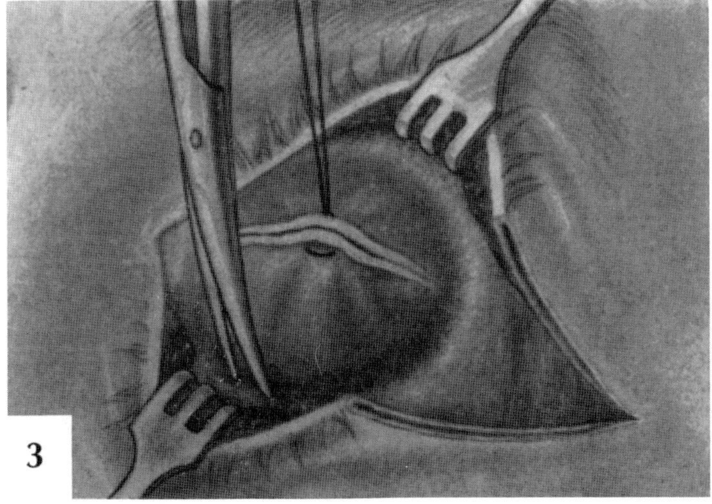

Figure 3. The margins of the posterior half of the lid have been sutured together by a double-arm suture in the interest of easier manipulation when the exenteration is done. A horizontal incision extending from the external canthus temporally exposes the lateral bony wall and the temporal fossa.

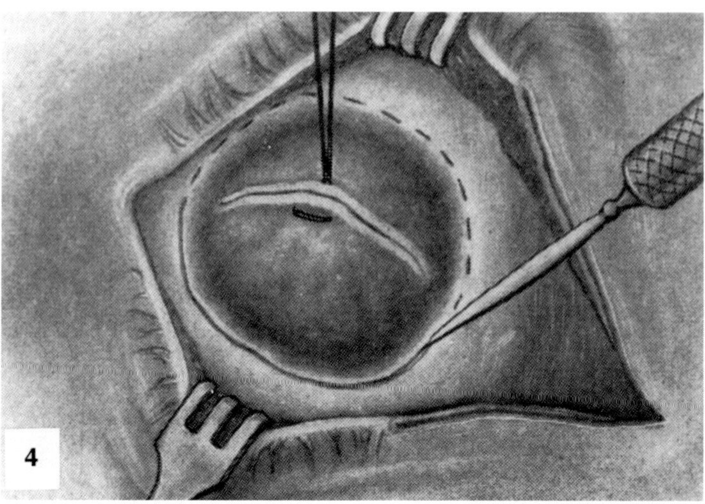

Figure 4. The periosteum is divided at the orbital rim and the contents are mobilized.

TECHNIQUE OF SOCKET RESTORATION

When sufficient time has elapsed after exenteration of the orbit so that a recurrence seems unlikely, then the socket may be restored. This has been done on two of the patients in the present report. The technique is as follows:

A knife cut is made between the two rows of cilia to a depth of 2 mm. The length of the incision and the placement of the lateral and medial ends are determined with the palpebral

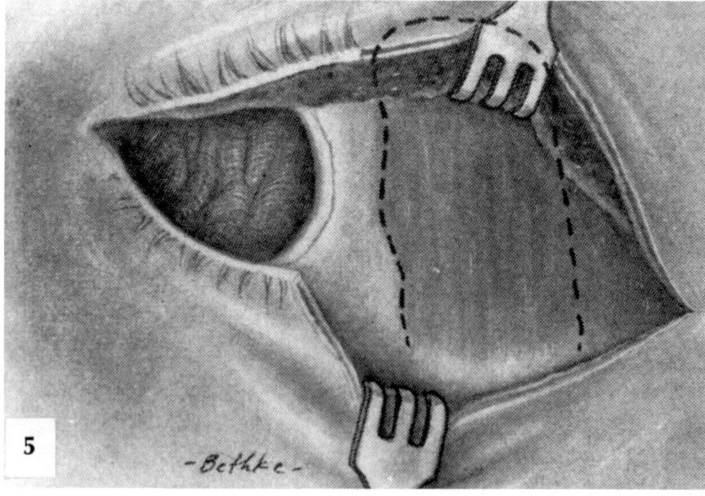

Figure 5. The position of temporalis muscle to be used as a graft is outlined.

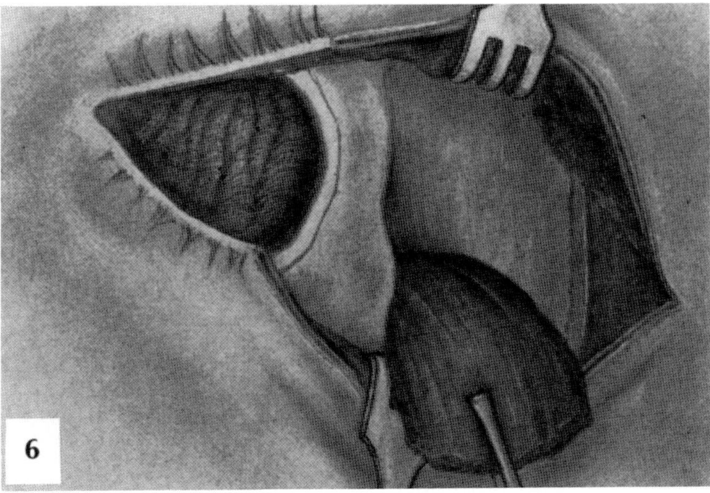

Figure 6. After exenteration of the orbit, the anterior half of the temporalis muscle is mobilized from its fossa and cut free from the zygoma.

fissure of the fellow eye in view so that a good match is obtained. At the 2-mm depth of the incision the surface of the underlying graft fascia is found and the lids can be separated from it by sharp and blunt dissection. This is carried above and below to the orbital rim. Two large plastic conformers are sutured back to back. A split-thickness skin graft measuring about 5.0 by 8.0 cm is taken from the abdomen with the Paget dermatome. This is placed around the previously prepared conformers with the cut surface out. The edges of the skin graft should

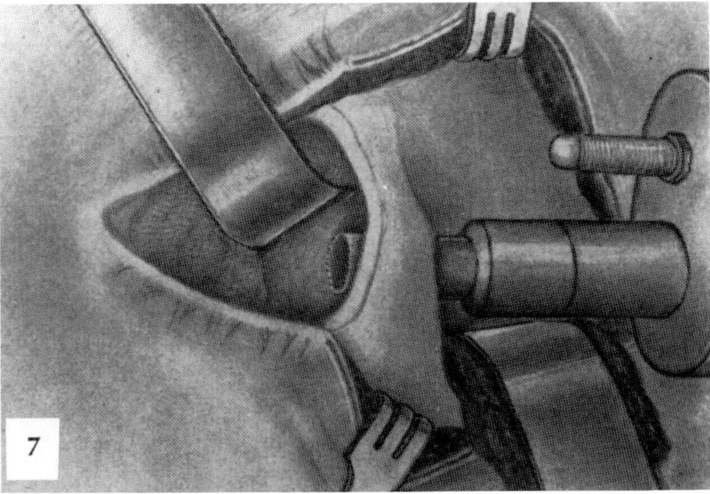

Figure 7. Lateral wall of the orbit is perforated by a trephine or a straight saw. The opening is then enlarged.

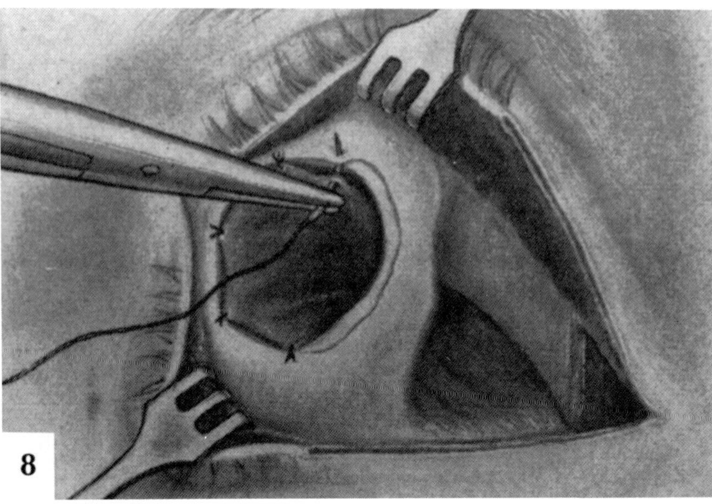

Figure 8. The temporalis muscle and deep fascia are passed through the hole in the lateral wall and sutured to the cut edges of periosteum. A gold or plastic sphere lies behind the muscles.

come together on the front surface of the plastic form. This is then placed under the lids and the upper and lower lid edges are drawn firmly toward each other. This is to push the skin graft as deeply into the fornices as possible. Excess protruding skin may be trimmed off. The conformers are removed in five to seven days, and a prosthesis can be fitted when all devitalized skin has been excised.

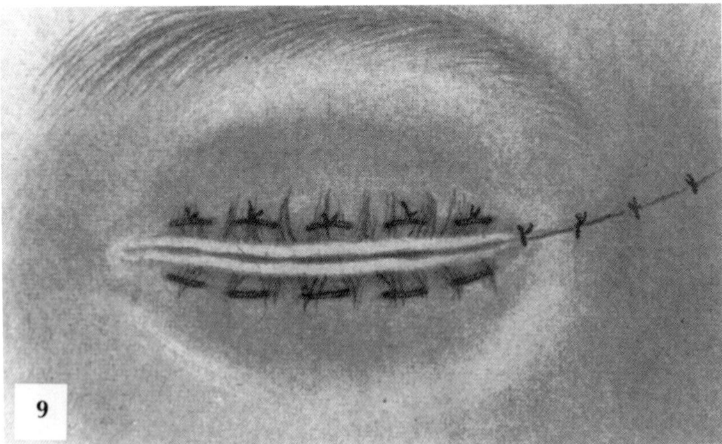

Figure 9. The remaining anterior leaf of each lid is sutured with the borders everted and the skin of the temple is repaired.

TECHNIQUE OF EXENTERATION WITH RETENTION OF THE CONJUNCTIVA

If the condition for which the exenteration is being done does not involve conjunctiva, then the technique can be modified. This has been done on one patient. The technique varies in the following manner. Instead of the lids being split in the gray line, the entire thickness of each lid is preserved. The conjunctiva is divided at the limbus and reflected to the fornices. The knife cuts to the orbital rim are then made under the conjunctiva and the exenteration proceeds in the usual manner. After the temporalis graft has been sutured in place, the conjunctival opening is closed as it would be after an enucleation. A conformer should be used and a prosthesis can be fitted in two weeks.

PRESENTATION OF CASES

Patient J. C., a white girl, aged 7 years, who was presented in the previous paper [1], was first seen nine days after the referring doctor had removed an orbital mass from the upper part of the left orbit through a conjunctival approach. Sections of the mass revealed a rhabdomyosarcoma so that prompt exenteration with temporalis muscle graft was carried out. Follow-up examination revealed a satisfactory cosmetic result with no sinking in the temporal fossa and an adequate number of cilia in the upper lid. It is now one year postoperatively and the patient will have a socket restoration at a future date. A photograph taken 12 months after surgery is shown (Fig. 10).

Patient S. A., a 50-year-old white man, was first seen because of slight redness of the right eye for one year, double vision for four months, and swelling of three months' duration. Studies including thyroid tests, X-ray films of skull and orbit, hands, and chest were carried out with negative results. The patient was discharged with a diagnosis of exophthalmos due to a pseudotumor or nonspecific granuloma. Fifteen months later the patient was again seen, with sight in his right eye reduced to hand movements at two feet. There was marked vascularity with atrophy of the optic nerve. A Krönlein procedure disclosed a large tumor mass below. This mass was excised and the pathology report was a carcinoma, primary site unknown. Subsequently, an exenteration with a temporalis muscle graft was performed. One year postop-

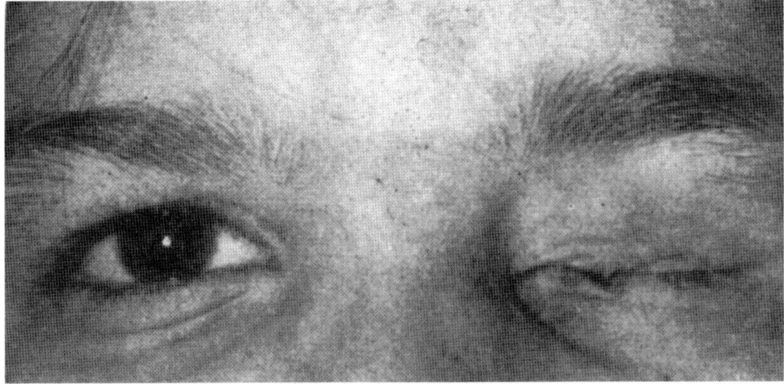

Figure 10. Patient J. C. was shown in previous paper [1]. The present photograph was taken one year after surgery.

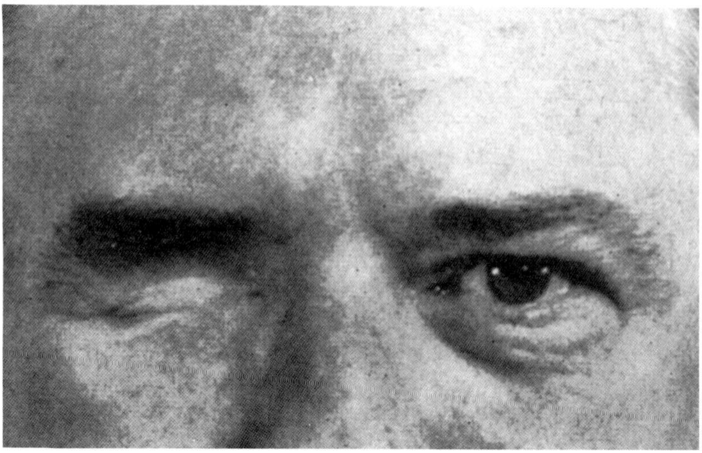

Figure 11. Patient S. A. Front view taken one year after surgery.

eratively no evidence of disease was found. One and one-half years after surgery there was no evidence of disease and the cosmetic result was good. Restoration with prosthesis is to be considered later. Photographs taken 12 months after exenteration are shown (Figs. 11 and 12).

Patient B. L., a woman, aged 47 years, noted a red spot on the conjunctiva of the left eye for 35 years. One year previously it became pigmented and was excised. There was recurrence of the pigmentation and the lesion was again excised. After one month ptosis was noted. The patient was found to have a 3-mm limbal pigmentation at the 3-o'clock position, ptosis of the left upper lid, and a pedunculated pigmented lesion of the conjunctiva of the left upper lid, 3 to 5 mm in size, at the upper tarsal border. Excision of these lesions was carried out. Microscopic examination showed malignant melanoma of the conjunctiva. Accordingly, an exenteration combined with a temporalis muscle implant was performed. On follow-up two months after the exenteration procedure, a fluctuant abscess in the left upper lid was incised

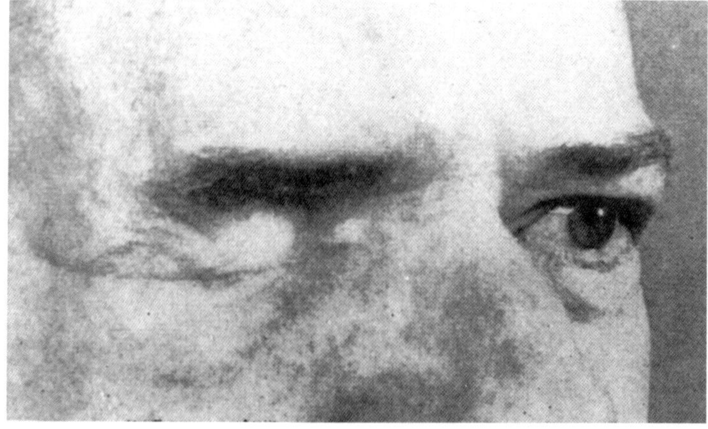

Figure 12. Patient S. A. Photograph taken one year after surgery.

and drained. Three weeks later the abscess was again incised and curetted. Three months post-operatively a biopsy of the left orbit was done. Along with the biopsy specimen taken at all levels, the edges of the sinus tract on the left were also removed for mircoscopic study and a border-to-border closure of the opening was carried out. The specimens were granulation tissue. Seven months after the exenteration, there was no evidence of disease. The cosmetic result was good with the exception of slight depression in the temporal region. One year post-operatively, there was marked sinking in the temporal fossa with a lump palpated through the lower lid at the orbital margin. One month after this nodule was palpated, a study of biopsy tissue from the lesion revealed recurrence of tumor. The cytology of this tissue showed a high degree of malignancy with many mitotic figures. Since that time, examination at monthly intervals has revealed marked sinking in the temporal region with a progressively downhill course. Four months after last biopsy, there was evidence of pulmonary metastases. A photograph taken three weeks after operation is shown (Fig. 13).

Patient R. H., a white woman, aged 53 years, had a pigmented conjunctival lesion on the right which had been excised four times over the previous six years. At the last excision a diagnosis of malignant change in a pigmented nevus was made. The orbit was exenterated and the defect repaired by transplantation of part of the temporalis muscle. Two years after this surgery, the patient remains well with a satisfactory cosmetic result.

Patient J. F., a 36-year-old white man, presented with blurred vision and proptosis of the right eye of six months' duration. A Krönlein operation under general anesthesia with excision of a tumor was performed. Tissue study revealed a hemangio-endothelioma. An exenteration with temporalis graft was advised and was subsequently executed. The patient had an uneventful convalescence and a plastic reconstruction of the fornix with a fitted prosthesis is to be considered at a later date.

Patient R. G., a 38-year-old white woman, complained of protrusion of the left eye of six months' duration and diplopia for three months. Two weeks prior to referral an orbital exploration was carried out through the left upper lid medially. A tumor was palpated at that time but was not biopsied. On examination a round, firm mass could be felt in the upper inner angle of the left orbit. X-ray films showed the left orbit to be larger in all dimensions than

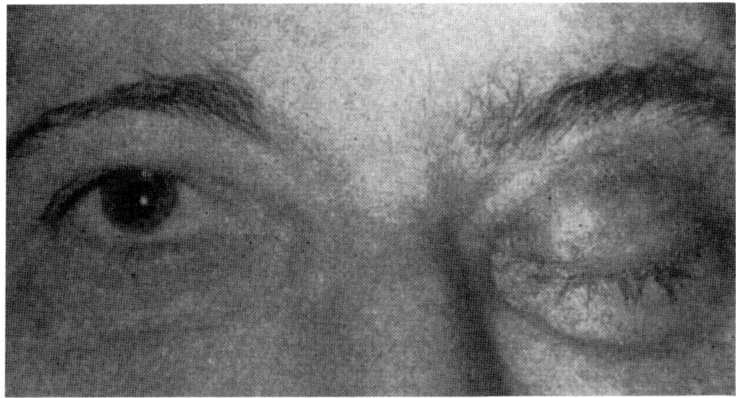

Figure 13. Patient B. L. shown three weeks after surgery. The minimal amount of reaction should be noted.

the right. Although the patient's main subjective symptom was diplopia, she also had pain in back of the left orbit and had noticed transitory blurred vision. A Krönlein and exploration procedure was carried out. A tumor was palpated nasally. On attempted removal the capsule proved to be fragile and the tumor came out as a friable poorly defined cellular mass. Pathologic sections of tumor tissue indicated a hemangiopericytoma. Accordingly, an exenteration with temporalis muscle graft was performed by means of the usual procedure. An 18-mm gold-sphere implant was used. The patient had difficulty in opening her mouth one month postoperatively. Two months after operation the patient was reportedly fine except that the gold sphere had extruded through the upper lid.

Patient B. H., a white girl, aged 13 years, had a history of recent episodes of blurred vision in the left eye. Examination revealed a proptosed eye with limitation of motion on upward gaze. Vision was reduced in that eye to counting fingers at one foot. Exploration and biopsy of the left orbit was made through a lateral canthotomy. Study of the mass confirmed the diagnosis of an intraorbital rhabdomyosarcoma. An exenteration was performed with the temporalis muscle graft. On initial follow-up, a good cosmetic result was noted; however, on subsequent visits there was a great deal of sinking of the lids with marked depression in the temporal fossa. Eight months postoperatively, examination revealed recurrence of tumor in the orbit with bone involvement so that no restoration of the socket could be carried out. One year and three months from the date of operation, the patient died.

Patient K. T., a 49-year-old white woman, was referred with a history of a nevus of the left bulbar conjunctiva which had been excised elsewhere. The specimen was diagnosed as precancerous melanosis and perhaps early malignancy. One year later examination revealed a recurrence of dark discoloration. Section again was taken and the diagnosis of precancerous melanosis was repeated. Exenteration with temporalis muscle graft was carried out using the usual procedure. A gold sphere was not used. The final pathology report revealed malignant melanoma of the conjunctiva. One month postoperatively, the patient complained of soreness in the jaw and difficulty in opening her mouth. One year postoperatively, considerable sinking in the temporal region was noted.

Patient L. B., a white girl, aged 5 years, was referred one month after removal of a tumor in the left orbit which was diagnosed as a rhabdomyosarcoma. On examination the eye was

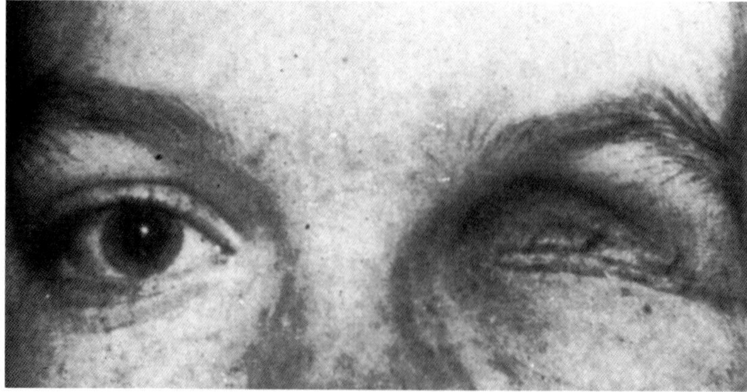

Figure 14. Patient V. W. Front view of patient taken three months after surgery.

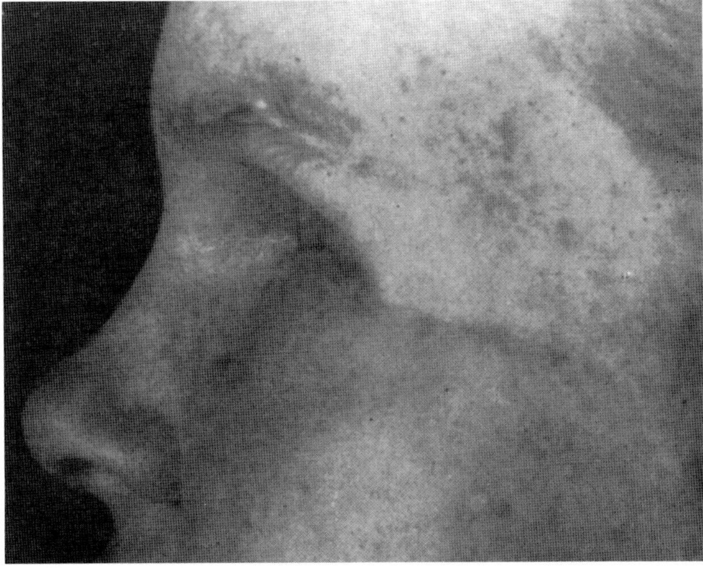

Figure 15. Patient V. W. Side view of patient taken three months after surgery.

found to be markedly proptosed laterally and down due to a firm mass in the orbit which presented itself, for the most part, in the upper lid nasally and at the inner canthus. Accordingly, an exenteration with the temporalis graft was done. Postoperative examination showed no sinking or depression in the temporal region and the patient, three months after exenteration, was well.

Patient V. W., a 14-year-old white girl, was referred with a history of painless swelling of

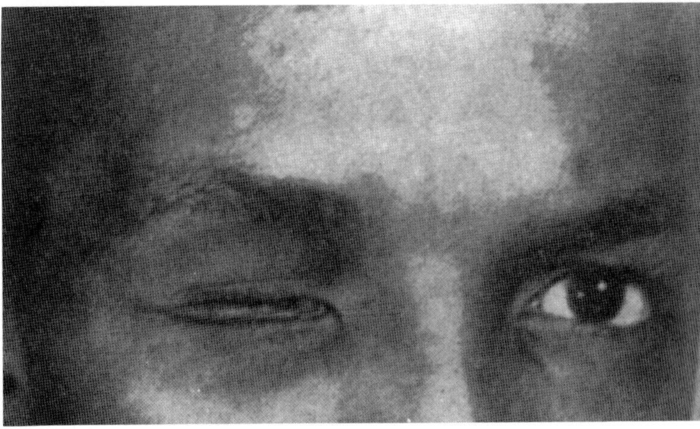

Figure 16. Patient I. R. Front view of patient taken two months after surgery.

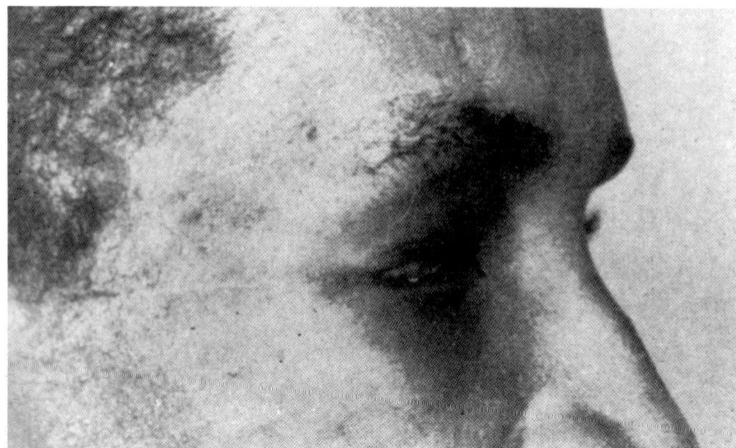

Figure 17. Patient I. R. Side view of patient taken two months after surgery.

the lids of the left eye. A biopsy had been carried out elsewhere and a diagnosis of rhabdo-myosarcoma of the orbit had been made. Accordingly, an exenteration with a temporalis muscle graft was performed. Three months postoperatively, the patient's physical condition was good. Photographs taken three months after surgery are shown (Figs. 14 and 15).

Patient I. R., a 33-year-old Puerto Rican woman, was referred with a progressive melanosis of the conjunctiva of the right lower lid, lower fornix, bulbar conjunctiva laterally and above, and palpebral conjunctiva above. A biopsy specimen revealed malignant melanoma of the conjunctiva. An exenteration of the right orbit with temporalis muscle graft was accordingly performed. The cosmetic result of the procedure was excellent on follow-up examination (Figs. 16 and 17); however, four months postoperatively, the patient developed enlarged

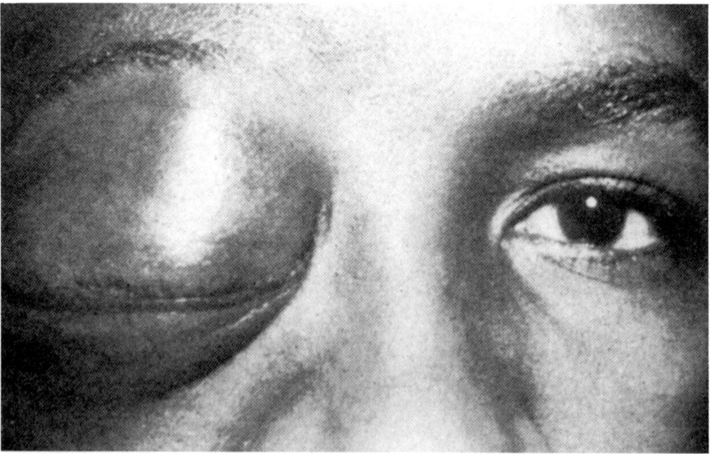

Figure 18. Patient I. R. Photograph taken six months after surgery, showing appearance after recurrence of melanoma within the orbit.

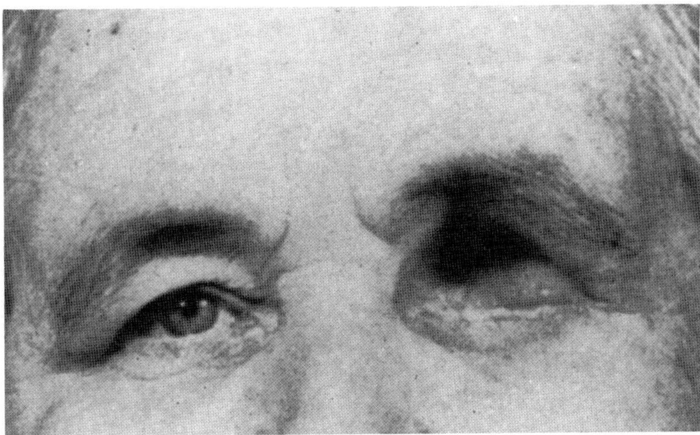

Figure 19. Patient H. A. Photograph taken five months after surgery. Insufficient filling of the defect is apparent.

regional lymph nodes which on biopsy proved to contain malignant melanoma. The orbit then began to show evidence of intraorbital growth of tumor tissue and the pressure became so pronounced that an exenteration of the remaining soft tissues in the orbit was carried out. When the patient was last seen, eight months postoperatively, the orbit again contained a fungating mass of pigmented tissue and the melanoma was judged to be inoperable. A photograph taken six months after surgery is shown (Fig. 18). The patient has since died.

Patient H. A., a 73-year-old white woman, presented with a history of glaucoma of the left eye of nine years' duration. The eye had recently become painful. On examination the tension

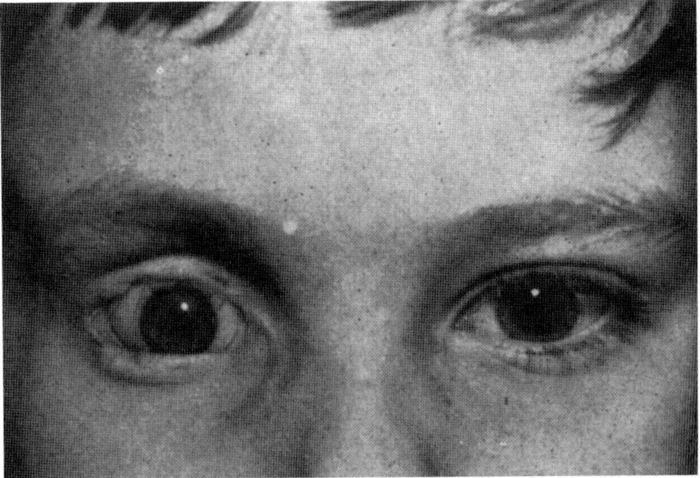

Figure 20. Patient S. M. who was shown in previous paper [1]. This photograph was taken after the second socket reconstruction and 12 months after the original surgery.

on the left was plus four and there was a left exotropia of 30 diopters. Vision in the left eye was reduced to no light perception and was not improved with correction. The clinical impression was malignant melanoma of the choroid with extraocular extension. An exenteration with temporalis muscle implant was performed in the usual manner. No gold sphere was used. The microscopic diagnosis revealed stromal cell melanoma. On follow-up examination one month postoperatively, the patient complained of some numbness on the left, but had no difficulty in chewing. Five months postoperatively, a negligible depression in the temporal region was noted and there was some numbness over the left forehead. A photograph taken five months after the surgery is shown (Fig. 19).

Patient A. G., a 67-year-old man, had a detached retina in the left eye six years previously. The eye became painful and was eviscerated. It proved to harbor malignant melanoma of the choroid. The orbit was exenterated including periosteum. The anterior half of the temporalis muscle was transplanted into the orbit over a plastic sphere. Convalescence is proceeding smoothly.

Patient P. G., a white woman, aged 60 years, had a two-year history of an enlarging spot on the conjunctiva of the right eye. Biopsy showed malignant melanoma. An exenteration including periosteum was done. The anterior half of the temporalis muscle was transplanted into the orbit over a gold sphere. Convalescence was uneventful and the present state of the patient is satisfactory.

Patient A. C., a white man, had an enlarging tumor under the left upper lid for two months. Biopsy showed this to be malignant melanoma of the conjunctiva. An exenteration including periosteum was done. Part of the temporalis muscle was transplanted into the orbit over a gold sphere. Convalescence was uneventful. Five months later the cosmetic result was satisfactory except for sinking of the temporal fossa.

Patient E. R., a 42-year-old white man, was seen with conjunctival pigmentation and a small nodule at the angle of mandible noted one year previously. An exenteration including periosteum was done. The anterior one half of the temporalis muscle was transplanted into the orbit over a 20-mm gold sphere. The patient had a rapid and uneventful recovery except for the presence of a small hematoma temporally corresponding to the dead space left by the removal of the portion of temporalis muscle. An insufficient amount of time has elapsed since this operation to assess the cosmetic result.

Patient M. S., a 60-year-old man, had drooping of the left upper lid for 10 months. Biopsy specimens from the caruncle revealed carcinoma. An exenteration including periosteum and the bone of the upper inner angle of the orbit was done. Part of the temporalis was transplanted into the orbit over a gold sphere. The convalescence was uneventful.

Patient S. M., a white boy, aged 6 years, was referred with a history of a tumor of the right upper lid. On examination a firm mass could be felt through the upper lid nasally which seemed to be attached to the bone and could be palpated quite deeply. No exophthalmos was present and no pre-auricular nodes were felt in the neck. A complete medical workup failed to reveal a primary tumor site elsewhere in the body. It was, therefore, felt that the orbital tumor was primary and accordingly, an exenteration with a temporalis muscle transplantation was carried out. A gold sphere was not used. Tissue study of the mass revealed a rhabdomyosarcoma. One and one-half years postoperatively, the patient had a plastic repair of the contracted right socket with insertion of a stent which was made up of dental wax to conform to the socket. This stent was covered with a Thiersch graft taken from the left thigh. Two weeks later the dental stent was removed. A good fornix was present above and below and the graft appeared to be viable. It was not possible to insert a conformer, of the size avail-

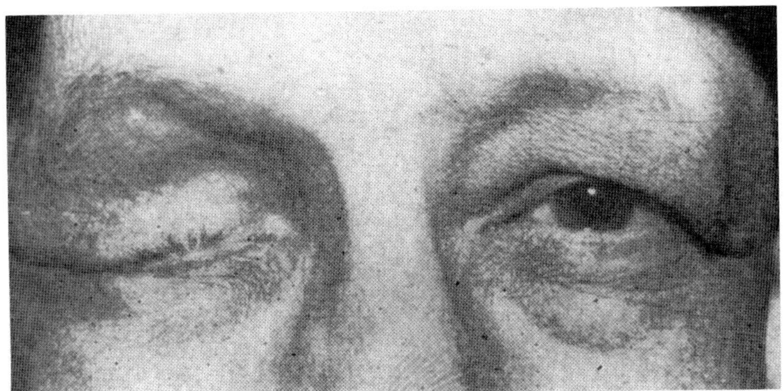

Figure 21. Patient F. B. Photograph taken six months after surgery.

able, between the lids. Thus, the eye was left open with an ointment applied to the macerated cheek. Five months after this procedure, the patient was noted to have a satisfactory result except for some sinking in the temporal region. On follow-up one year and three months after the first reconstruction of the socket, the patient was in good health. He had a good cilia line but had lost part of the upper and lower cul-de-sac. A second reconstruction of the socket was accordingly done. A split-thickness skin graft was taken with the Paget dermatome from

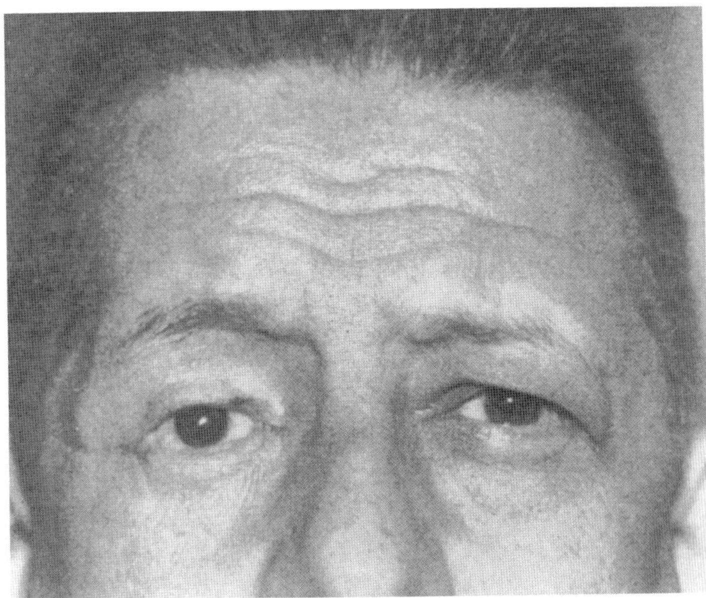

Figure 22. Patient F. B. Photograph taken seven months after restoration of socket with a split-thickness skin graft (approximately 23 months after exenteration procedure).

the left side of the abdomen. The old contracted skin graft from the right socket was removed. Blunt and sharp dissection was carried down to a point inside the orbital rim above and below and the fissure was lengthened especially at its nasal end. The previously prepared lucite molds were found to be too large. Therefore, two large conformers were sutured together back to back and the skin graft was wrapped around these conformers on all sides. The conformers were then placed between the lids which were sutured together over the graft and the conformers. One month after this restoration procedure, the conformer was removed and the socket appeared adequate except temporally where more canthus was desirable. Two weeks later a beautiful cosmetic result was noted. Earlier photographs of this patient were shown in a previous paper. One photograph of this patient is shown taken 12 months after the original surgery (Fig. 20).

Patient F. B., a 47-year-old white man, had a rupture of the right globe which subsequently proved to contain a malignant melanoma of the choroid. Accordingly, the orbit was exenterated with a temporalis muscle transplant performed in the usual manner. Approximately 17 months after this surgery, a reconstruction of the fornices with a split-thickness skin graft was carried out. Subsequent to this procedure, the lower fornix was deepened on one occasion and the lower lid was shortened. The upper fornix is still to be made deeper. Photographs are shown after the temporalis transplant and after the reconstruction of the socket with the patient wearing a prosthesis (Figs. 21 and 22).

Patient D. D., a 10-year-old white boy, was seen with a tremendous exophthalmos of the right eye. Nodes were palpable in the neck. Biopsy tissue from the orbit revealed leiomyosarcoma or hemangiopericytoma. Accordingly, an exenteration and a temporalis muscle trans-

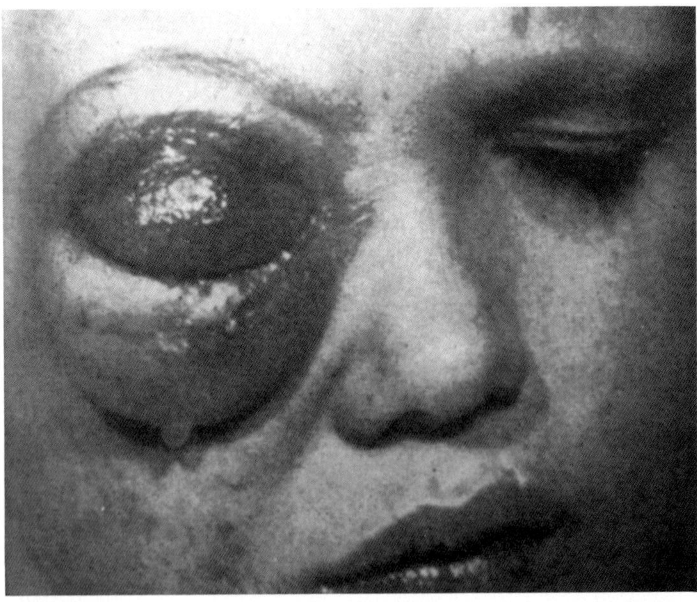

Figure 23. Patient D. D. Photograph taken prior to surgery, showing the enormous protrusion of the skin and conjunctiva of the right lower lid. The mass is so large it pushes the globe under the upper lid.

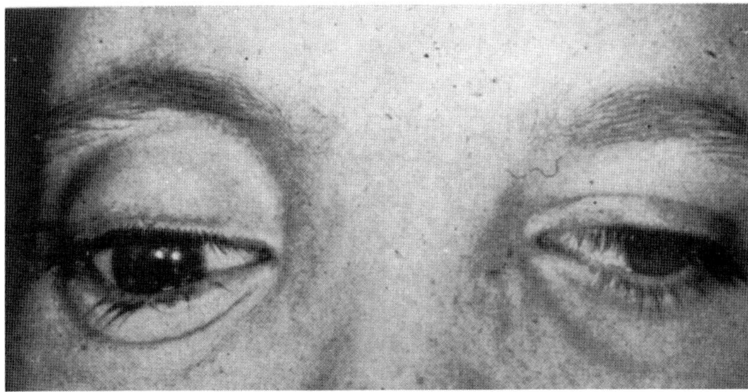

Figure 24. Patient D. D. Photograph of patient taken six months after exenteration and temporalis transplantation with preservation of the conjunctiva. Further procedures will be done to elevate the socket.

plant were carried out. This procedure varied from the usual one in that the conjunctiva and the full thickness of the lids were saved. Early in the convalescence, the prosthesis was fitted but the best result will only be obtained after the lower fornix has been elevated. A photograph taken before surgery (Fig. 23) and one taken six months after surgery (Fig. 24) are shown.

DISCUSSION

When confronted with the necessity of an exenteration there may be five surgical courses open to the surgeon: (1) ordinary exenteration without graft; (2) exenteration with split-thickness skin graft; (3) exenteration with temporalis muscle transplant; (4) exenteration with temporalis muscle transplant and reconstruction of the socket; (5) exenteration with temporalis muscle transplant and preservation of the conjunctiva.

If there is extension to bone or if radiation is to be given, the ordinary exenteration is the procedure of choice. In our opinion it is always preferable to do the exenteration without skin graft. The final defect is smaller and the convalescence is often shorter. If it is felt that exenteration is clean, then an even better procedure is to follow the exenteration with a temporalis muscle transplant. The after-care is much reduced and the operative site is dry in one week. The cosmetic result is superior. There remains the possibility of a socket reconstruction and the wearing of a prosthesis at a later date. If the case is such that the conjunctiva can be preserved, then a prosthesis may be worn within two weeks after surgery. One such case is included in this study.

To date, only two socket reconstructions have been done at long intervals after the original temporalis transplant, but there seems to be no reason why the reconstruction of the socket cannot be done at the same time as the exenteration and temporalis muscle transplant. This technique is now being worked out.

The advantages of the technique deserve reiteration. Foremost is the superior cosmetic result. Even without the restoration of the socket, the result is more acceptable than the usual exenteration. Furthermore, the continuing refinement of the technique for restoration of the

Table 1. Summary of Cases

Case	Diagnosis	Surgery	Repair	Present status
J.C. Previously reported [1]	Rhabdomyosarcoma	Exenteration with temporalis muscle transplant	–	Good. To have socket restoration
S.A. New	Metastatic carcinoma	Exenteration with temporalis muscle transplant	–	Good. To have socket restoration
B. L. New	Malignant melanoma of conjunctiva	Exenteration with temporalis muscle transplant	–	Living with disease
R. H. New	Malignant melanoma of conjunctiva	Exenteration with temporalis muscle transplant	–	Good
J. F. New	Hemangiopericytoma	Exenteration with temporalis muscle transplant	–	Good. To have socket restoration
R. G. New	Hemangiopericytoma	Exenteration with temporalis muscle transplant	–	Good. To have socket restoration
B. H. New	Rhabdomyosarcoma	Exenteration with temporalis muscle transplant	–	Died of metastases 15 months after surgery
K. T. New	Malignant melanoma of conjunctiva	Exenteration with temporalis muscle transplant	–	Good
L. B. New	Rhabdomyosarcoma	Exenteration with temporalis muscle transplant	–	Good. To have socket restoration
V. W. New	Rhabdomyosarcoma	Exenteration with temporalis muscle transplant	–	Good. To have socket restoration
I. R. New	Malignant melanoma of conjunctiva	Exenteration with temporalis muscle transplant	–	Died of recurrence one year after surgery
H. A. New	Orbital extension of choroidal melanoma	Exenteration with temporalis muscle transplant	–	Good
A. G. New	Orbital extension of choroidal melanoma	Exenteration with temporalis muscle transplant	–	Good
P. G. New	Malignant melanoma of conjunctiva	Exenteration with temporalis muscle transplant	–	Good
A. C. New	Malignant melanoma of conjunctiva	Exenteration with temporalis muscle transplant	–	Good
E. R. New	Malignant melanoma of conjunctiva	Exenteration with temporalis muscle transplant	–	Good

continued

Table 1 continued.

Case	Diagnosis	Surgery	Repair	Present Status
M. S. New	Carcinoma	Exenteration with temporalis muscle transplant	–	Good
S. M. Previously reported [1]	Rhabdomyosarcoma	Exenteration with temporalis muscle transplant	Restoration of socket with split skin graft	Wears prosthesis
F. B. New	Orbital extensin of chloroidal melanoma	Exenteration with temporalis muscle transplant	Restoration of socket with split skin graft	Wears prosthesis
D. D. New	Hemangiopericytoma	Exenteration with temporalis muscle transplant	–	Wears prosthesis

socket promises good prosthetic results. Not the least of the advantages lies in the shortened hospital stay and the greatly abbreviated convalescence.

The only major disadvantage of a temporalis muscle transplant which has been recognized to date is that it may mask a recurrence. One patient in the present series had a recurrence which was not immediately appreciated. This patient had distal as well as local recurrence of tumor, but in some cases there might be a masking of a solitary local recurrence. This is probably of theoretical rather than practical importance. Minor drawbacks are temporary difficulty in jaw movement, and, in some cases, a sinking of the temple from which the muscle was transplanted.

SUMMARY

1. The technique of orbital exenteration and repair by temporalis muscle transplant is described.
2. Twenty cases are presented.
3. The advantages and disadvantages of the technique are discussed.
4. The improved cosmetic result is illustrated.

REEFERENCE

1. Reese AB: Exenteration of the orbit: With transplantation of the temporalis muscle. *Am J Ophthalmol* 1958; 45:386.

Frontalis Muscle Transfer in the Reconstruction of the Exenterated Orbit

Giulio Bonavolontà, M.D.

ABSTRACT

A technique using the frontalis muscle to reconstruct the exenterated orbit is described. The technique is simple and does not leave a depression in the temporalis fossa.

INTRODUCTION

The cosmetic rehabilitation of an exenterated orbit is difficult to achieve because of the absence of deep well-vascularized tissues. There is no vascular bed to support external reconstructive procedures. Some authors have described the use of temporalis muscle to provide a vascularized bed, allowing for further socket reconstruction. Although this technique gives satisfactory results, it is not easy to perform; it obliges the surgeon to make a wide osteotomy in the lateral wall of the orbit, and it produces a secondary depression in the temporalis fossa. For these reasons, I prefcr to use the frontalis muscle. The transfer of this muscle into the orbital cavity has allowed the reconstitution of a satisfactory socket in those cases that underwent partial exenteration with the preservation of both eyelids.

SURGICAL TECHNIQUE

Orbital exenteration is performed reaching the orbital rim by a conjunctival approach through the upper and lower fornix, sparing both eyelids. A lateral cantolysis may be necessary to increase surgical exposure (Fig. 1).

The frontalis muscle is approached with a frontal midline incision (Fig. 2). A rectangular muscular flap (5 × 8 cm), which includes the galea capitis, is undermined, taking care to preserve the muscle's blood supply that comes from the superficial temporal artery (Fig. 2). The flap is rotated anteriorly into the orbital opening and behind the eyelids; it remains attached to its insertion onto the dermis under the eyebrow. Its posterior surface then faces anteriorly.

The flap is then sutured to the periosteum of the inferior orbital margin (Fig. 3). The skin is sutured using 3–0 prolene interrupted sutures. At the end of the operation both eyelids will lie over the periosteum attached to the muscular flap. A sterilized symblepharon plastic ring is applied into this reconstructed cavity to maintain the upper and lower fornices; a temporary tarsorrhaphy is advisable.

When the physiological shrinkage of the muscular flap and the scarring process of the deep

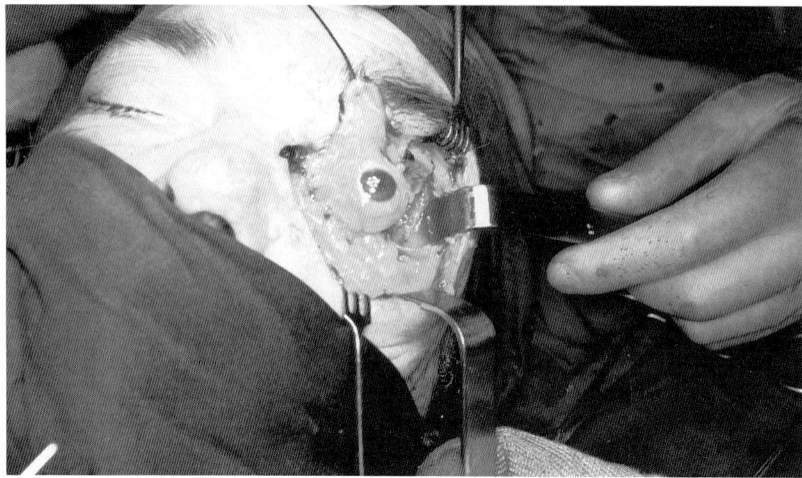

Figure 1. Subtotal exenteration preserving upper and lower eyelids. The intraorbital contents are better exposed performing a wide lateral cantholysis.

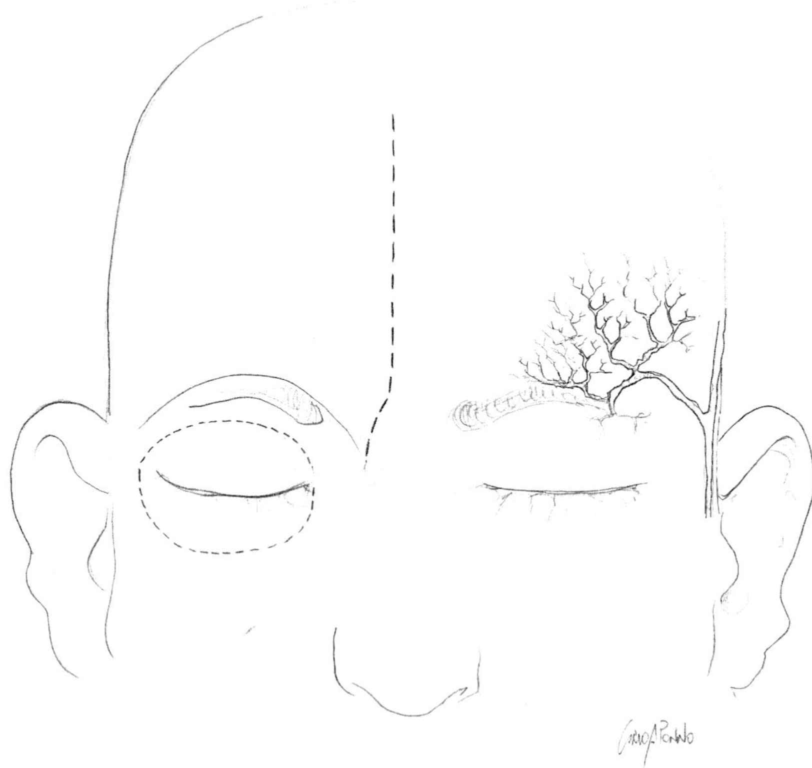

Figure 2. Lines of surgical incision for approaching the frontalis muscle (– –) and for transconjuntival exenteration (--). Localization and vascularization of the frontalis muscle.

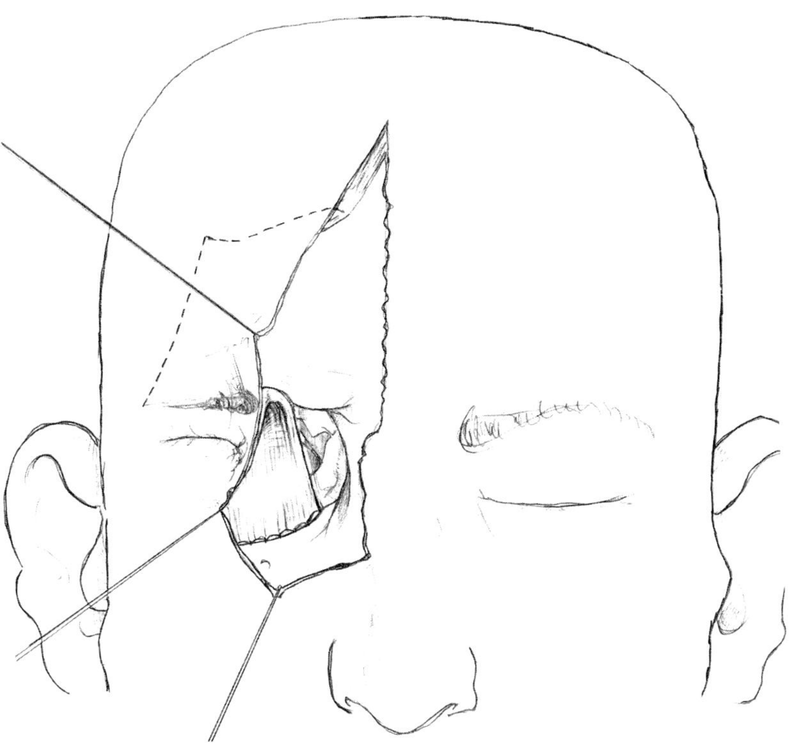

Figure 3. After a frontal midline incision, the frontalis muscle is rotated down behind the eyelids.

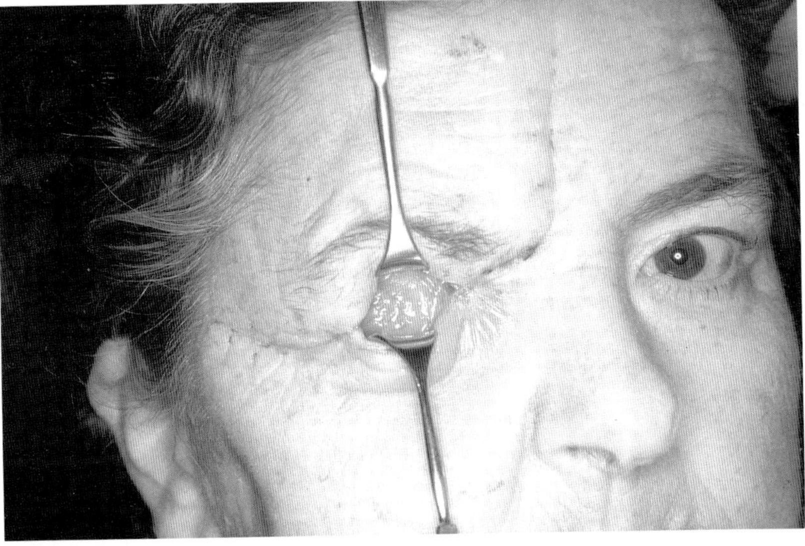

Figure 4. Following exenteration of the orbit, this socket has been reconstructed with a frontalis muscle flap. Note the generous lining and the appropriate shape of the rebuilt socket.

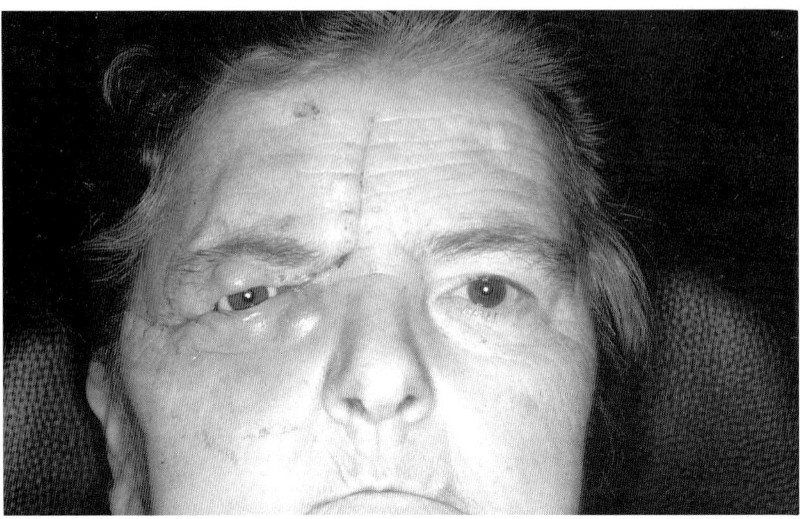

Figure 5. Final result. The patient is wearing a prosthesis in the right side one month after the exenteration.

tissues is complete, the lids are opened and fornices are examined (Fig. 4); if some shrinkage has occurred they will be deepened using free mucous membrane graft. A silicone sterilized conformer of the appropriate size is applied at this stage. The permanent prosthesis will replace the conformer two weeks later (Fig. 5).

DISCUSSION

Orbital exenteration is the only possible surgical approach in management of some orbital tumors. Nevertheless the disfiguring results with traditional techniques often cause psychological disorders for the patient. To deal with these problems, complex surgical techniques or special orbital prostheses have been proposed.

In recent years the good results obtained in the reconstruction of the severely contracted socket with temporalis muscle transfer convinced us to use muscular flaps, also on exenterated sockets. The frontalis muscle represents a good alternative to the use of temporalis muscle as a vascularized bed on which to rebuild a socket capable of supporting a prosthesis.

The main advantages of transferring the frontalis muscle into the orbit, instead of the temporalis muscle, are that this technique is easier and there is less of a risk of damaging the blood supply.

REFERENCES

1. Bonavolontà G: *Temporalis muscle transfer in the treatment of severe contracted socket.* Orbital Society, Vancouver, June 17 to 18, 1989.
2. Reese AB: *Orbital Tumours,* 2nd Ed., Philadelphia, PA, WB Saunders.
3. Rougier J, Tessier P, Hervouet F, Woillez M, Lekieffre M, Derome P: *Chirurgie plastique orbito-palpébrale.* Paris, Masson, 1977; 47–53.
4. Tessier P, Krastinova D: La trasposition du muscle temporal dans l'orbite anophtalme. *Ann Chir Plast.* 1982; 3:213–220.

The History and Development of Facial Prostheses

Augustus J. Valauri, D.D.S.

ABSTRACT

This paper includes the historical development of the modern-day facial prosthesis, the various materials used from the early days to the present, and the historical input of various people and their contributions towards the development of the qualities in fabricating a lifelike facial prosthesis.

At what point in history prosthetic restoration was first attempted to disguise the presence of congenital or acquired facial deformities is not clear. Facial disfigurement of an acquired or congenital origin has been present from the beginning of time. There is historical evidence that the major causes of these deformities were wounds sustained during hunting or tribal wars, injuries, disease, and punitive mutilations. Archaeological excavations of tombs pre 2,500 B.C. have illustrated material found in carvings, sculptures, which provides evidence of fabrication of nasal, orbital, auricular prostheses, and dental restorative treatment being carried out.

Many clinical and technical writers have reported that dental restorations and facial prostheses found in mummies to have been for therapeutic function and aesthetic reasons; conversely, Egyptologists have reported that such prosthetic appliances were, in probability, inserted after death to meet the religious beliefs of the time.

X-ray examination of mummified remains from the Egyptian period often shows the presence of metal inserts in the orbital region that resemble artificial eyes. The eye prostheses found in recent years [1], are apparently of a sheet of metal swaged to convex shape and painted with enamel to resemble the coloring and detail of the eye. Other historians and archaelogists have reported the discovery of facial prostheses fabricated in wood, wax, and clay in tombs from the early Chinese period [2] which no doubt were also inserted after death [3–11].

Note that amputation of facial parts, for example, the tip of the nose or an ear, was used in early times as a form of punishment. This was a well-established legal procedure in the early years of "civilization," used particularly by the Indians, Romans, Egyptians, and Babylonians. Whether such unfortunate individuals were able to obtain some form of prosthetic replacement is unknown, but no doubt persons with such a deformity would have wished to hide the evidence of their past infringement of the law. Regarding the Greek and Roman period (1,000 B.C.) Popp [2] states that artificial eyes of quartz, rock crystal, and enamel were made for the statues; thus arose the idea that artificial eyes could be used in living humans who have lost one or both eyes.

Popp [2] further states that artificial eyes were first known in Egypt and China. Nasal prostheses were made of lacquer in India and likewise in China in the second century of the Christian era.

In recent years, excavations of burial grounds in Bulgaria have unearthed some interesting relics from the Thracian period, one of which takes the form of a silver face mask joined to an iron helmet. Because the mask is of a thin silver plate construction which would not have afforded much protection in battle, leads one to believe that the mask may have been intended to disguise the presence of a facial defect acquired as a war injury or as a result of disease [3].

Paschke [12] reported in 1957 that Kaiser Otto III, a German Emperor, born 983, died 1,002 A.D. wore a golden nasal prosthesis to disguise a nasal defect. Lufkin [13] reported in 1939 that Abulcasis of Cordova fabricated facial prostheses from ivory in the 10th century.

The first well-documented account of facial prosthetics is provided by Ambroise Paré (1509–1590) [14], a French military surgeon of great ability who made many and varied contributions to the development of surgery and medical science. He is considered by many to be the father of modern surgery—no doubt the father of "facial prostheses." Paré was one of the first to approach the problems of physical deformity in relation to designing realistic and functional replacements.

Paré's famous book, *The Opera*, published in 1579, shows many examples of facial prosthetic replacements. Paré also provides information regarding the indications for facial prosthetic treatment and the various materials that could be used to fabricate a prosthesis, citing such examples as gold, silver, papier maché, linen cloths glued together, and leather. He also mentions methods of retention. For example, he says that an ear prosthesis could be retained by means of a metal band passing over the patient's head (Fig. 1). He suggests ways of retaining a nasal prosthesis by means of a series of linen tapes (Fig. 2). In his book he shows the feasibility of facial prosthetic rehabilitation and also provides guidelines regarding the choice of material and design. The text that accompanies these illustrations is of particular interest because of the manner in which Paré so clearly sets facts, the reasons why use of a prosthe-

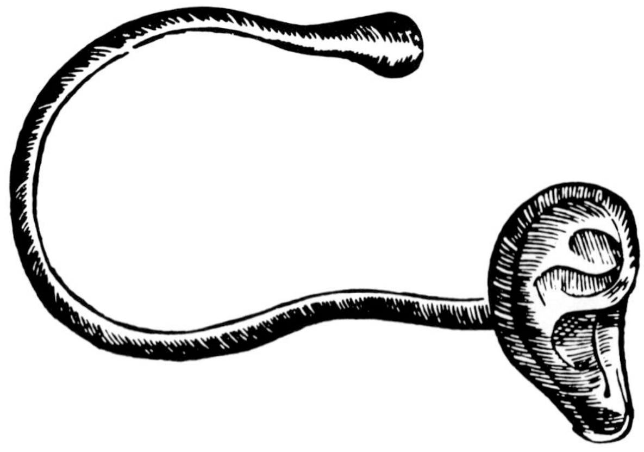

Figure 1. Ear prosthesis illustrated by Paré, A.

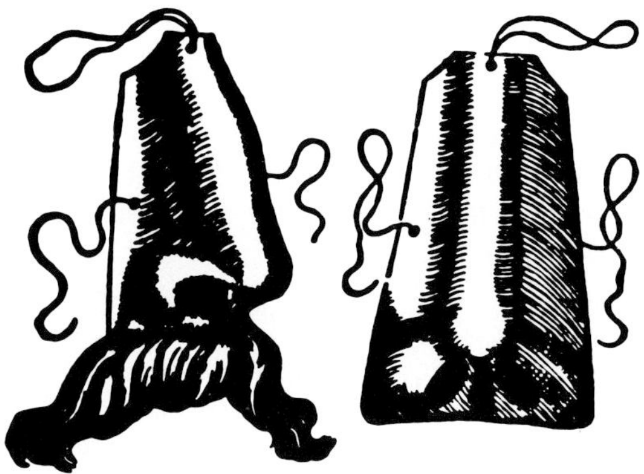

Figure 2. Nasal prosthesis illustrated by Paré, A.

sis should at times be considered the method of choice. He points out two of the chief obstacles to total reconstruction of the nose by plastic surgery.

Jalen [3] provided the following information in 1606: "There are men in Calabria who are accustomed to building up mutilated noses (surgically); others shape noses from papier maché

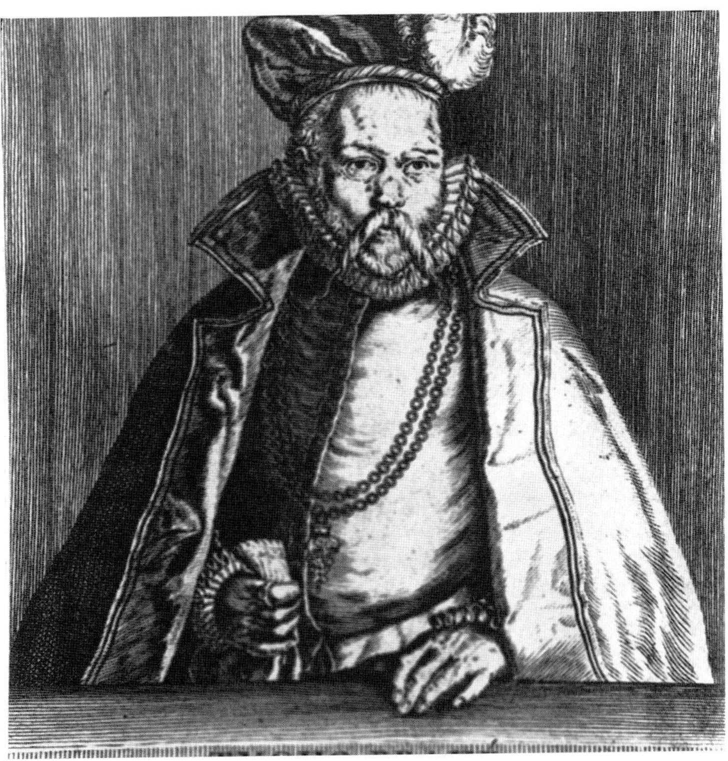

Figure 3. Portrait of Tycho Brahé wearing his nasal prosthesis.

of stuff of which masks are made, or silver, and cover them with the same flesh-coloured pigment and attach them with glue or other sticky substance, and when they go to sleep they remove them; the next morning, however, they put them on again."

During the 16th century Tycho Brahe (1546–1601), the famous Danish astronomer, was obliged to wear a nasal prosthesis during the latter part of his life (Fig. 3). In 1890, Dreyer [15] explained fully the cause of the deformity, which happens to have been the outcome of an argument that had to be settled by a duel.

"An event took place at Rostock soon after this, which was a good deal more unfortunate for Brahe, and which become more widely known than many others and much more important incidents in his life. On the 10th of December 1566 there was a dance at Professor Bachmeister's house to celebrate a betrothal, and among the guests were Brahe and another Danish nobleman, Manderup Parbjerg. These two got into a quarrel, which was renewed at a Christmas party on the 27th, and finally they met (whether accidentally or not is not stated) on the 29th, at seven o'clock in the evening, 'in perfect darkness,' and settled the dispute with their swords. The result was that Tycho lost part of his nose, and in order to conceal the disfigurement, he replaced the lost piece by another made of a composition of gold and silver. Gassendi, who recounts all these details, adds that William Jansson Blaev, who spent two years with Tycho at Hveen, had told him that Tycho always carried in his pocket a small box with some kind of ointment or glutinous composition, which he frequently rubbed on his nose . . . The various portraits which we possess of Tycho show distinctly that there was something strange about the appearance of his nose, but one cannot see with certainty whether it was the tip or the bridge that was injured, though it seems to be the latter. A very venomous enemy of his, Reymers Bar, of whom we shall hear more farther on, says that it was the upper part of the nose which Tycho had lost."

Brahe is said to have commissioned a silversmith to construct a silver cover-prosthesis that he used to disguise his acquired loss for the remainder of his life.

Pierre Fauchard [16], a French surgeon-dentist, made a special contribution to the field of maxillofacial prosthetics by designing and constructing many ingenious intra- and extraoral prostheses. His facial restorations were mainly fabricated in papier maché and silver.

DEVELOPMENTS IN THE 17TH THROUGH THE 19TH CENTURY

A well-known case of facial prosthetic rehabilitation is that of the "Gunner with the Silver Mask." The mask was designed by Dr. Forget and executed in silver by a M. Verschuylen of Antwerp. A full description of the very extensive maxillofacial prosthesis was published in the London Medical Gazette in 1833 [17].

"The patient, a private by the name of Alphonse Louis, a native of St. Laurent, Pas de Calais and a soldier in the 2nd Regiment of Artillery, received his injury during the siege of Antwerp in 1832. The battle involved the French and the Dutch forces. The mode of battle was trench warfare but Private Louis was injured while standing forward of his gun emplacement.

His injury was caused by a large shell fragment that weighed 7 lb. This carried away, as already said, most of the lower third of the face and jaw, leaving only remnants of the ascending rami. There was also an associated alveolar fracture involving the left side of the maxilla, lacerations of the carotid duct and the left side of the tongue, extending to the vicinity of the Hyoid bone.

Private Louis was transported to a field hospital at Hoboken where a surgeon major attempted to close the wound by drawing the remaining tissues together. It is reported that the right forearm was amputated at the same time. Apparently, scant hope was given by the attending surgeon to the patient of surviving his extensive injuries. The patient did, however, recover, despite gangrene and large portions of tissue in and around the face and jaw sloughing away.

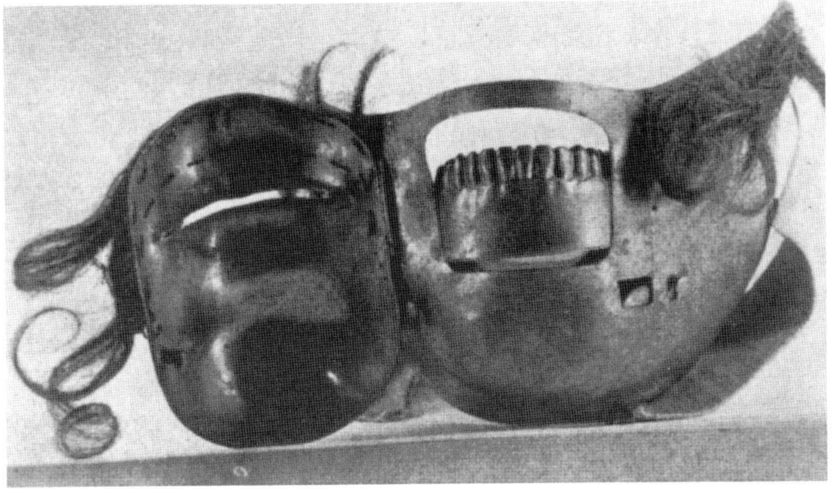

Figure 4. "Silver Mask" illustrating the ingenious device.

In due course, Private Louis came under the care of a Doctor Forget, surgeon-dentist, who it is reported showed great interest in the patient's treatment and rehabilitation. After many weeks of care, the patient made sufficient recovery to allow a plaster cast to be taken of the face, on which Dr. Forget designed a half-facial mask.

The design and model made by Dr. Forget was passed to a M. Verschuylen, a master crafts-man, who fabricated the facial mask in silver. This was supported on the face by means of leather straps that fitted around the neck and the back of the head (Fig. 4). Within the mask, a hinged mandibular section with gold teeth was sited under which a drainage chamber was also provided. The external aspect of the mask was painted with oils."

The clinical details of the case, together with ingenuity exercised by Dr. Forget and M. Ver-schuylen, attracted the attention of Sir William Whymper of the Grenadier Guards, who translated the report from French into English and published it in the London Medical Gazette [17]. A duplicate of this prosthesis is now housed in the museum of the Department of Anatomy at the University of Edinburgh.

Saunders [18] wrote a detailed account of the prosthesis of the Gunner with the Silver Mask in 1941:

"... it was a half mask, without nose or cheeks, that enclosed the whole extent of the edges of the contrivance, where they came in contact with the face, were skillfully obscured by mustachios and whiskers, and it was to his fortune that these were the fashion of the day. The external aspect of the mask was painted in oils so as to correspond with his complexion, and it was said of it that the illusion was so strong that 'unless forewarned, he might be steadfastly examined at a short distance without betraying his misfortune.' The lower part of the mask was obscured by his cravat. The straps which held it in place were hidden by his hair, and altogether, judging from the quaint wood-cut in Ballingall's Military Surgery, he must have presented quite a fine appearance.

A trap carrying the lips and chin could be sprung by pressing a small button which had thoughtfully been placed on the left side of the face. This when opened revealed a second or internal chin and a row of metal teeth, as well as a complete buccal cavity. This, and the aperture between the artificial lips, provided free communication between the pharynx and the exterior, permitting him to breathe quite freely without taking off his mask . . . Strongly built of silver, the different portions were so arranged that they could be taken apart and cleaned. The mask weighed about three pounds, and cost approximately twelve pounds sterling . . . It apparently did much to improve his existence, for it not only served to hide his deformity, but relieved him of what must have otherwise been troublesome secretions, and provided a considerable measure of support for his tongue. In addition it must have assisted his speech, for although his larynx had in no way been damaged he had had difficulty in articulation owing to the absence of the front of his mouth, and had found sibilants and labials particularly troublesome.

What happened to him eventually I do not know. He was apparently at the Hotel des Invalides in Paris, where he was known as the 'Gunner with the Silver Mask,' and then Whymper says of him: 'On our last visit to Alphonse Louis, the day previous to his departure for Lille, he appeared in high spirits; he walked about with agility; used the stump of his forearm with address; took off and readjusted his mask with his left hand; spoke not only intelligibly but easily; he was high coloured, and fatter, as he stated, than he had ever been prior to his misfortune. He played at cards and seemed to be as proud of showing the mechanism of his artificial jaw, as he was of the crosses of the Legion of Honour and Leopold, that glittered on his bosom."

Delabarre [19], a French surgeon-dentist, published a book in 1820. This clinician introduced many innovations that had a definite application to the development of maxillofacial prosthetics.

In 1876 the sultan of Turkey had organized for nasal prostheses to be made for soldiers who had lost their noses due to amputation by their Burganon captors. These mutilations occurred following fighting between the Sultan's troops and the Russian forces. In 1868 John Wesley Hyatt [3], an American chemist, prepared the first organic plastic molding compound which was called celluloid. In fact it was a cellulose nitrate. This may have been the beginning of the plastic era and this material was used quite extensively for maxillofacial prosthesis. However, due to its poor physical properties the material was destined to be replaced by newer, more durable material such as vulcanite, acrylics, and more recently with silastics.

William Morton [20] who was the first to discover the advantages of sulphuric ethers as a general anesthetic for dental anesthesia, was apparently a man of many talents and interests. He constructed a number of facial prostheses, mostly noses made of porcelain and enamelled to the exact color of the patient's complexion.

Among those of the 19th century who made notable contributions to the field of maxillofacial prosthetics, Norman W. Kingsely [21], an American and Claude Martin [22], a Frenchman, stand out with their classic textbooks. Kingsely's book, *A Treatise on Oral Deformities* is a comprehensive well-detailed text on the art of treating oral and facial deformities caused by trauma, disease, or congenital causes, dedicates a section to facial prosthesis and illustrates a number of cases of both intraoral and extraoral prostheses. An example is:

"Artificial Nose. — In July, 1869, a gentleman from a distant city, a lawyer by profession, applied to me for advice. His face presented the appearance indicated in [Fig. 5]. An examination showed the loss by disease of the soft palate, a portion of the hard palate, the vomer and turbinated bones, the nasal walls of the antra, portions of the nasal and maxillary bones, and the cartilage of the nose.

A rhinoplastic operation would not be submitted to, for various reasons — among which were, the suffering and inconvenience attending it, the disfigurement caused by it, the uncertainty of the result, and the doubt of making by such process a nose which should resemble to any extent the original appendage. An artificial nose being the only alternative, a case of the face

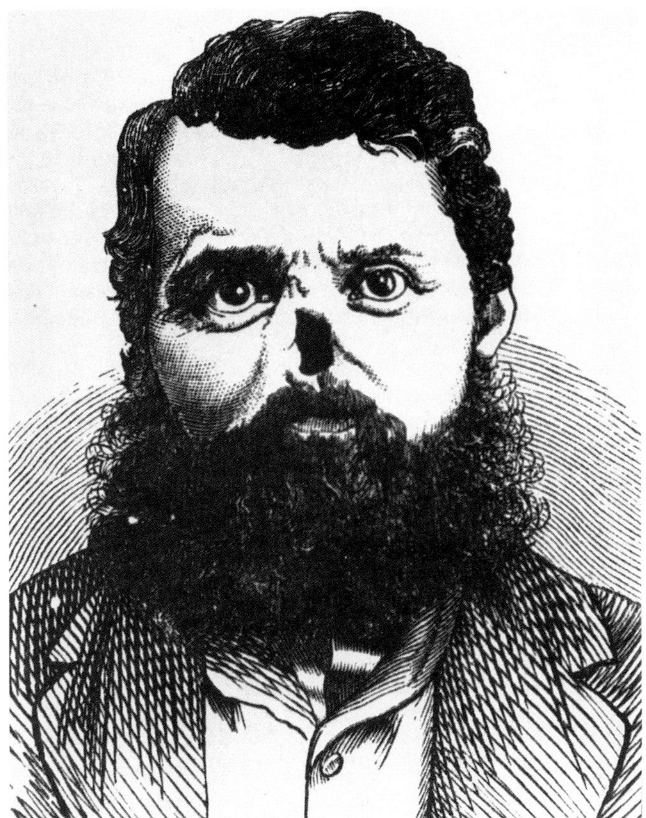

Figure 5. Patient with nasal deformity.

and nasal cavity was taken in the following manner: The nasal cavity was filled to the orifice with plaster—not in one mass, but in sections, to facilitate its removal. Before removal, however, the cast of the face was taken, the plaster coming in contact with that already in the nasal cavity at the orifice, the precaution having been taken to soap the surface to prevent the two masses from adhering. After the removal of the external mask, the sections in the nasal cavity were pushed backward, and brought out through the opening caused by the loss of the soft palate.

The sections being all brought together, a cast was made which showed the surface of all the parts adjacent to the nasal orifice both internal and external. Upon this plaster cast there was modeled a form of the new nose in wax, made to resemble the color of the flesh, this wax model being tried on the living face from time to time for criticism. The object of using flesh-colored wax for this model is, that the operator is enabled to judge better of the effect of his art than he could were the material in contrast with the surrounding parts. It is herein that art and mechanism triumph over surgery—it being within the power of the artist by such means to restore this feature so that, in its individual character, it shall be in perfect harmony with the surrounding features, which it is not possible to accomplish by surgery. The extra large mass which must be cut from the forehead in a rhinoplastic operation to provide for shrinkage, renders it difficult to preserve the physiognomical relations of the nose with the face.

The model in wax having been determined upon as described, a duplicate must be made of such material as shall closely resemble the flesh and prove durable. Of all substances heretofore employed for this purpose, I know of none which are durable that are not decidedly objectionable in appearance. All opaque substances, no matter how beautifully they may be painted in imitation, do not look like flesh. Porcelain or enamel has an advantage in its transparency, but it reflects the light, and looks like a piece of crockery. For these reasons collodion was used in this case with remarkable success — the preparation being that known to dentists under the name of 'rose pearl,' with some modifications in color to suit the case. With this substance a nose was made, which had the color, tone, and translucency of flesh, giving also the delicate little tracery of veins which are so often observable in the nose toward the tip. This substance possesses also the qualities of elasticity, strength, and durability; it is not easily broken, nor affected by exposure to the elements or thermal changes. The wax model, after being completed externally, was scooped out inside, so as to leave a mere shell of not more than a line in thickness. The collodion duplicate was produced by making a die of fusible metal, pressing the mass into shape, and curing it in substantially the same manner in which 'rose pearl' base is worked.

[Figure 6] gives a view of the nose complete, with the attachments for securing it in place. Labels A and A are pads made of vulcanite, adapted to depressions in the nasal cavity and connected with the nose by flat gold springs. The gentle pressure of these springs is sufficient to keep the nose firm in its place; at the same time their elasticity will permit its removal at pleasure. The border of the nose is brought to a thin, beveled edge, wherever it comes in contact with the cheek, and the adaptation is so accurate that at a short distance no mark of separation is visible. In many cases of the application of an artificial nose, the attachment has been so insecure as to require the patient to wear a pair of spectacles to keep it from moving. Some artificial teeth and a palate, which were also required in this case, were made independent of the nose, and it is always desirable that they be disconnected. The movement of the muscles of the face is such that the nose should be permitted to yield with them. Besides, a nose secured by an unyielding connection to a plate of teeth through an opening in the roof of the mouth must necessarily show all the movements of mastication."

Figure 7 represents the patient with the nose attached.

The success in this case may be inferred from the following extract from a letter received from the patient soon after his return home:

"Every one here is delighted with my improvement; it gives me, I am glad to say, no discomfort, and I feel no weight. Many of my most intimate friends, after being in company with me several hours, both indoors and in full light of the sun, believed it genuine flesh, so deceptive

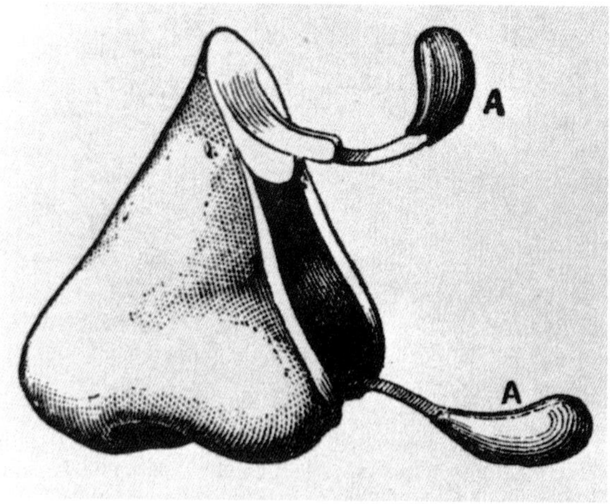

Figure 6. Nasal prosthesis with retentive pads A and A.

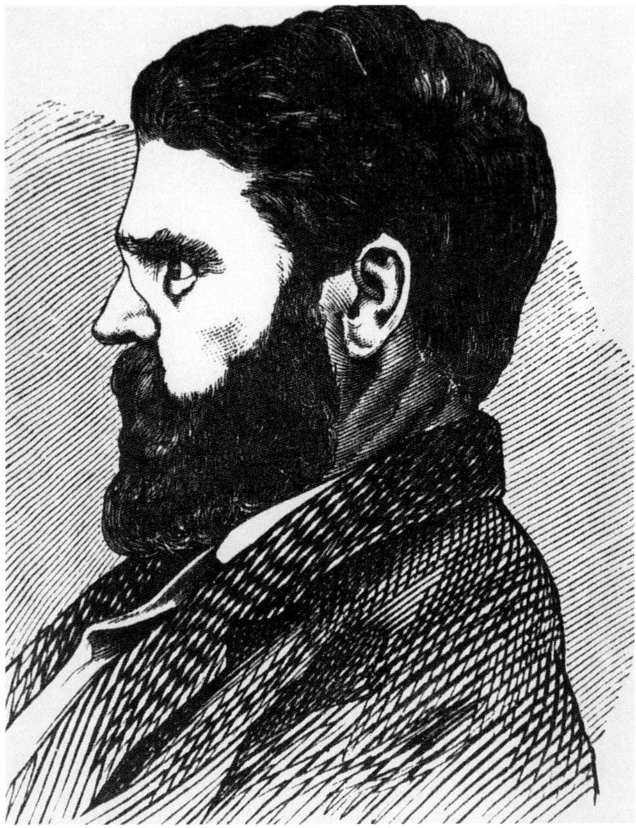

Figure 7. Patient wearing nasal prosthesis.

is it. Several medical gentlemen who have seen me have said that, in all similar cases to mine, they should never again advise an operation when such a thing can be made."

Claude Martin published a comprehensive book on the maxillofacial prosthetics in 1889 [22]. Martin, as Kingsley indicated, demonstrated many ingenious combinations of appliances both intraoral and extraoral.

At the 9th International Congress held in Washington, D.C. in 1887, Martin read a paper entitled "Artificial Nose Made of Ceramic and Retained Without the Aid of Spectacles." In his book he illustrates the treatment of a patient with an orbital deformity:

Observation IV
"Julie L . . . forty years old. The patient entered the Hotel Dieu for a recurrence of epithelioma of the eyelids which had spread into the conjunctiva, a part of the nose and the left cheek.
During the operation, everything that seemed suspicious was removed. The eye and the upper eyelid which was affected in its inner third were enucleated.
To cover this hole, a prosthetic device was fitted. This was 46 millimeters high and 67 millimeters wide. It closely approximated the missing soft parts [Fig. 8], that is to say, the surfaces above and below the eye socket and the area around the nose starting on the left side and proceeding down to the tip.

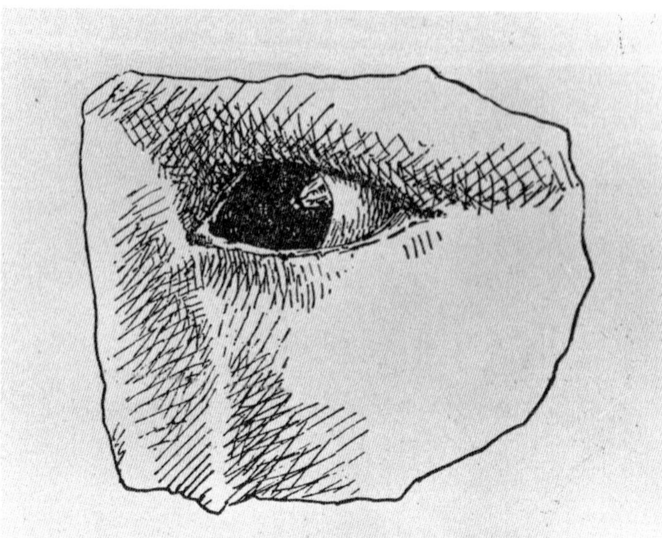

Figure 8. Orbital prosthesis.

An artificial eye fills the quivering crack that was left in the orbital cavity after the operation and in the scar tissue there are a certain number of depressions that we have used to attach our prosthesis. To this end, we have built out of rubber a small device that consists of three prongs in the shape of a "Y" and that fits into the the three depressions, one of which is located below the eye socket and the other two to the left and right above it (Fig. 9).

In the middle of this device there is a stem which holds the artificial eye in place.

We ought to mention that the central portion of the device is made of hard rubber while the ends of the branches (after the first centimeter and a half) are constructed out of soft rubber which can be molded to fit in the depressions that were mentioned, adapt closely to their shape and which carefully support the existing system.

The exterior of the prosthesis is made of ceramic which is sculpted to look like the parts it will replace.

This patient, after the prosthesis was applied to her, was presented by Professor Gayet to the Medical Board of the hospital on February 13, 1885.

The photographs shown (Figs. 10 and 11) represent the result of this restoration.

In 1894, Tetamore [23] described prosthetic rehabilitation of a number of patients with loss of nose and parts of face which he had reconstructed prosthetically. He used the spectacle frames to a great advantage in retaining and disguising the margins of the facial prosthesis usually made of light plastic material, that is, cellulose nitrate, introduced during that period.

THE 20TH CENTURY

"The nineteenth century ushered in an era of many improvements, in particular in plastic and rubber materials used in industry and brought into dental technology and particularly in prosthetic dentistry. The discovery of the principle of vulcanization of raw rubber when combined with proper amounts of sulfur by Goodyear in 1851 had already been placed at the disposal of the dentist. This versatile material appeared to have possibilities not only in the pure dental field but also in maxillofacial prosthetics. For this reason, during this period there are numerous references in the literature to the prosthetic reconstruction of nose, ears, and palates with this new material." [24,25] (Bulbulian AH, oral communication, Fall 1954.)

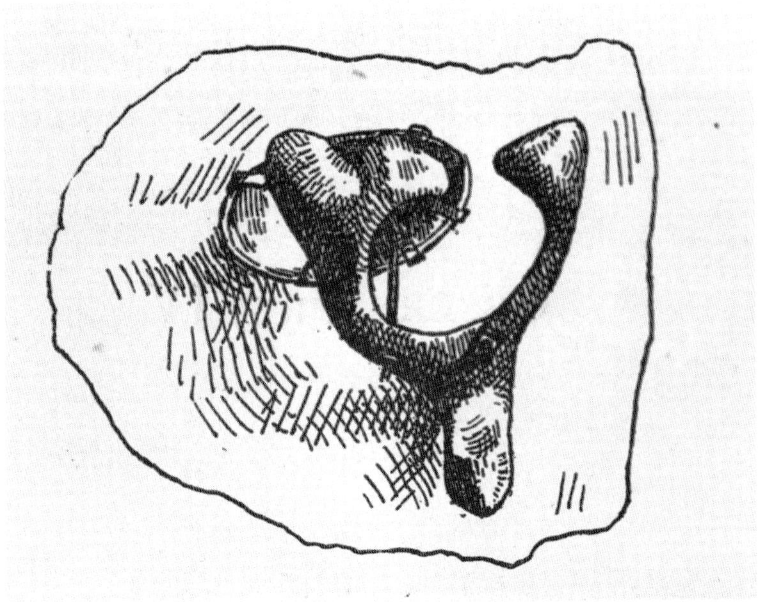

Figure 9. Prosthesis illustrating retention prongs in shape of Y.

In 1901, Upham [26], a Boston dentist, reported that he had made plates, noses, and ear prostheses for some 20 years. He stated that vulcanized rubber is the best material to use. It is easily worked, has no odor, and is not easily broken. Celluloid is harder to work, is easily broken, and readily catches fire if the wearer of a nosc happens to be an absent-minded smoker. Aluminum is too hard to work, and so is silver. Soon after Upham's paper a number of independent articles were published obtaining similar results with the same materials.

Hunting [3,25] developed a new facial prosthetic material in Germany. This was a combination of gelatin, glycerin, and coloring matter. To rend the material somewhat opaque, carbon-carbonate was added. This formula produced a very flexible, semi-translucent and lightweight restorative material which permitted fabrication of aesthetic prostheses; however, the material had a short life and deteriorated in 10 days. Zinsser, a colleague of Heening also used this material which became known as Elastin. This material was discontinued by most clinicians by the mid- and late 1920s.

The period of the First World War brought about a renewed interest in rehabilitation of the facially deformed caused by war injuries. Kazanjian's pioneering work during and after the First World War provided an impetus for dental surgeons, maxillofacial prosthodontists, and plastic surgeons to work together for the successful rehabilitation of the facially injured or deformed patients [27–31] (Kazanjian VH, oral communication, October 1972). Various types of maxillofacial appliances and extraoral prosthetic restorations were used, and basic principles were outlined. In the treatment of casualties of the wars of this century, prosthodontic and facial prostheses were constructed mainly to serve as temporary supports for the soft tissue of the face when deprived of this skeletal framework; such prostheses were indispensable for the rehabilitation of the patient.

In France, Ladd [3] became famous for using Vulcanite to fabricate facial prostheses in

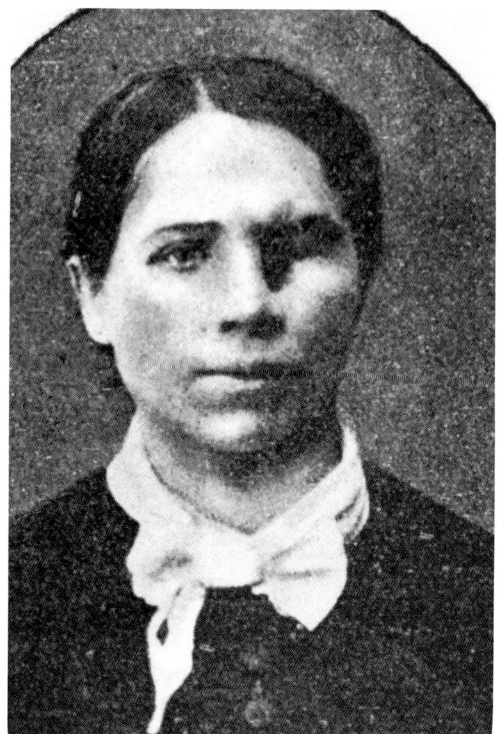

Figure 10. Patient with orbital deformity.

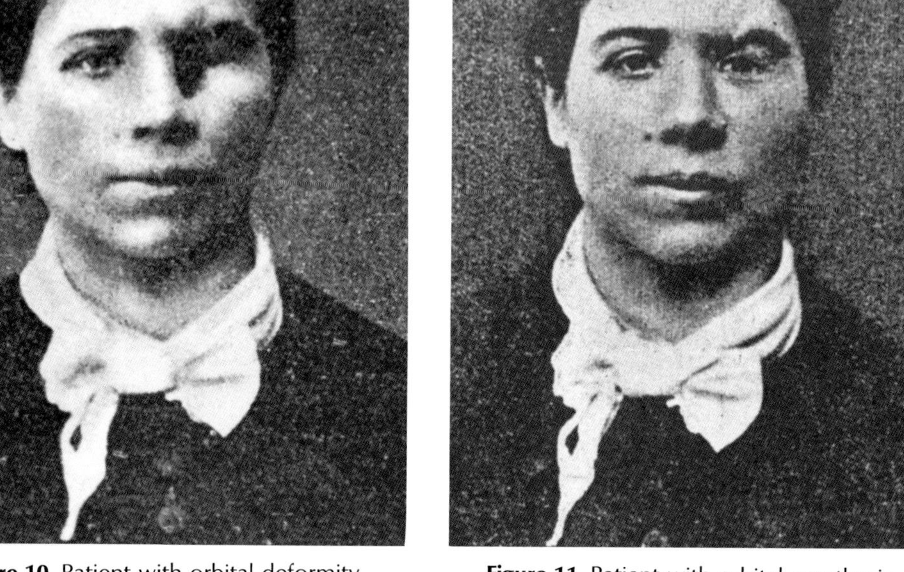

Figure 11. Patient with orbital prosthesis.

restoring war torn faces. In England, Derwent Wood, a sculptor, fabricated facial prostheses for the war injured. Vulcanite and glass eye ocular prostheses were constructed by an optician and dental surgeons working together in Glascow in the 1920s. The orbital prostheses were supported by wire spectacle frames; similar prostheses were made by Kazanjian in the U.S.A.

The use of prevulcanized latex for pliable prosthetic facial restorations was an outstanding contribution of an American dental surgeon, Arthur Bulbulian [24,25], and by Clarke. Bulbulian in 1939 published two papers describing in detail the application of latex compound in the fabrication of certain types of extraoral prostheses. It had the advantage of fabricating lightweight prostheses. The latex prosthesis had a much longer life than Elastin, the gelatin-glycerin prosthesis, but it also deteriorated in time.

It is a well-known fact that materials used in industry such as vulcanized rubber, plastics, and so on, have become significant in the field of restorative dentistry especially prosthodontics. Methyl-methacrylate (acrylic), owing to its advantages over vulcanite, had already replaced the latter as a denture base by the late 1930s. Because of its various advantages over other material used for extraoral prostheses, methyl-methacrylate became the material of choice for many maxillofacial clinicians, during World War I and for a period of time afterwards.

Note also, that during World War II, the fabrication of glass ocular prostheses (the glass eye) which had been known to many for centuries, was replaced by an acrylic resin eye which

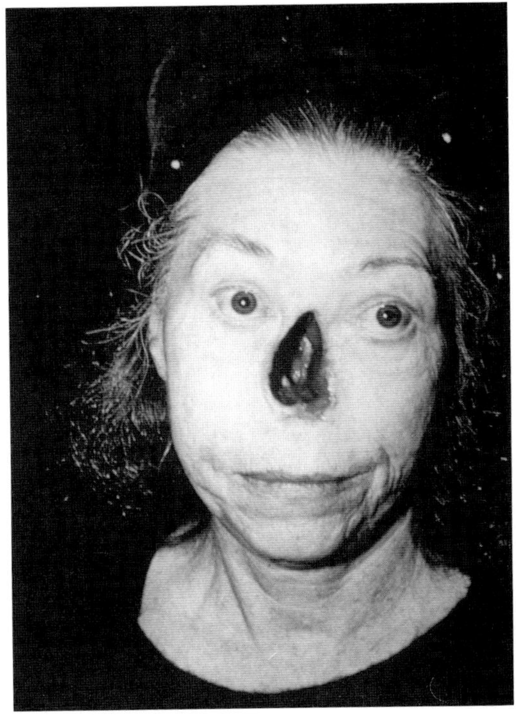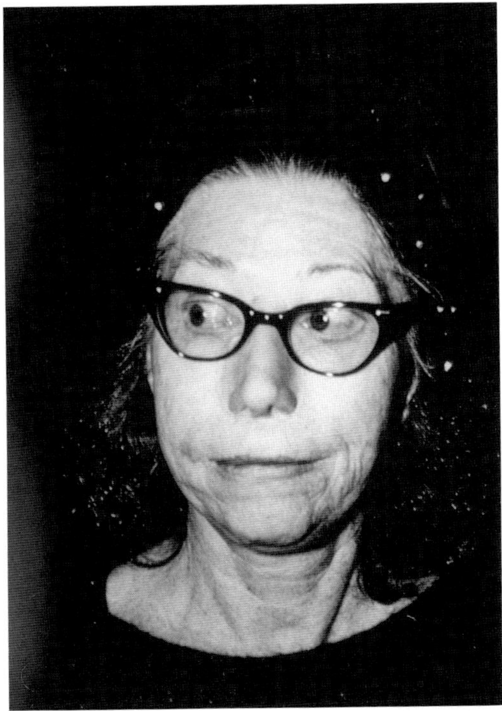

Figure 12. (A) Patient with nasal deformity. (B) Patient wearing silicone nasal prosthesis.

is much easier to manufacture and more importantly, much safer to wear. Acrylic was the material of choice by many clinicians throughout the world.

Pliable plastics came into the market between 1940 and the 1950s. Some of them were known as Dicor, Skintex, Flexiderm. These materials were widely used but still fell short of being the ideal material for facial prostheses.

Poly-vinyl chloride (PVC) powder plasticized by one of several plasticizing agents, following incorporation of opacifying or coloring pigments in the powder, has been one of the more popular types of plasticized plastics used for facial prostheses, especially used with sponge filler for bulk. One of the major innovators and developers of PVC was Dr. Cleaver and his technician at the Veterans' Hospital in New York [32] (Cleaver M, oral communication, 1953). More recently, PVC-type materials have been rejected because it is thought to be a health hazard material during processing.

Because of a revitalized interest in the rehabilitation of the facially disfigured patient in the late 1940s and early 1950s in the United States and Europe, maxillofacial prosthetics became an important branch of major medical centers, veteran's hospitals, and cancer centers throughout the United States.

The American Academy of Maxillofacial Prosthetics was formed in 1953, for the purpose of pooling the scientific, clinical, and technical knowledge and experience of its members, and to provide a center of information that may be needed by other workers interested in this field.

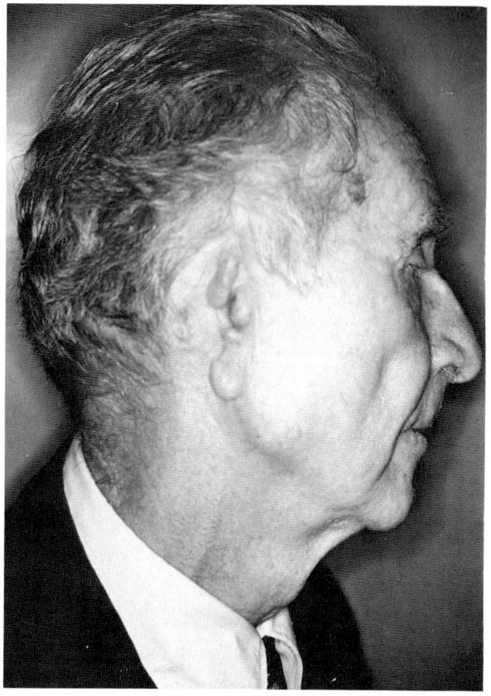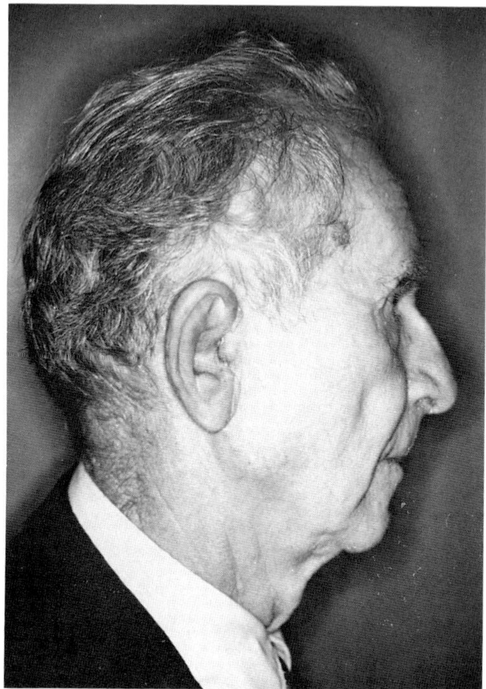

Figure 13. (A) Patient with ear deformity. (B) Patient wearing a silicone ear prosthesis.

In the 1950s Corde, a derivative of PVC, was developed by Dr. Cleaver (Cleaver M, oral communication [1952]) and Mr. J. Peruski, as a facial prosthetic material.

In 1960, a completely new material, silicone, was introduced by Dow Corning Co. This material which has many of the properties desired for extraoral facial prostheses is at the present the material of choice.

The properties of the ideal material for external maxillofacial prostheses have been enumerated by various authors and were reconfirmed at the American Academy of Maxillofacial Prosthetics Workshop in Washington, in 1966 [33]. These include:

1. Tissue compatibility. The material must not cause irritation or discomfort to the tissues upon which it must rest.
2. Reproduction of true skin tones. The prosthesis should be soft and pliable, easily colored, and textured to simulate true skin tones.
3. Translucency. It should have the characteristics of translucency to give a lifelike appearance.
4. Flexibility. It must be flexible and resilient to simulate the feeling of real soft tissue.
5. Durability. It must be durable to withstand sunlight, cold and heat and not be affected by body fluids such as perspiration. It should be resistant to the effects of air pollution and chemicals for a reasonable length of time.
6. Low thermal conductivity. It should be a poor or low conductor of heat or cold.

7. Lightness of weight. It should be light in weight so it does not dislodge and fall easily. Adhesives should be able to retain it.
8. Moldability. It should be easy to mold into the desired anatomical shapes and forms of the ear, nose, and other facial features.
9. Ease of processing. It must be simple to process without the need for expensive equipment.
10. Easy to duplicate. Duplication should be possible to produce identical or duplicate prostheses.
11. Easy cleaning. It should be easily cleaned without damage or deterioration.
12. Chemical and physical inertness and patient comfort. It should be comfortable for the patient to wear, and it should not chemically or physically irritate the patient.

No material in use today fulfills all of the criteria. At present, there are a few materials, such as silicone, rubber, and vinyl plastics, which show promise and are used extensively for external prosthetic restoration (Figs. 12, 13, 14). These prosthetic restorations have a number of advantages of the hard acrylics in that they tend to produce a more natural skin tone. They are flexible, similar to soft tissue, and light in weight: they may be self-retentive, using undercut areas such as the orbit, and they provide patient comfort (Figs. 15 and 16).

Several methods have been developed for coloring and tinting: these may be intrinsic, extrinsic, or a combination of both, which in many cases is desirable to obtain the more natural effect. The greatest disadvantage of the flexible materials is the deterioration of the prosthesis because of the perishable nature of the available materials and the consequent need for periodic replacement. This problem, however, can be easily rectified by retaining the mother mold used in the duplication of the prosthesis. Proper color records and charts should be maintained and adjusted at the final fitting of the prosthesis.

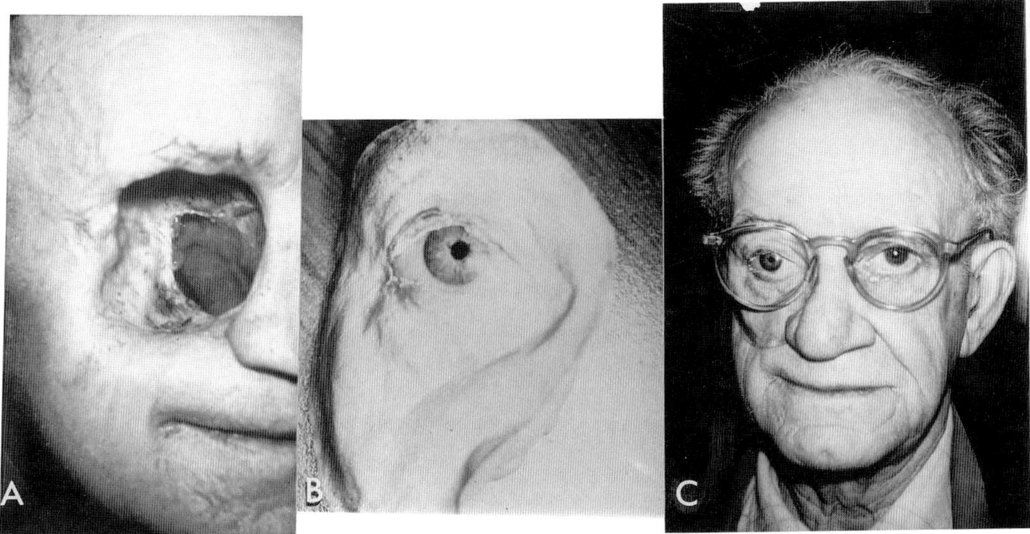

Figure 14. (A) Patient with extensive orbital deformity. (B) Facial prosthesis made of silicone. (C) Patient wearing orbital prosthesis.

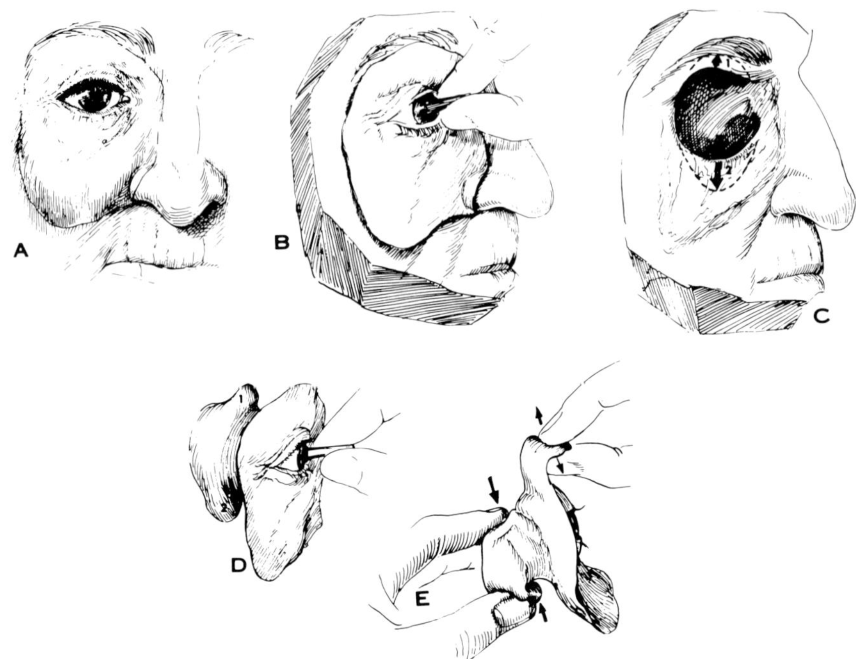

Figure 15. (A) Orbital prosthesis in position. (B) Prosthesis is removed with a suction cup applied to the ocular prosthesis. (C) Recesses 1 and 2 behind the supraorbital and infraorbital rim are used for retention. (D) Addition of a posterior extension which will fit into the recesses 1 and 2. (E) Demonstrating the resiliency of the silicone prosthesis.

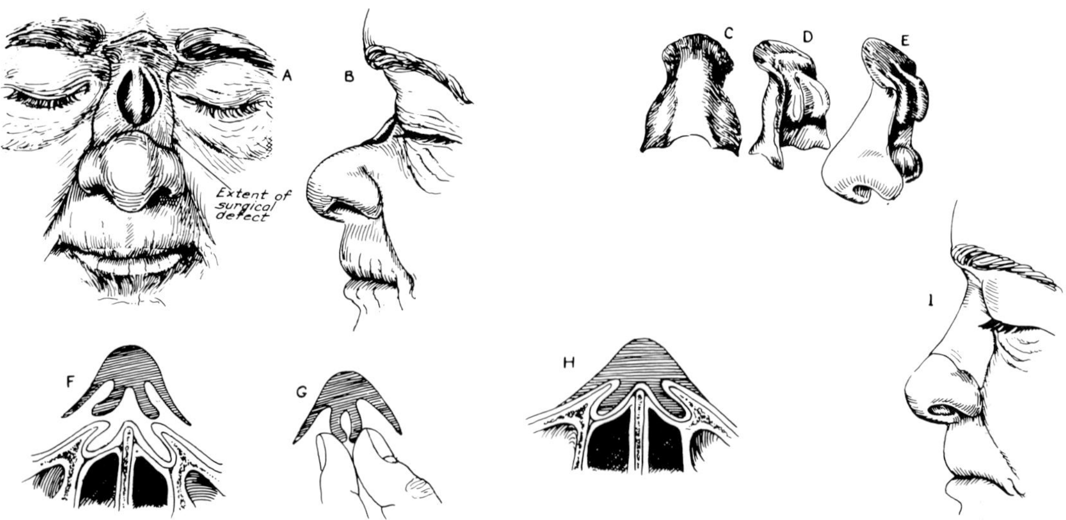

Figure 16. (A,B) Extent of nasal deformity. (C,D) Views of the partial nasal prosthesis. (E) Side view of a complete nasal prosthesis. (F,G,H) Illustration of retention obtained with flexible plastic material which is easily adapted to the remaining anatomical areas. (I) Partial flexible nasal prosthesis in position.

CONCLUSION

The magnitude of the accomplishments in fabricating lifelike facial prostheses over the years becomes apparent when reviewing the art and science of materials and techniques developing to their present state. The prosthestist who in past centuries made his usual contrivance did not have at his disposal the numerous versatile materials and elaborate equipment that are now readily available.

Retention of the prosthesis was always a problem. Today we have developed better adhesives. Because of the strength and flexibility of our silicones we have designed more mechanically retentive prostheses (see Figs. 15 and 16).

More recently osseointegration implantology [34] has been introduced for better retention. The quality of material has been improved so that it is difficult to tell where the deformity ends and the prosthesis begins (see Fig. 16). Cases like the Gunner with Silver Mask today would probably be treated by means of microvascular surgery replacing both bone and soft tissue from other parts of the body, aided by intraoral prosthesis stabilized with osseointegrated implants.

Facial deformities such as noses and ears are also replaced by surgical means with acceptable results. However, these are cases where surgery is contraindicated and facial prostheses are of a great value to the patient.

Orbital prostheses are best used for patients who are deformed by trauma or disease or congenital malformations beyond the scope of surgical correction. No surgical procedure exists that can entirely replace the eye and eyelids. Orbital prosthetic therapy throughout history has been the most difficult problem to solve, especially since the eye and lids must move to function. The prosthetic replacement has no movement. What will the future bring?

Note — I am sure that during the development of facial prosthetics many prosthodontists, chemists, and technicians have been involved; if they do not see their names in this chapter, the omission was not intentional.

REFERENCES

1. Gray PHK: Radiograph of ancient Egyptian mummies. *Med Radiogr Phot* 1967;43:2–36.
2. Popp H: Zur Geschichte Der Prothesen, Med. Welt, 1939; 13:961–964.
3. Controy B, Hulterstrom A: The history and development of facial prosthetics. *Dent Tech* 1978; 31(3):11–12.
4. Valauri AJ: Principles of maxillofacial prosthetics. In: Kazanjian VH and Converse JM (ed): *The Surgical Treatment of Facial Injuries.* 3rd Ed. Baltimore, MD, Williams & Wilkins Company, 1974: 1408.
5. Valauri AJ: Maxillofacial prosthetics: In theory and practice. *Dermatol Surg* 1975; 1:52.
6. Valauri AJ: Maxillofacial prosthetics: In Epstein E. (ed): *Skin Surgery.* Springfield, IL, Charles C Thomas, 1977; 253–271.
7. Valauri AJ: The orbit. In Converse JM (ed): *Reconstructive Plastic Surgery.* 2nd Ed. Philadelphia, PA, WB Saunders Co., 1977: 962.
8. Valauri AJ: Maxillofacial prosthetics. In Converse JM (ed): *Reconstructive Plastic Surgery.* 2nd Ed. Philadelphia, PA, WB Saunders Co., 1977: 2917.
9. Valauri AJ: *Diagnostico e tratamento das lesoes adquiridas da face.* In I Simposio Latino Americano De Reabilitacao Da Face E de Prostese Buco-Maxilo-Facial. Proceedings First Latin-American Symposium of Maxillofacial Prosthetics Rehabilitation of the Face, Sao Paolo, Brazil, 1979: 5.
10. Valauri AJ: Maxillofacial prosthetics. *Aesth Plast Surg* 1982; 6:159.
11. Valauri AJ (ed): Maxillofacial prosthetics. In: McCoy FJ, et al. (eds): *The Yearbook of Plastic and Reconstructive Surgery, 1984.* Chicago, IL, Year Book Medical Publishers, 1984: 82.
12. Paschke H: Die Epithetische Behandlung Von Gesichtedefekten Johann Ambosius Barth Verlag Munchen, 1957.
13. Lufkin AW: *A History of Dentistry.* Philadelphia, PA, Lea and Febiger, 1939: 69–70.
14. Pare A (1579): "The Opera". The Workes of That Famous Chirurgien Ambrose Pare, Translated out of the Latin and Compared with the French by Tho: Johnson, London, Richard Cotes and Willi Du-Gard (1649), 578.

15. Dreyer JLE: *Tycho Brahe*, New York, The Macmillan Company, 1890.
16. Fauchard P: Quoted by Kingsley NW: *Oral Deformities*, N.Y., Appleton, 1880, 218.
17. Whymper, W: The Gunner with the Silver Mask, *London Med Gaz* 1833; 12:705–709.
18. Saunders RL de CH: The Gunner with the Silver Mask. *Ann M History* 1941; volume 3 8s:283–287.
19. Dellabarre CF: Traite de Portie Mecanique de L'art du Chirurgien-dentiste, Paris: 1820; Vol. 2.
20. Woodward GS: *The Man Who Conquered Pain — a Biography of William Thomas Green Morton*. Boston, MA, Beacon Press, 1962; 30.
21. Kingsley NW: *A Treatise on Oral Deformities*. New York, D. Appleton and Co., 1880: Book Chapter XIV, 306–360.
22. Martin C: *De La Prosthèse Immediate*, Paris, Masson, Libraire De L'Academie de Medecine Boulevard Saint-Germain et rue de l'Eperou, en face de l'Ecole de Medecine, 1889: 259–373.
23. Tetamore FLR: *Deformities of the Face and Orthopedics*. Brooklyn, NY, Press of the Adams Printing Co., 1894.
24. Bulbulian AH: *An Improved Technic for Prosthetic Restoration of Facial Defects by Use of a Latex Compound*. Proc Staff Meet, Mayo Clin 1939; 14:433–439.
25. Bulbulian AH: *Facial Prosthesis*. Philadelphia, PA, WB Saunders Co., 1945.
26. Upham RH: *Artificial Noses and Ears*. Boston, MA, 1901: 145, 522–523.
27. Kazanjian VH: Prosthetic restoration of acquired deformities of the superior maxillo. *J Allied Dent Soc* 1915; 10:1423.
28. Kazanjian VH: Modern accomplishments in dental and facial prosthesis. *J Dent Res* 1932; 12:651.
29. Kazanjian VH, Converse JM: *The Surgical Treatment of Facial Injuries*. Baltimore, MD, Williams & Wilkins Co., 1959: 30, 1041–1070.
30. Kazanjian VH: Problems of prosthetic restoration following injuries of the face and jaw. *Mil Dent J* 1922; 5:69–86.
31. Kazanjian VH: Treatment of nasal deformities. *JAMA* 1925: 84; 177–181.
32. Cleaver M: *Prosthetic Treatment of Facial Defects Proceedings*, Facial Disfigurement, A Rehabilitation Problem. A Conference of the I.R.P.S. of the N.Y.U. Medical Center, New York, U.S. Dept. of Health, Education, and Welfare, 1963.
33. *Maxillofacial Prosthetics* — Proceedings of an Interprofessional Conference. Sponsored by the American Academy of Maxillofacial Prosthetics. Washington, D.C., September, 1966.
34. Parel SM, Branemark P-I, et al: Osseointegration in maxillofacial prosthetics. Part II: Extraoral applications. *J Prosthet Dent* 1986; 55:600–606.

Three Dimensional Imaging and Computer-Designed Prostheses in the Evaluation and Management of Orbitocranial Deformities

Don S. Ellis, M.D., Bryant A. Toth, M.D., and William B. Stewart, M.D.

ABSTRACT

Three dimensional images reconstructed from two dimensional CT scans allow improved analysis of complex orbitocranial bony deformities. This evaluation may be useful in patients with defects resulting from trauma, tumor, congenital abnormalities, or developmental disorders. Diagnosis, surgical management, and long-term follow-up evaluation may be aided by improved understanding of bony contour and volume analysis. Computer designed prostheses can be fabricated to precisely match bony defects and may be used as an alloplastic implant or as a model to aid intraoperative contouring of an autogenous bone graft. The limitations of three dimensional imaging include artifacts in the reconstructed images, increased radiation exposure, and increased cost. The technology is still evolving and the indications and benefits remain undefined at the present time.

INTRODUCTION

Complex bony anatomy makes analysis of orbitocranial abnormalities difficult. Analysis of three dimensional images reconstructed from two dimensional computerized tomographic scanning can facilitate the understanding and evaluation of normal and abnormal bony anatomy. This technology has been discussed and evaluated with increasing frequency in recent years [1–10].

Three dimensional imaging may be useful in selected patients with complex orbitocranial bony deformities due to trauma, congenital processes such as craniosynostosis, neoplasms, and developmental disorders such as fibrous dysplasia. This imaging can be useful for diagnosis [7], formulation of a management plan or surgical approach [1,2,6,8,11], evaluation of postoperative results, and for longitudinal evaluation with serial studies. For example, longitudinal evaluation may be especially useful in monitoring the growth and change of the anophthalmic socket in a child undergoing treatment with progressively larger ocular prostheses or conformers. Furthermore, contour and volume analysis are qualitatively aided by a dramatic pictorial display of the bony anatomy. Efforts have been made to quantitatively determine orbital volume with the use of sophisticated computer analysis [12–14].

A computer-guided milling device can be used to fabricate prostheses corresponding to the orbitocranial bony defect defined in the three dimensional scan [3,8,15]. Alternatively, a three dimensional model of the skull can be constructed for preparation of a custom prosthesis [9]. Prostheses can be used as an alloplastic implant or as a template to fashion autogenous bone

261

grafts [8,16]. Three dimensional images and models can be used for graphic illustration during discussions with the patient and family.

MATERIALS AND METHODS

An array of computer software programs are available for three dimensional image construction from CT or magnetic resonance imaging (MRI) data [1,2,4–8,10,14]. Most programs are designed to reconstruct bony anatomy and to accept information from a variety of CT scanners. Serial cuts of 1.5 mm on a high resolution scanner are usually needed to create three dimensional images of adequate resolution. Although it is possible to reconstruct soft tissue contours from CT or MRI data, the computer software for these applications is not as well-developed and the results are less satisfactory [10]. Marsh and Vannier have developed a computer program to show the position of the eye within the bony anatomy [7]. Software is available to perform surgical simulation directly on a computer terminal [14].

The patients studied in our experience and the example images presented in this text were constructed with the computer hardware and software of Cemax Medical Products Inc. (Mountain View, California) and data obtained from a General Electric (Milwaukee, Wisconsin) 8800 CT scanner. The three dimensional image is viewed on a high resolution video monitor and can be rotated through 360°. Sections can be removed from the image to allow an improved view of underlying structures. The source of illumination can also be rotated through 360°.

Prostheses to closely match orbitocranial defects can be created by mirror imaging tech-

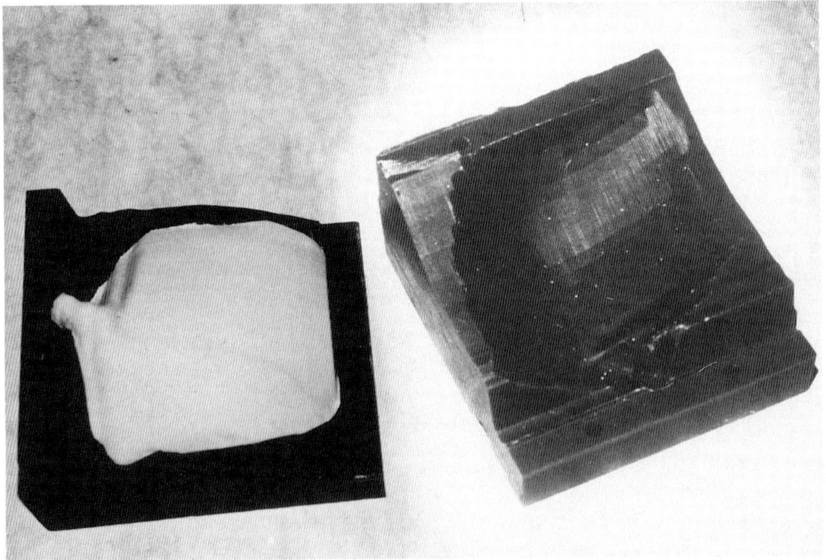

Figure 1. A wax mold, created by the computer-guided milling machine, and a resin model are shown. The resin model is used as a guide to make a methyl-methacrylate prosthesis. (Reprinted with permission from Toth BA, Ellis DS, Stewart WB: Computer designed prostheses for orbitocranial reconstruction. *Plast Reconstr Surg* 1988; 81:317–322.)

niques which subtract the defective side from a superimposed normal side. A computer-designed prosthesis is displayed on the monitor, over the bony image and in a contrasting color. Prostheses for midline defects can also be constructed with subjectively selected contour. The images can be photographed and are stored on cartridge tape for subsequent viewing at any time.

A computer-controlled three-axis milling machine can construct a mold corresponding to the computer designed prosthesis. The mold is used to make a resin model from which a methyl-methacrylate or silicone prosthesis is fabricated (Fig. 1).

CASE REPORTS

CASE 1

A 17-year-old girl had previously undergone multiple resections of facial neurofibromatoses and right enucleation. Our preoperative examination was notable for facial soft tissue asymmetry with multiple subcutaneous masses and a large orbital mass displacing the right ocular prosthesis inferotemporally (Fig. 2). There was right upper eyelid ptosis without levator function, right lower eyelid entropion, and right seventh nerve paresis. Three dimensional images showed an enlarged right orbit with defects in the medial, lateral, superior, inferior, and posterior walls. The images were used to aid the planning of reconstructive surgery (Figs. 3 and 4).

Surgical reconstruction consisted of resection of orbital and subcutaneous facial neurofibromatoses, right facial rhytidectomy, right orbital floor reconstruction with split-thickness

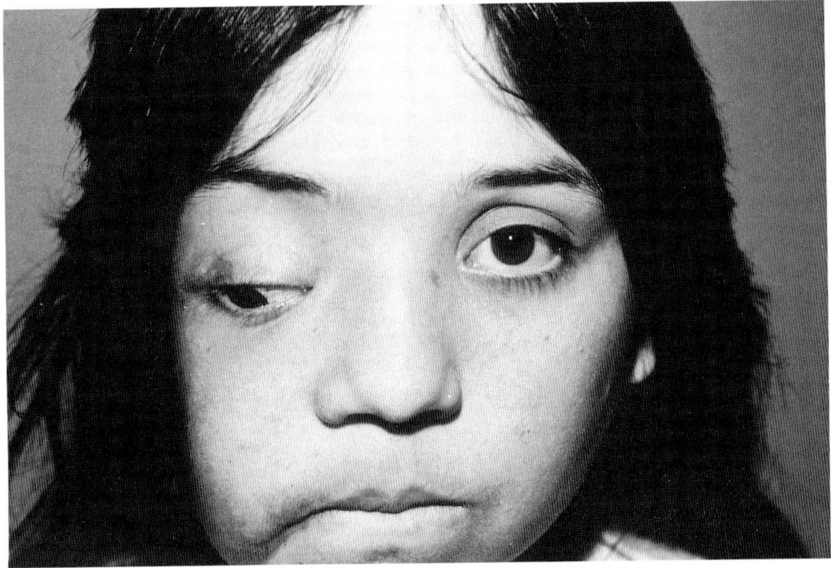

Figure 2. Case 1. Preoperative photograph of a 17-year-old girl with neurofibromatosis. Facial soft tissue deformity, ocular dystopia, and right upper eyelid ptosis are present.

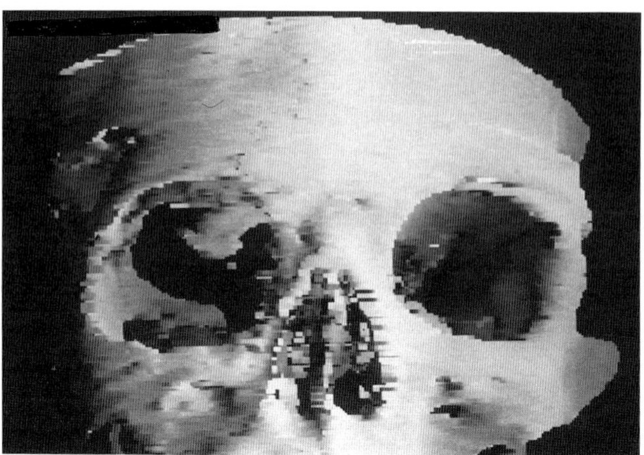

Figure 3. Three dimensional image of Case 1 shows an enlarged right orbit with defects in the lateral, medial, posterior, and inferior walls. Asymmetry of the malar complex is evident.

autogenous cranial bone, and lateral canthoplasty. A second procedure consisted of further excision of facial neurofibromatoses with scar revision, repair of upper lid ptosis with a silicone frontalis suspension, and full-thickness everting sutures for repair of lower lid entropion. The postoperative course was uncomplicated and results were satisfactory (Fig. 5).

CASE 2

A 47-year-old man, previously reported [8], sustained a gun-shot injury to his left orbit and maxillary sinus. Left enucleation was performed at the time of his original injury; the eyelids

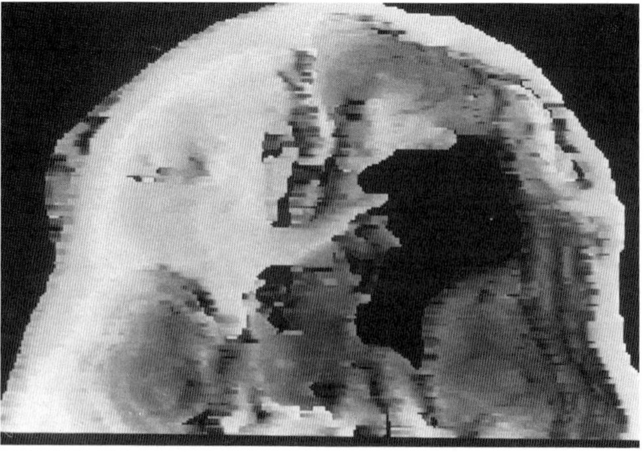

Figure 4. Axial view of Case 1 shows the orbit from above with the superior cranium removed. An extensive defect in the orbital roof is evident.

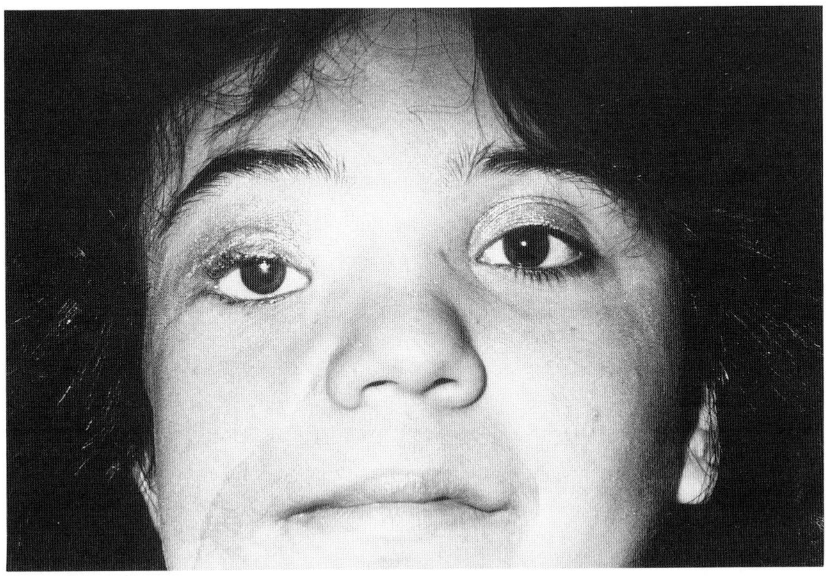

Figure 5. Postoperative photograph of Case 1 shows improvement in facial symmetry with improved soft tissue contour, eyelid position, and ocular alignment.

and deep orbital tissues were preserved. The maxillary sinus communicated with the orbit (Fig. 6).

Three dimensional images were used for evaluation of bony contour and orbital volume (Fig. 7). The medial, lateral, and inferior walls of the orbit were disrupted. A computer generated prosthesis was fabricated for use in reconstruction of the inferior and lateral orbital rims (Fig. 8). Reconstruction of the bony orbit is necessary prior to attempting orbital volume replacement and the fitting of an ocular prosthesis. The patient was lost to follow-up before reconstructive surgery was performed.

CASE 3

A 5-year-old boy, previously reported [8], had undergone exenteration of the right orbit, including the eyelids, at one week of age (Fig. 9) because an extensive blue nevus affecting the right globe and periocular soft tissues was clinically suspected to be a malignant melanoma. Three dimensional images at 5 years of age showed marked hypoplasia of the right orbit (Fig. 10). A computer designed prosthesis was created to show the extent of bony deficiency in the orbit and malar complex (Fig. 11).

CASE 4

A 33-year-old man sustained severe facial trauma in an automobile accident one year prior to exam. The right ocular prosthesis was enophthalmic and displaced inferiorly. There was a depressed right malar complex and a saddle deformity of the nose. CT scan showed a comminuted fracture of the right frontal bone, a depressed fracture of the right malar complex,

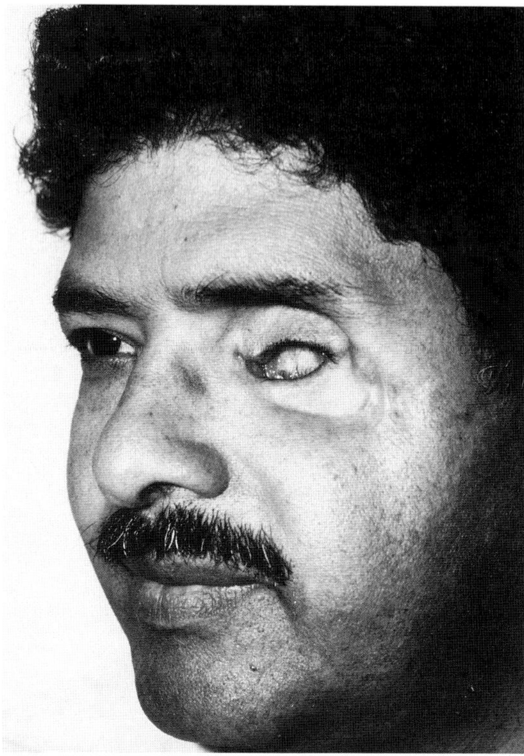

Figure 6. Case 2. This 47-year-old man has posttraumatic anophthalmos with a fistulous tract connecting the maxillary sinus to the orbit. Asymmetry of the malar complex is evident.

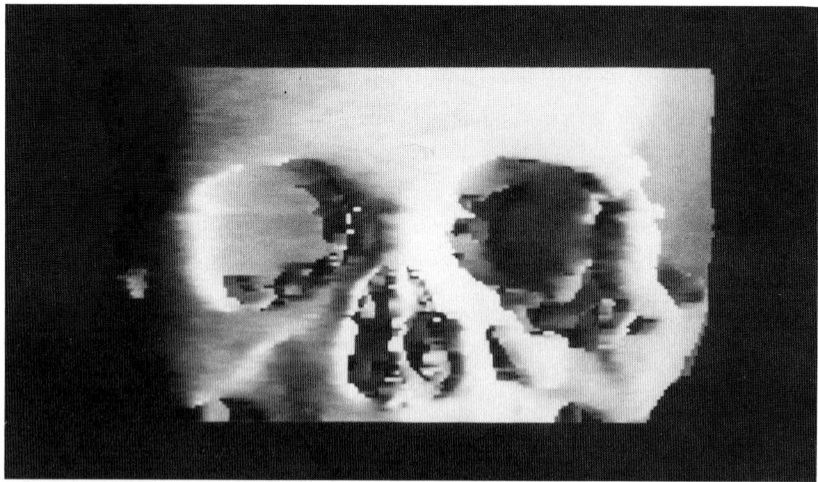

Figure 7. Three dimensional image of Case 2 shows a depressed malar complex. The obital floor defect is not apparent in this view.

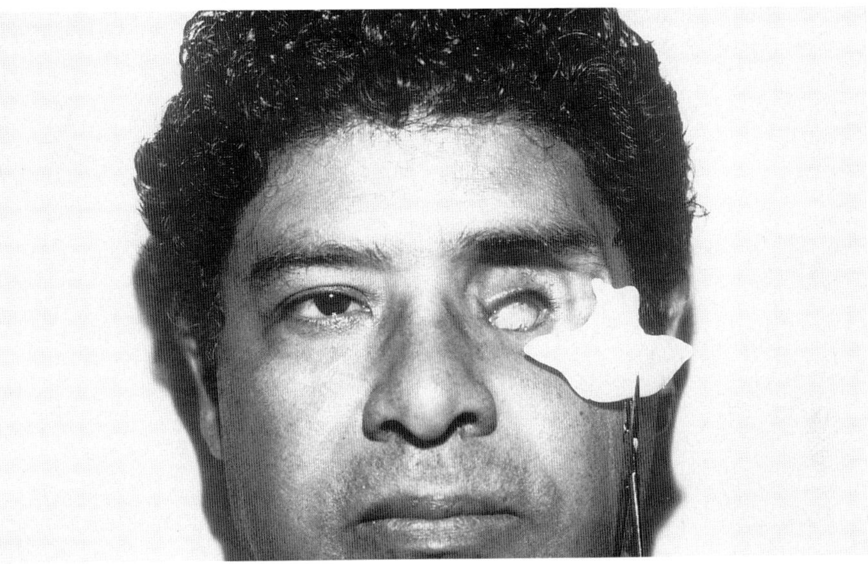

Figure 8. Case 2. The computer-designed prosthesis is shown overlying the malar complex deformity, demonstrating the requirements of bony orbital reconstruction.

and defects in the orbital floor and roof. Three dimensional images were reviewed prior to a staged reconstruction (Fig. 12) but were of minimal use for preoperative planning of a multistaged reconstructive effort. The first stage of reconstruction was the placement of a methylmethacrylate sphere implant wrapped with eye bank slcera and was then followed by

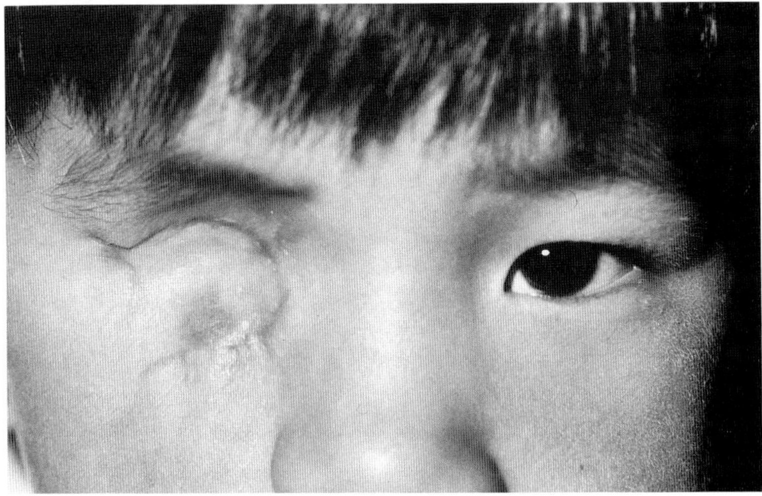

Figure 9. Case 3. Photograph of a 5-year-old boy who had exenteration at age one week.

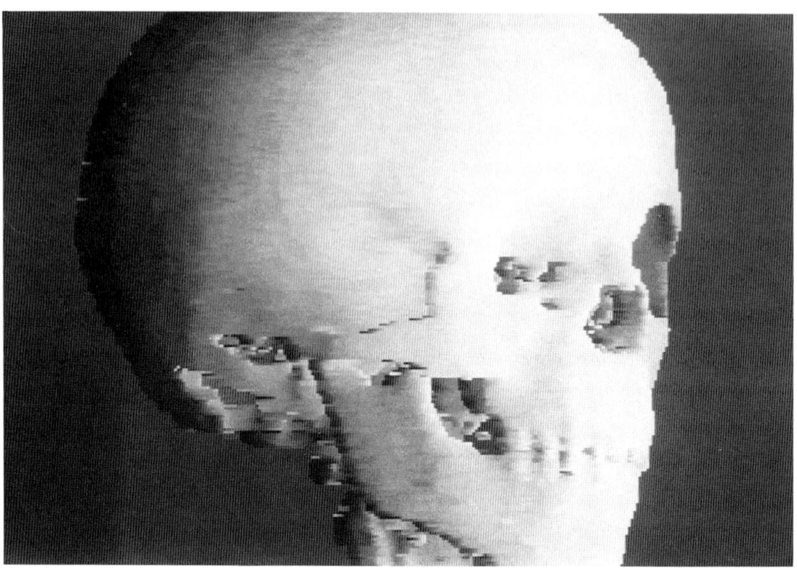

Figure 10. Three dimensional image of Case 3 shows marked right orbital hypoplasia with decreased orbital volume.

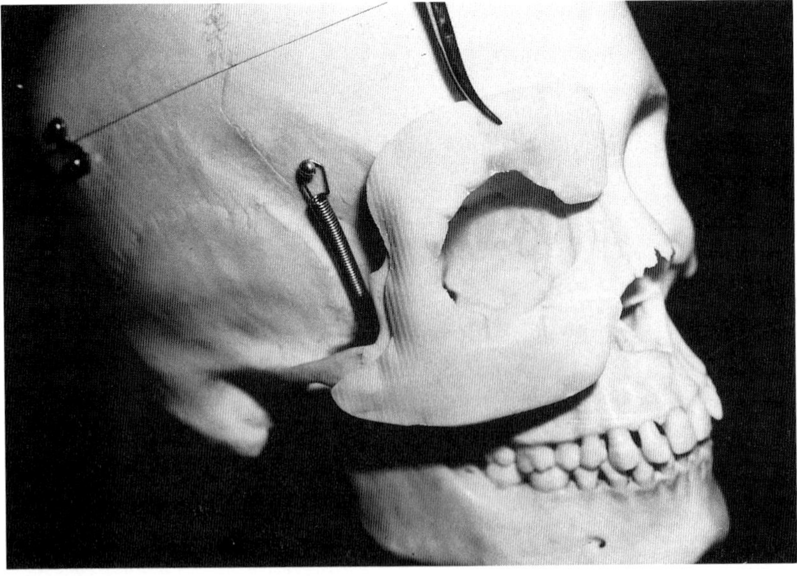

Figure 11. The computer-generated prosthesis for Case 3 is shown overlying a normal adult human skull. The prosthesis shows the contour and volume of bony deficiency and indicates the requirements of orbital bony reconstruction.

frontocranial recontouring with the high speed burr, autogenous split-thickness cranial bone graft to the orbital floor, and rhinoplasty with autogenous split-thickness cranial bone graft. The third stage of reconstruction required repair of lower lid ectropion by a lateral tarsal strip, revision of the rhinoplasty, and forehead scar revision.

CASE 5

A 24-year-old man sustained a LeForte II fracture, comminuted left orbital floor fracture, and left scleral laceration in an automobile accident. He underwent multiple ophthalmic surgeries, including vitrectomy and retinal reattachment procedures, in the left eye. When evaluated at 31 years of age, he was wearing an ocular prosthesis over a phthsical eye with light perception vision. Three dimensional images showed a depressed fracture of the malar complex and a large orbital floor fracture (Fig. 13). The orbital floor was repaired with autogenous split-thickness cranial bone. In this patient, three dimensional images were no more useful than the standard two dimensional CT scan in contributing to the development of the surgical plan.

CASE 6

A 66-year-old man, previously reported [17], had an orbitocranial deformity after resection of a squamous cell carcinoma. He had undergone left exenteration and hemimaxillectomy. The orbit communicated with the oropharynx. Three dimensional images graphically

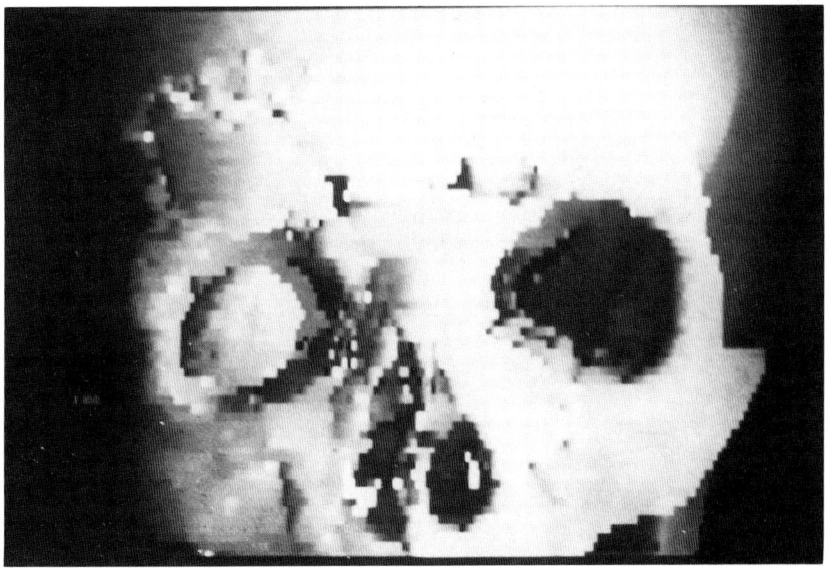

Figure 12. Three dimensional image of Case 4. Depressed fracture of right malar complex is shown. There is right lateral orbital wall irregularity and right frontal bone discontinuity. Right ocular prosthesis is shown, displaced inferiorly.

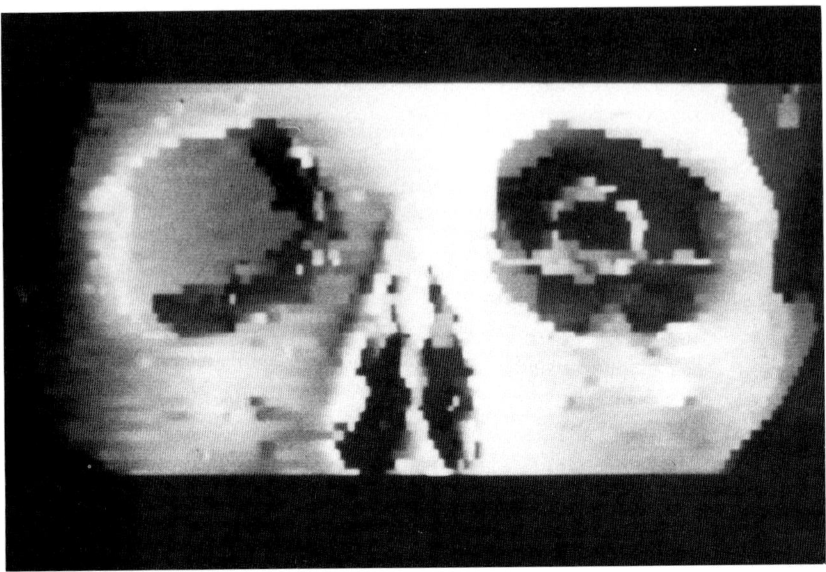

Figure 13. Three dimensional image of Case 5. Depressed fracture of left malar complex is shown. Scleral band from previous repair of retinal detachment is seen. The large left orbital floor fracture readily seen on CT is not easily seen on this three dimensional image.

showed the extensive area of bone and soft tissue loss (Fig. 14), and were an aid to formulating a reconstructive plan. Reconstruction was accomplished with a free flap of the latissimus dorsi muscle.

DISCUSSION

We have used three dimensional imaging to study over 50 patients with a range of orbital problems. Patient evaluation and surgical management can be aided, in selected cases, by three dimensional image analysis and computer-assisted prosthesis manufacture. Preoperative planning is easier because complex reconstructive requirements may be better understood. This is illustrated by Cases 1 and 6. Surgical results may be improved and the length of surgery may be reduced by using an accurate prefabricated prosthesis. The prosthesis is used as an alloplastic implant when use of an autogenous bone graft is not desirable, such as when donor material is not available. When the patient is young or when postoperative infection is a concern, an autogenous bone graft is preferred and a predesigned prosthesis may facilitate the selection of a donor site and the intraoperative contouring of the graft.

The shortcomings of three dimensional analysis and computer-designed prostheses have been discussed [7,10]. The reformatted images may have missing or incorrect information, because structures may be smaller than the 1.5 mm CT slices. Errors in volume averaging may create pseudoforamina (defects in bony contours where there actually are none) or the obliteration of true foramina, small fractures or narrow sutures (such as in the evaluation of craniosynostosis) [7]. The increased radiation exposure (especially with repeated scans), the increased time necessary to perform adequate scans with multiple closely spaced slices and

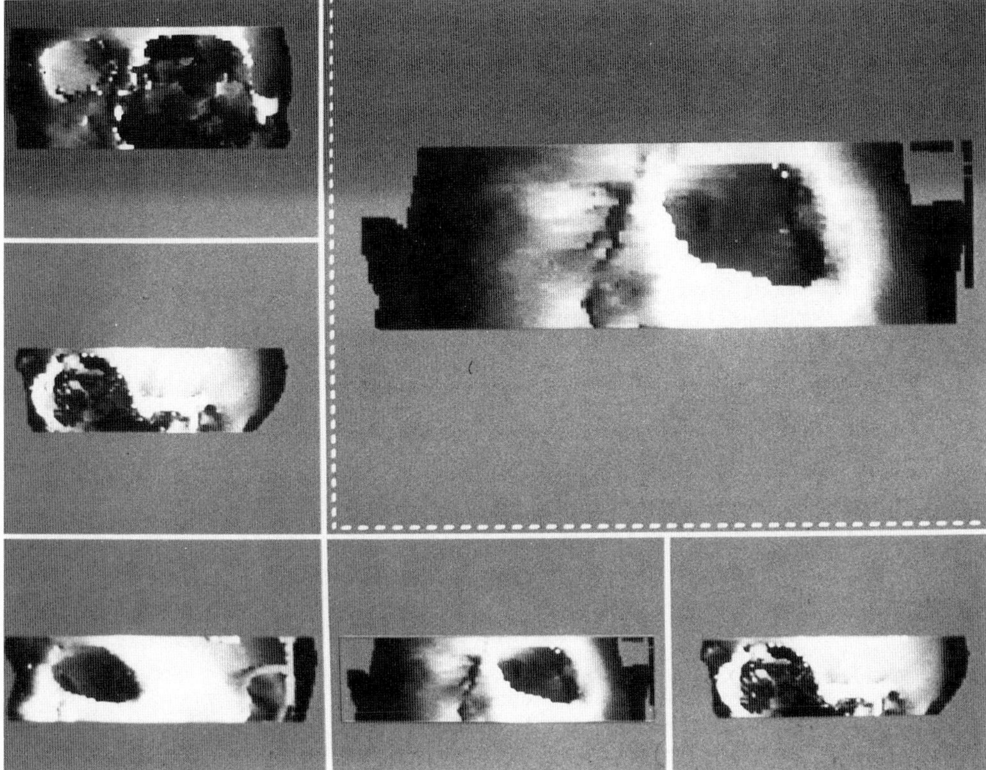

Figure 14. Three dimensional images of Case 6. Clockwise from upper right: frontal view of soft tissue contours shows enlarged exenterated left orbit and maxillary sinus; left three-fourths view of bony contour; frontal view of soft tissue contour; left three-fourths view of soft tissue contour; left three-fourths view of bony contour; frontal view of bony contour shows extensive bone loss.

the increased cost may not be justified. Distortion induced by metallic objects may preclude the usefulness of this technology in certain patients. The three dimensional images provide dramatic pictures but it must be remembered that those skilled in analyzing two dimensional studies may gain no additional information. In Case 4 there was no clear benefit obtained from the three dimensional images.

The techniques, software, and applications of three dimensional analysis and computer-assisted prosthesis manufacture are evolving. The appropriate selection of patients for these modalities is undefined at present and surgery may not be indicated in all patients studied. Adequate long-term follow-up is lacking. These techniques need validation as determined by prospective studies with comparison to standard evaluation and treatment methods.

REFERENCES

1. Hemmy DC, David DJ, and Herman GT: Three dimensional reconstruction of craniofacial deformity using computed tomography. *Neurosurg* 1983; 13:534–541.
2. Marsh JL and Vannier MW: The "third" dimension in craniofacial surgery. *Plast Reconstr Surg* 1983; 71:759–767.

3. Woolson ST, Dev P, Fellingham LL and Vassiliadis A: Three dimensional imaging of bone from computerized tomography. *Clin Orthopaedics* 1986; 202:239–248.

4. Knapp RH, Vannier MW and Marsh JL: Generation of three dimensional images from CT scans: Technological perspective. *Radiol Technol* 1985; 56:391–398.

5. Arridge S, Moss JP, Linney AD and James DR: Three dimensional digitization of the face and skull. *J Max-Fac Surg* 1985; 13:136–143.

6. Jackson IT and Bite U: Three dimensional computed tomographic scanning and major surgical reconstruction of the head and neck. *Mayo Clin Proc* 1986; 61:546–555.

7. Marsh JL and Vannier MW: The anatomy of the cranio-orbital deformities of craniosynostosis: Insights from 3-D images of CT scans. *Clin Plast Surg* 1987; 14:49–60.

8. Toth BA, Ellis DS and Stewart WB: Computer-designed prostheses for orbitocranial reconstruction. *Plast Reconstr Surg* 1988; 81:315–322.

9. Marsh JL: *Advanced radiologic technology in the evaluation of facial trauma.* Presented at the annual meeting of the American Society of Plastic and Reconstructive Surgeons, November 1, 1983, Dallas, Texas.

10. Katowitz JA, Herman GT, Whitaker LA and Welsh MG: Three-dimensional computed tomographic imaging. *Ophthalmic Plast Reconstr Surg* 1987; 3:243–248.

11. Vannier MW, Marsh JL and Warren JO: Three dimensional CT reconstruction images for craniofacial surgical planning and evaluation. *Radiology* 1984; 150:179–184.

12. Hemmy DC and Tessier PL: CT of dry skulls with craniofacial deformities: accuracy of three dimensional reconstruction. *Radiology* 1985; 157:113–116.

13. Forbes G, Gehring DG, Gorman CA, Brennan MD and Jackson IT: Volume measurements of normal orbital structures by computed tomographic analysis. *Am J Neuroradiol* 1985; 6:419–424.

14. Cutting C, Grayson B, Bookstein F, Fellingham L and McCarthy JG: Computer-aided planning and evaluation of facial and orthognathic surgery. *Clin Plast Surg* 1986; 13:449–462.

15. Young SW, White DN, Kaplan EN, Dev P, and Wood S: CT and NMR contour-finding algorithm for automated organ volume calculation, 3-dimensional CRT scan display and prosthesis milling. *Radiology* 1983; 149(p):275.

16. Toth BA, Stewart WB, Elliot LF: Computer designed prostheses for orbitocranial reconstruction. In: Marchac, D (ed): *Craniofacial Surgery.* Proceedings of the First International Congress of the International Society of Cranio-Maxillo-Facial Surgery. Cannes-La Napoule, 1985: 19–24. Berlin Heidelberg, Springer-Verlag, 1987.

17. Stewart WB, Toth BA: A multidisciplinary approach to orbital neoplasm. *Clin Plast Surg* 1988; 15:263–272.

Impressions for Oculofacial Prosthetics

Donald Mitchell, D.D.S., and Barry Shipman, D.M.D.

ABSTRACT

Primary to the development of an acceptable and functional facial prosthesis *is the* impression procedure. *The fabrication of a facial prosthesis combines the art and science of anatomy, cosmesis, and function, to develop a nonliving substitute to replace altered, missing, or defective regions of the head and neck area. Success depends on patient's cooperation, motivation, and commitment to treatment as well as the technical and artistic scope of the facial prosthetic service.*

INTRODUCTION

The construction of an orbital or oculofacial prosthesis involves the art and science of anatomical, cosmetic, and functional reconstruction by the use of nonliving substitutes to replace those areas of the head and the face that are traumatically or congenitally missing or surgically lost. Successful maxillofacial rehabilitation depends on the patient's cooperation, motivation, and commitment to treatment as well as the technical skills and artistic talents of the maxillofacial prosthodontist. Of primary importance to the development of an acceptable and functional orbital prosthesis is the impression procedure. Appropriate prosthesis form and function can only be obtained when the orbital prosthesis is accurately fitted to the supporting tissues. It must blend with the adjacent anatomical structures in a smooth and harmonious nature. The importance of selecting the appropriate impression material and making an accurate facial impression is apparent when the facial prosthesis accurately fits the supporting tissues and meets the aesthetic and functional requirements of the patient.

Historically the construction of orbital and facial prostheses dates to the ancient civilizations of Greece, Rome, and Egypt. Archeological excavation of ancient Egyptian graves has revealed mummies with artificial eyes, noses, and other facial parts. During the 2nd century reports of the fabrication of lacquer noses have been noted but descriptions of impression techniques and impression materials are unavailable. Writings during the 16th century record the recommendations of Ambroise Paré, describing facial prosthetic restorations and the methods of attachment. Claude Martine devoted much time and energy to facial prosthetic construction and to the use of new and innovative retention techniques. In 1894 Tetamore described the fabrication of a nasal prosthesis using facial impressions made at different head positions. This recorded for the first time the impression technique and indicated its importance to the overall development of the facial prosthesis [1].

When reviewing the history of facial prosthetics a lack of investigation and standardization of impression materials and impression techniques is clearly evident. Descriptions of impression procedures are difficult to find and when available, they generalize and incompletely describe the clinical procedures. Most often, impression techniques are directly related to operator preference and the working properties of the material.

This article will organize the facial–orbital impression process into a concise, practical, and accurate step by step process. The critical factors for clinical success with orbital and facial impressions include the following factors: a knowledge of orbit and facial anatomy; an understanding of the properties of the impression materials; a knowledge of the impression procedure; the evaluation of tissue tolerance; and an understanding of the psychology of facial disfigurement.

IMPRESSION MATERIALS

The selection of an impression material used for facial and orbital impressions will vary; variables such as cost, operator preference, tissue topography, and the mechanical and physical properties of the impression material are considered. The choice of materials for the facial impression process should depend primarily on those qualities that allow the development of accurate impression and accurate master casts.

A classification system for facial impression materials is important to an understanding of their selection and clinical use. Impression material can be classified as either flexible or rigid. The flexible materials presently used for facial impression procedures include: reversible and irreversible hydrocolloid, polysulfides, silicones, and polyethers. A variety of brands are available in each category and material selection primarily reflects properties of the material and operator preference. In addition to the flexible impression materials there are the rigid or nonflexible impression materials. The use of a rigid impression materials for facial and orbital impressions is somewhat limited. In certain situations a rigid impression plaster may be used to record nonmoveable facial structures. This method is appropriate when facial and orbital tissues are not easily distorted and present no tissue or bony undercuts. The rigid material most often used is impression plaster. It is highly accurate and on occasions may be a welcome addition to the impression armamentarium.

The flexible impression materials are the most common impression materials used today for both facial and orbital impressions. They vary considerably in their physical and mechanical properties. The evaluation and selection of an impression material is improved when the clinician can compare the properties of the selected material with the properties of a theoretical "ideal" material. Table 1 compares five flexible and one rigid impression material with a theoretically "ideal" material. The parameters used are primarily applicable to the extraoral impression process. The score of 5 designates the "ideal" material and represents the highest score for all standards. A review of Table 1 indicates that the material which best equals the "ideal" material with a score of 57/65 is the reversible hydrocolloid. Note that the data in Table 1 should only serve as a guide to clinical selection and represents the clinical observations of one author.

The choice of impression material for the construction of orbital prosthesis should reflect both an inherent accuracy for reproduction as well as an adaptability for a variety of clinical situations. A second set of parameters for determining the appropriate impression material is dictated by the local conditions of the tissue as well as the physical and esthetic requirements of the final prosthesis. The quality and the quantity of the surrounding tissue is important to the overall process. When the floor of the orbit is missing or when tissues are

Table 1. Comparison of Impression Materials

Properties of Ideal Material	"I" Ideal Material	Reversible Hydrocolloid	Irreversible Hydrocolloid	Silicone	Polysulfide	Polyether	Impression Plaster
Ease of preparation	5	4	4	4	4	4	4
Accuracy in clinical use	5	5	3	3	3	3	5
Setting characteristics	5	5	3	3	3	3	3
Strength	5	2	4	5	5	5	5
Dimensional stability	5	3	3	5	4	5	5
Ease of application	5	5	3	2	2	2	3
Heat transfer	5	4	5	5	5	5	3
Working time	5	5	3	3	3	3	3
Weight of material	5	5	2	2	2	2	2
Ability to add to	5	5	2	2	2	2	5
Cost of material	5	5	5	4	4	3	5
Tissue tolerance	5	5	5	5	3	5	3
Elastic properties	5	4	5	5	5	5	1

5 = Excellent; 4 = Good; 3 = Fair; 2 = Poor; 1 = Reject.

easily distorted, an impression material that causes minimal tissue movement and accurately records tissue is necessary. It is important that the placement of the impression material cause minimal tissue distortion, disengage from undercuts without distortion, and incorporate all tissue dimensions. The impression material should be able to be placed in thin layers, avoiding a large bulk of material that can easily distort moveable tissues. Setting time must be adequate to allow material application at functional head and chair positions. A material with a low viscosity and prolonged setting time is useful to allow the selective placement of impression material in areas that require great detail and have limited access. Elastic impression materials offer the ability to impress tissues with anatomical undercuts without significant permanent deformation. The degree of undercut must be evaluated according to the tissue tolerance, impression material properties, and retention needs of the prosthesis.

The accuracy of fit of facial prosthesis is, in part, determined by the accuracy and suitability of the impression material. The development of an accurate master cast, which duplicates the orbital defect is the first step in the fabrication of an oculofacial prosthesis. A simplified acrylic shell technique is one method available to ensure this accuracy. The fabrication of a clear, thin acrylic resin shell is used to verify the similarity in marginal fit of both the master cast and the patient [2]. This is accomplished by first blocking out of undercuts in the defect with wax or a water-soluble noncontaminating clay and applying a separating medium to the cast. A thin autopolymerizing polymethyl-methacrylate acrylic resin shell is fabricated with extensions 1 to 2 mm short of the proposed borders of the prosthesis. The acrylic resin shell is seated on the patient to verify marginal fit. Contour and inaccuracies are observed clinically and marked on the acrylic resin shell. Inaccuracies are corrected with wax or impression material. The stone cast is modified where the acrylic shell is marked. This is repeated until the acrylic resin shell and wax modification are well adapted to the patient. This simple step will help to verify the accuracy of the master stone cast before valuable time and effort is spent in fabricating the oculofacial prosthesis.

The acrylic resin shell can be used both to verify the accuracy of the stone cast as well as to help positioning the ocular portion of the oculofacial prosthesis. Orientation lines are located on the patient before the impression begins and transferred from the patient to the stone cast. An indelible marker and ridged ruler are used to score three vertical equidistant lines that meet the following criteria: travel through the pupil of the remaining eye while the patient is in a conversational position; transect the midline of the face; and travel through the proposed pupil position which lies equidistant from the midfacial line and the existing vertical pupil line. The three vertical lines are connected by a horizontal line drawn through the existing pupil of the remaining eye. The orientation lines are located on the patient's face before the impression begins. The orientation lines will be transferred to the stone cast by the impression. An additional aid in the location of the ocular position of the oculofacial prosthesis is accomplished by tracing with a wax pencil on a 5 × 5 inch acetate sheet (0.020 inch thick) the orbital anatomy of the remaining eye and the orientation lines directly from the patient [3]. The acetate tracing is inverted over the surgical defect to verify that all orientation lines are superimposed providing the correct location of the ocular portion of the oculofacial prosthesis. The use of orientation lines will help to position the ocular portion of the orbital prosthesis. The acrylic resin shell is stabilized by using clay or Play-doh (Kenner Products, Cincinnati, Ohio), which allows repositioning because of the plasticity of the material. With the correct position of the ocular portion verified on the patient, it is stabilized and secured with wax. The orientation lines are located on the patient's face before the impression begins and can be removed with soap and water.

IMPRESSION PROCEDURE

An accurate clinical technique for making facial impressions is essential for the development of accurately fitting orbital and facial prosthesis. This next section will describe specific impression techniques and discuss some basic parameters in the selection of materials to the impression process. Bulbulian [4] noted that one of the basic requirements for all facial prosthesis is a normal appearance during use. To achieve this natural appearance, facial impressions must reproduce the soft tissue topography of the orbital or facial defect in as normal and natural state as possible. Regardless of the choice of impression material, patient preparation is the first step in the impression process. The preparation includes body and head position as well as the preparation of the tissues at the impression site.

PATIENT PREPARATION

Whether the etiology of the defect is traumatic, surgical, congenital, or developmental, the impression site preparation is similar. All tissue surfaces should be cleaned with a mild detergent to remove any skin oils, topical medications, dried or dead tissues. Scaly and crusty areas of facial hyperkeratosis should be debrided, removing any accumulation of sloughing skin or mucosa. Facial hair that will hinder accurate margin reproduction or fit of the prosthesis should be removed. Hair accumulations such as eyebrows, lashes, mustaches or beards that engage the impression material and cause deformation on removal should be lubricated or taped. Paper tape can be used to hold large pieces of hair out of the impression site facilitating the accuracy and removal of the impression. The use of bacteriostatic water soluble lubricant (Surgilube, E. Fougera & Co., New York) will aid impression release and will not interfere with the setting characteristics of the water-soluble impression materials such as reversible and irreversible hydrocolloid. The lubricating jelly can also be applied over areas of early healing to prevent the rupture of new granulation tissues. Irradiated tissues can be coated with lubricant to reduce tissue irritation and discomfort during the impression procedure.

Close inspection of undercut areas with bony prominence and thin epithelial coverings is important. Lubrication and block out of these areas may be necessary if they are undesirable undercuts. Diagnostic evaluation for path of removal of the impression is necessary prior to the impression process. A prominent zygomatic bone, if impressed unilaterally, allows easy removal of the impression, but bilateral engagement without lubrication and block out could present tissue and bony undercuts which result in difficulty with removal and possible distortion of the impression. Tissue tabs and redundant tissue should be surgically removed allowing as stable a supporting tissue base as possible.

Chair position and the position of the patient's head are also critical to the development of accurate impressions. In a clinical study [5], significant facial tissue distortion is seen with variation in head and chair position during the impression process. As chair position becomes obtuse, facial tissues distort. In addition, as the weight of impression material and chair position increase, this distortion is enlarged. It becomes evident that the clinical positions of patients during the impression procedure should be upright, simulating a normal functioning head position.

REVERSIBLE HYDROCOLLOID IMPRESSIONS

The impression technique used for reversible hydrocolloid is a simple and uncomplicated process. It is applicable for most impression situations for orbital and facial defects. The reversible hydrocolloid material is prepared over a hot plate or double boiler and melted to a liquid state. It is then cooled to 140° Fahrenheit and stored in a water bath until application. The defect is prepared, orientation lines are marked with indelible pencil, and the chair position determined with respect to functional requirements for prosthesis use (Fig. 1).

The material is stored at 140° Fahrenheit and reduced in temperature to 120° for application. Reversible hydrocolloid impression material is applied with a fine bristle brush to the appropriate tissue areas (Fig. 2). The material is painted in thin layers beginning at the superior border of the defect and moving in an inferior direction until the entire border of the defect is covered with material to a thickness of 1 to 2 mm. The rest of the area is covered to a similar thickness and the material is allowed to cool. The surface is inspected and thin areas are thickened with fresh hydrocolloid. No adhesive is necessary to join the layers of reversible hydrocolloid. The material will not layer and separate as is seen with other impression materials. The surface of the hydrocolloid should be left irregular during application to improve the mechanical retention of the plaster base which acts as a tray. Additional retention, if necessary, can be developed by adding gauze to a second layer of impression material. An alginate adhesive (Getz Hold, Getz Company, Elk Grove Village, IL) is then applied to the reversible hydrocolloid and allowed to dry. After adequate drying, a thin layer of laboratory plaster is painted over the reversible hydrocolloid impression material. Application of the plaster in thin layers not to exceed .5 to 1 mm at the first application is required (Fig. 3). After the initial thin application has set, a second application of plaster should be added to build the base to 3 to 4 mm (Fig. 4). An initial thin application of plaster reduces the heat generated by the setting reaction and prevents the distortion of the reversible hydrocolloid.

When the final set of plaster is completed, the entire impression is removed (Fig. 5). Moist air is blown around the peripheries of the impression. The head is bent forward and the patient is instructed to activate the facial muscles to reduce the adhesion of impression material

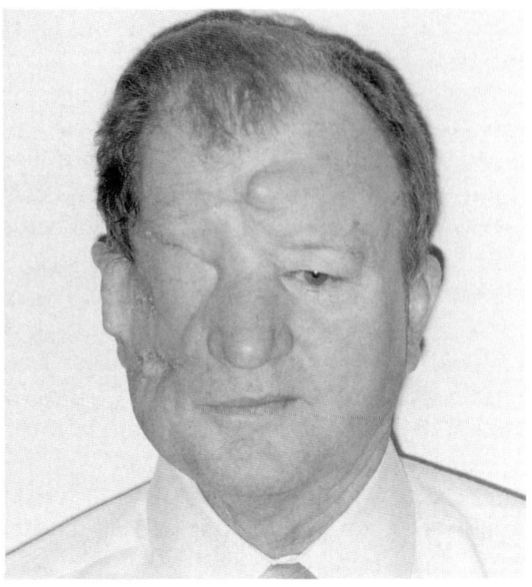

Figure 1. Impression procedure with reversible hydrocolloid: Patient ready for the impression.

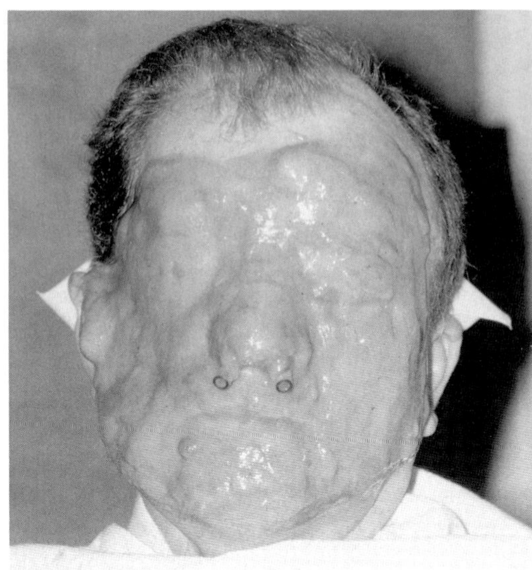

Figure 2. Hydrocolloid painted on the facial tissues.

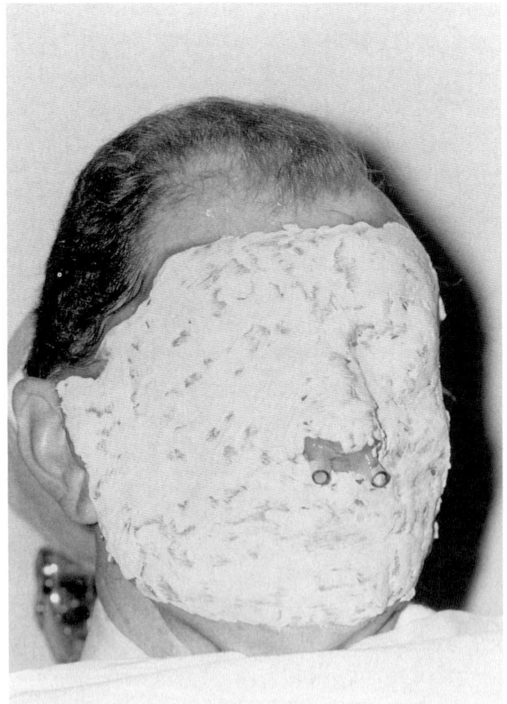

Figure 3. Thin plaster matrix painted over the hydrocolloid impression.

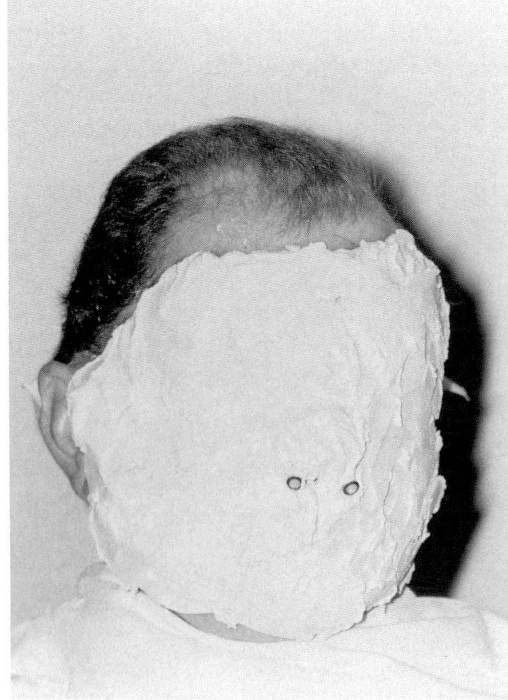

Figure 4. Plaster matrix supported with additional plaster.

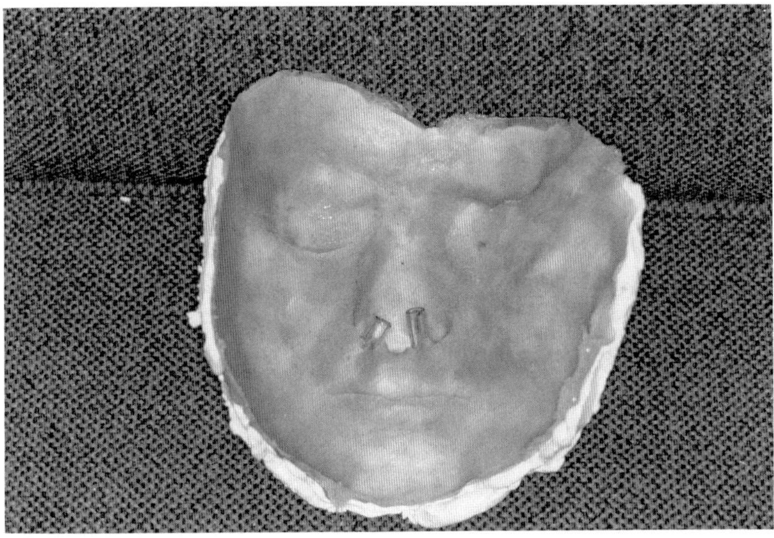

Figure 5. Hydrocolloid impression after removal from the patient.

to skin. With the aid of gravity, the impression seal is slowly broken and the impression is teased off the face and placed in a solution of 2.5% potassium sulfate for three to five minutes (Fig. 6). Any facial landmarks marked with an indelible pencil are readily transferred to the reversible hydrocolloid impression (Fig. 7) and eventually to the master cast. The impression is poured in improved stone according to manufacturer's directions. A thin layer is applied with a brush to cover the entire impression surface and allowed to set initially. Additional stone is added to a thickness of 1 to 1.5 cm to develop a strong working master cast (Fig. 8). When the cast has set, the impression is removed and the master cast trimmed accordingly (Fig. 9).

IRREVERSIBLE HYDROCOLLOID IMPRESSIONS

Another material suitable for making impressions of orbital or facial defects is irreversible hydrocolloid commonly known as "dental alginate." The base material is a fine powder to which a measured amount of water is added and mixed to a creamy homogenous mix. Irreversible hydrocolloid is a commonly used inexpensive dental impression material. Modification of the manufacturer's directions is necessary to allow proper clinical handling of the material for use in facial impressions. Approximately 25% more water should be added to the alginate powder to decrease viscosity and to increase the flow characteristics [6,7]. Patient preparation remains the same as with the reversible hydrocolloid. Excessive undercuts are blocked out with petrolatum gauze and the impression material is flowed onto the patient displacing any trapped air. The irreversible hydrocolloid can be syringed into undercuts and difficult access areas to ensure its flow. The thin irreversible hydrocolloid will capture both defect and as much surrounding tissue as the operator desires. The impression is then supported and backed with plaster of paris in a manner similar to that used with the reversible hydrocolloid.

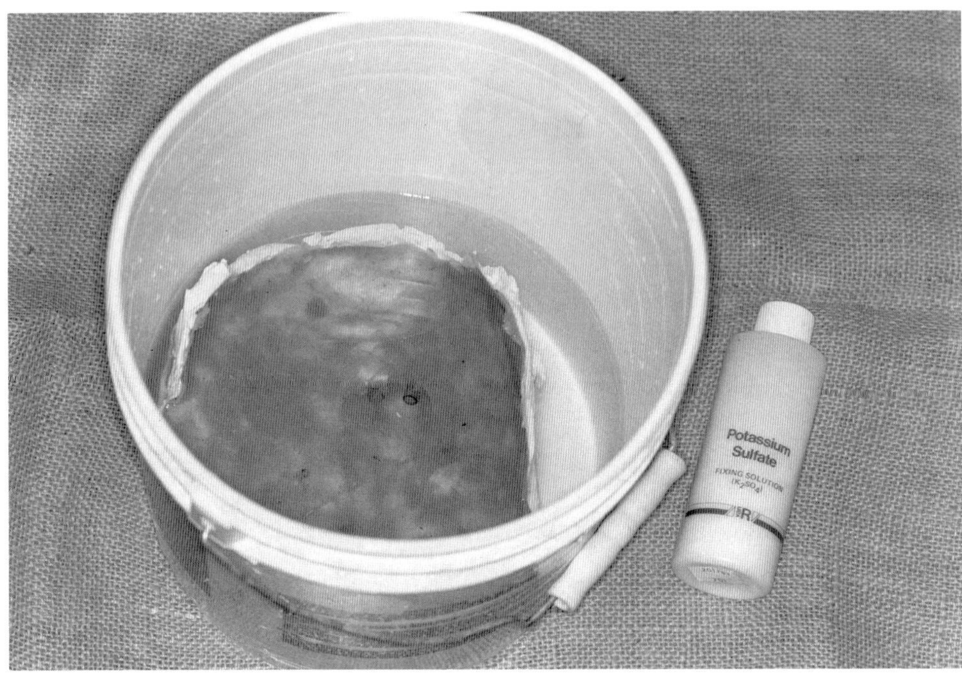

Figure 6. Impression soaking in potassium sulfate bath.

LIMITING FACTORS TO ACCEPTABLE FACIAL IMPRESSIONS

In evaluating tissue tolerance to facial impressions the clinician must critically examine and evaluate the supporting tissues for their use with facial and orbital prosthesis. Radiation therapy in conjunction with surgery alters tissues used to support the prosthesis. Tissues can become sensitive, and friable as a result of concomitant therapies. Patient tolerance to treatment will vary accordingly. The area in and around the orbit reacts to radiation as do other body tissues. The orbital tissues can become erythematous followed by desquamation with possible telangiectasis of the skin and alopecia of the lashes. These reactions vary according to the dosage, fractionation, and ports of radiation [8]. Skin grafts, myocutaneous flaps, and pedicle flaps may improve tissue conditions for prosthesis support, yet on occasion they may complicate the impression procedure. Grafted tissues do not move functionally as well as normal tissues. If the resection is confined to the contents of the orbit, the defect is easier to restore because the margins can be camouflaged with glass and are on a nonmovable base [6].

The bony orbit should be lined with skin at the time of the surgery because mucosa does not tolerate functional pressure or long-term contact with a prosthesis. On the other hand, the orbit should not be obliterated completely with skin, for that usually results in little or no room for proper ocular position and an inadequate prosthetic replacement [6]. Various methods have been used to reconstruct an orbital defect. One common method is the use of split-thickness skin grafts, which can offer support for the prosthesis, yet does not totally obliterate the ocular space. All of the surgical reconstructive procedures have both advantages and disadvantages. When a partial maxillectomy accompanies the orbital resection, a lack of bony

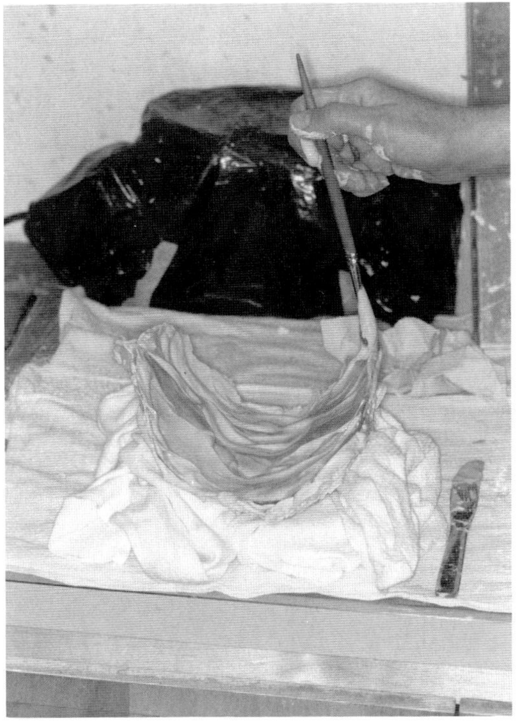

Figure 7. Initial thin matrix pour of final hydrocolloid impression.

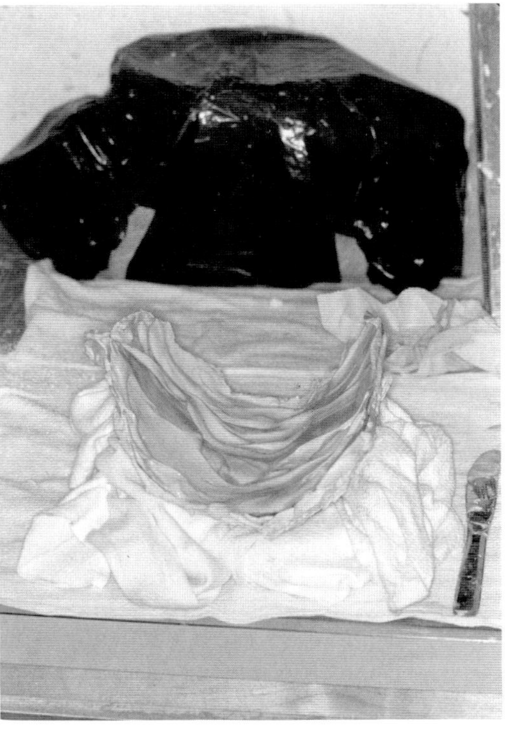

Figure 8. Impression thickened with additional stone for final set.

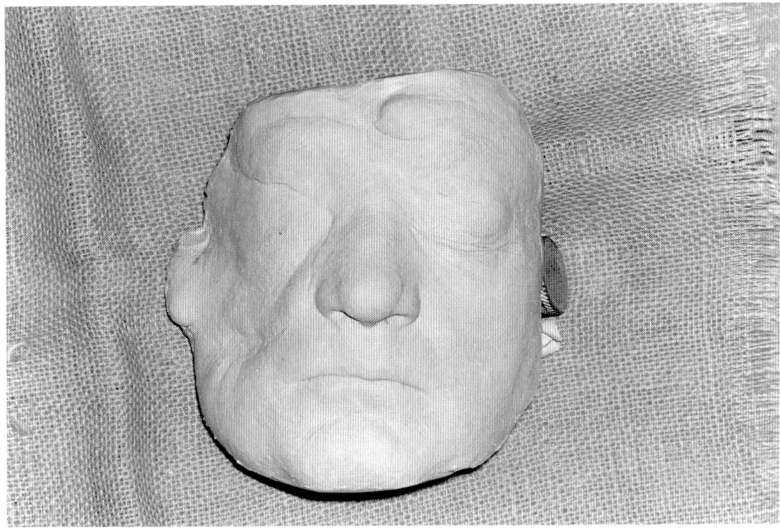

Figure 9. Final master cast in cast stone.

support is seen in the cheek region because of the loss of the maxilla and orbital floor [6]. The result is usually a concave or sunken appearance to the lateral, inferior malar and orbital areas. It is critical to replace the intraoral tissues with a definitive obturator before making the final impression of the orbital defect, as the intraoral prosthesis will serve as the underlying support for the prosthesis.

The first choice of restoration for most surgical defects is surgery. Yet because of the complexity of the orbital area and the additional loss of the eye, the rehabilitation treatment of choice in this situation is usually prosthetic. The prosthetic restoration of orbital and facial defects has several advantages unique to this particular anatomic area [9]:

1. Immediate restoration with a prosthesis that can be modified or changed as the tissue heals and matures.
2. Decreased hospitalization and fewer surgical procedures, because the prosthetic modification and prosthetic replacement can be done on an out-patient basis.
3. Economically advantageous, as the cost for prosthetics is less than surgical reconstruction.
4. Physiologically beneficial to the patients who do not have to submit to multiple surgical procedures.
5. The application of prosthetics is noninvasive and reversible; it can be a definitive or an interim process. Some surgeons prefer to wait at least one year after radical maxillofacial surgery before surgical reconstruction [6].
6. Prosthetic replacements allow direct visualization of the surgical site. This is especially beneficial when there is questionable tumor involvement at the margins of resection.

PSYCHOLOGY OF FACIAL DEFECTS

One important yet often overlooked aspect of orbital and facial prosthetic restorations is the psychological implication of facial disfigurement for the patient. Careful psychological evaluation of the patient must be an integral part of the restoration process. Explanations of procedures and the expectations of result must be part of the overall process. Postsurgical shock to the loss of a body part can be devastating to patients and their families. If patients are not prepared for their "loss" they can become depressed and exhausted physically, financially, and emotionally [10].

The size and location of the facial defect is an important influence in the rehabilitation of the patient. The rehabilitation of a facially disfigured patient requires the highest degree of skills of both the surgeon and the maxillofacial prosthodontist. There must be cooperation and a mutual effort before the first surgical procedure is begun [5]. Even though the smallest defect may be restored aesthetically with a simple ocular prosthesis, the psychological trauma for the patient is unpredictable and may result in a greater depression than a patient with a large orbital defect [5]. Aesthetically even though an ophthalmos may be successfully camouflaged, it may be devastating for the patient.

CONCLUSION

Whether the loss of facial tissues includes a simple orbital exenteration or a large composite facial resection, the impression process is critical to the development of an aesthetic, realistic, and functional prosthesis. Whether the defect is confined within the orbit with bony support surrounding the defect or extends to the nose, cheek, and forehead, a variety of problems such as moveable tissues, additional weight of the prosthesis, lack of bony support, lack of movement, and the difficulty of camouflaging the margins of the prosthesis are inevitable.

Although the primary objective of treatment is the removal of the tumor, significant disabilities are associated with this "cure." Both the surgeon and the maxillofacial prosthodontist must remember the importance of planning the surgical treatment both for cure as well as for effective rehabilitation. Knowledge of the blood supply, location and size of the defect, and the positional requirement of the ocular/orbital prosthesis must be understood by all. Primary emphasis must be placed on the quality of life for the patient [9]. Accurate impressions and well-fitting orbital and facial prosthesis play a vital role in improving the quality of cancer rehabilitation.

REFERENCES

1. Bulbulian AH: *Facial Prosthetics.* Springfield, IL, Charles C Thomas, 1973:40–67.
2. Nusinov NS, McCartney JW, Mitchell DL: The orbital shell: An aid in positioning the ocular component and verifying margin contours for oculofacial prostheses. *J Prosth Dent* 1989; 61:337–339.
3. Nusinov NS, McCartney JW, Mitchell DL: Inverted anatomical tracing: A guide to establishing orbital tissue contours for the oculofacial prosthesis. *J Prosth Dent* 1988; 60:483–485.
4. Bulbulian AH: *Facial Prosthesis*, Philadelphia, PA, WB Saunders Co., 1945:67–103.
5. Shipman B: *Proceedings from the International Congress of Maxillofacial Prosthetics and Technology.* Southampton, United Kingdom, Millbrook Press Totron, 1983:219–224.
6. Beumer, J, III, Curtis TA, and Firtell DSN: *Maxillofacial Rehabilitation Prosthodontics and Surgical Considerations.* St. Louis, MO, CV Mosby Co., 1979:311–323.
7. Laney WR: *Maxillofacial Prosthetics*, Postgraduate Dental Handbook Series, Vol 4, Littletown, MA, PS 6 Publishing Co. 1979:28–30.
8. Fletcher GH: *Textbook of Radiotherapy*, 3rd ed. Philadelphia, Lea and Febiger, 1980:18–87.
9. Myers EN, Barofsk I, and Yates JW: *Rehabilitation and Treatment of Head and Neck Cancer.* Bethesda, MD, NIH Publication #86-2762, 1986:1–47.
10. Rosen RD, Orway DE, Curtis TA, and Cantor T: Psychological aspects of maxillofacial rehabilitation Part I, The effects of primary cancer treatment. *J Prosth Dent* 1972; 28:423–28.

Comment: Calculation of the Conjunctival Area
in an Anophthalmic Socket

Virginia Lubkin, M.D.

The other day, as we all stood around in Plastics Clinic at the New York Eye and Ear Infirmary, contemplating a contracted anophthalmic socket, it occurred to me that we must devise a method to register the topography of the cavern to know more conclusively the area of the conjunctival sac, and additionally, to have accurate measurements of the state of the upper and lower fornices. So that the true need for replacing tissue, as well as the reasonably correct area required, would be in our grasp. How should we do this?

The obvious first step is to make a mold, presumably out of alginate. Our laboratory has been operating at high-tech levels beyond compare. Our official genius suggested using our laser topographic device in some modification. Yes, of course, but let us look backward (and simultaneously forward) to a low tech and clinically simple device. The answer was immediately forthcoming. Paint the mold with polyurethane, cut off the new thin skin, and "Presto!", the areas are before us.

Now, to complete the answer, we need the following: (1) a series of normal sockets as models; (2) models of the bony orbit in these normals, measured by the orbit-volume technique developed in our Aborn Eye Laboratory, from CTs of the orbit; (3) having a series of these, and knowing the relationship between socket/conjunctival sac and bony orbit surface area, we can derive the remaining data from a CT of the patient's orbit. This seems to me a rather good idea.

Impression Making, Sculpting, and Coloring of Orbital Prostheses

*Luis R. Guerra, D.D.S., Israel M. Finger, D.D.S.,
Juan Echeverri, D.D.S., and Barry Shipman, D.M.D.*

ABSTRACT

The replacement of any anatomic structure by artificial means remains a challenge. This is particularly true in the facial area. The replacement must be one which blends with the adjacent tissues as well as replaces the missing structures. Careful planning and meticulous attention to detail in fabrication of a prosthesis can enable the maxillofacial prosthodontist to make a major contribution in the rehabilitation of the patient with an orbital defect.

INTRODUCTION

If the eyes are the mirror of the soul, it is the eyelids and soft tissues around the eyes which give us an insight into a person's thoughts and innermost feelings. The watchful eye of the mother, the wisdom in the gaze of the elderly, the worried expression of the leader, are all related by means of the periorbital structures. Capturing these features in an orbital prosthesis is the challenge faced by maxillofacial prosthodontists.

The foundation for any facial prosthesis is achieved by accurately reproducing in a working model the anatomic structures involved. There are a variety of materials available for this purpose [1,2]. Most of these are dental impression materials that have been modified for use on facial structures. The two materials most often used are: (a) irreversible hydrocolloid (alginate) and (b) reversible hydrocolloid. Care must be taken so as not to distort the existing tissues with the weight of the materials used. Both materials require the use of a mother mold, that is, a hard material to back the flexible impression material to prevent distortion as the impression is removed and handled in the laboratory. Neither material bonds to the mother mold (plaster). Therefore, mechanical retention between the plaster and the impression material must be provided.

If dental alginate is used, it is mixed with approximately 50% more water by volume than recommended by the manufacturer. This allows for the smooth flow of the material onto the defect site. The water used should be slightly cooler than room temperature to retard the setting time. However, the use of *cold* water should be avoided unless a prolonged setting time is required. The material is mixed to a smooth, creamy consistency. Mixing in a Vacu-Spat (Whipmix Corp., Louisville, KY) or using a bell jar and vacuum to remove air from the mixture will assure a smooth surface on the master cast.

The mechanical retention to the plaster mother mold can be achieved by either embedding bent paper clips into the unset impression material leaving one loop of the clip exposed to be incorporated into the plaster of the mother mold or by embedding pieces of gauze before the irreversible hydrocolloid is set and leaving areas of the gauze exposed to attach to the plaster.

After the impression material is set a thin layer of plaster is added. After this thin layer has set, more plaster of Paris is added to achieve the desired thickness. A thickness of 1 cm will give adequate support. As the plaster sets it will draw moisture from the impression material. It is necessary to keep the mother mold moist during this period to prevent cracking and tearing of the impression material.

To achieve superior accuracy and minimize distortion in patients with large anatomic defects, the use of a reversible hydrocolloid impression is preferred. This is a gel type material which when heated can be flowed or painted over the tissue in a relatively thin layer. The material should be tested on the ventral aspect of the wrist of the prosthetist to assure it will not burn the patient. The material will set rapidly as it cools.

Gauze squares or paper clips are also used with this material to secure it to the plaster mother mold. The plaster should be added on top of the impression material in a two-layer technique to prevent distortion, as previously described.

The impression should be poured in dental stone as soon as possible. Both impression materials exhibit imbibation if left exposed to moisture, or dehydrate if allowed to dry. The master cast should include areas adjacent to the defect site to allow for proper sculpting of the missing anatomy.

SCULPTING

Prior to sculpting, the master cast must be modified. The modification consists of changing the model topography to take advantage of those areas of the defect which can support and provide mechanical retention to the prosthesis and still allow for removal without engaging excessively bony–soft tissue undercuts (Figs. 1 and 2) [3,4]. The block-out consists of using wax of various thicknesses to specific areas of the cast. A hard, nonsticky wax is preferred so that it will not distort or adhere to the sculpting medium. The tissue undercuts are generally minimal in cases where the bony boundaries of the orbital cavity have not been included in the resection. Where an orbital exenteration has been combined with a maxillary resection the inferior boundary of the orbit has been violated and little or no support exists for the final prosthesis. It is in impressioning this type of a defect that excessive unusable undercuts are duplicated at the inferior aspect of the defect as the impression material flows into the resected maxillary space. Because the facial (orbital) prosthesis must fit or be adapted to the tissue contours it is imperative that any intraoral prosthesis that might change the facial contours be completed and placed prior to the making of an orbital impression.

After the block-out is completed, talcum powder is dusted on the working master cast. This will act as a separating medium to allow easy withdrawal of the sculpting pattern. A layer of 0.002 foil is then intimately adapted to the dusted master cast.

The ocular portion of the orbital prosthesis will usually require some modification to assure its fit into the orbital cavity. The ocular prosthesis will require removal and placement into duplicate orbital prosthesis. Its shape must be such that undercuts can be developed to retain the rigid ocular prosthesis within the flexible orbital prosthesis. This is accomplished by developing a "V" shape to the superior and inferior margin of the ocular prosthesis as viewed in a sagittal plane. The undersurface of the ocular prosthesis should be marked so that it can be keyed at a later stage in the processing procedure. Three circular depressions are

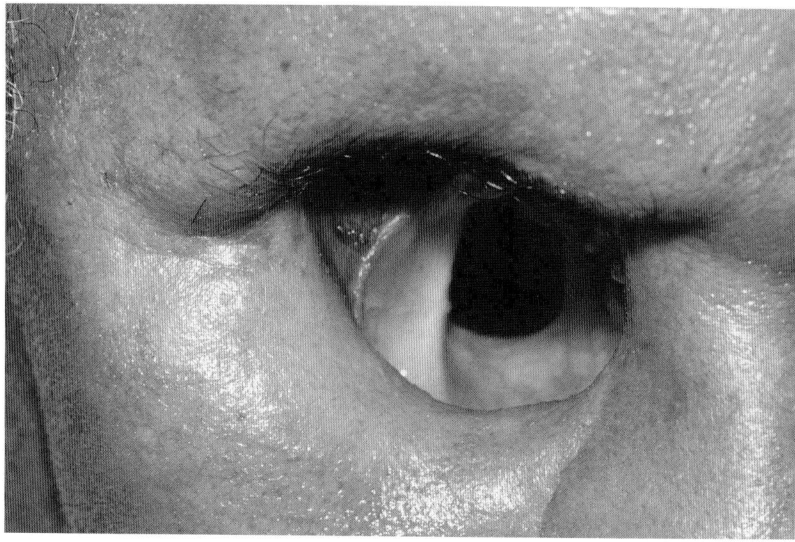

Figure 1. Orbital lesion, undercuts should be captured in final impression.

placed with a #8 round burr in a triangular position with one marking the superior aspect of the eye. This will adequately key the portion of the orbital prosthesis during processing.

One of the most difficult and time-consuming procedures in fabricating an orbital prosthesis is achieving the correct gaze [5–8]. The remaining eye and the prosthetic restoration

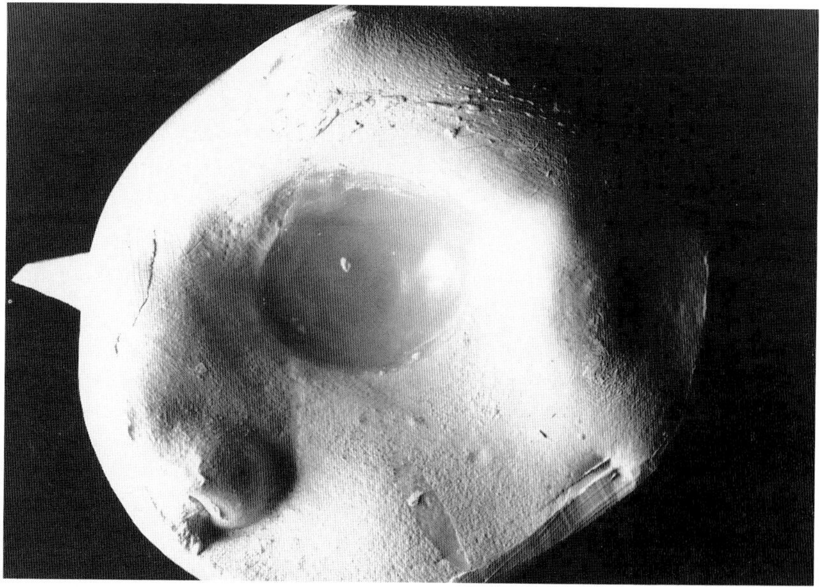

Figure 2. Wax block-out of undercuts on the cast.

should appear to be "looking" and focusing at the same point in space anterior to the face (Fig. 3). This can be accomplished by first placing a layer of wax or clay on the foil. The choice of sculpting material depends on the prosthetist. Either wax or clay can be used. An oil based clay is preferable because it will not dry out during the sculpting even if this extends over a prolonged period of time. A hard wax is preferred if this is the medium of choice. A hard dental base plate wax has proven to be quite suitable.

The initial sculpting pattern is removed and fitted to the patient. At this point the accuracy of the model can be verified by assuring that there is contact all around the periphery between the sculpting pattern and the working cast. Where there is no contact the cast may be trimmed and the sculpting recontoured. With the periphery corrected, attention is then directed to the ocular portion of the prosthesis.

With the sculpting pattern in position, the position of the ocular prosthesis is finalized. The horizontal position is verified by comparing the distance of the pupil of the remaining eye and the pupil of the ocular prosthesis to the midline of the face. The distance should be the same for both. The vertical position of the prosthetic eye is verified by holding a straight edge on the inferior rim of the pupil of the natural eye and assuring that the inferior rim of the pupil of the ocular prosthesis lies on the same plane. The anterior curvature of the globe should be reviewed in relation to other facial structures. This is best achieved by viewing the area from above. The ocular prosthesis is then placed in the same plane. Lastly, the eye is rotated up and down and to either side until the gaze is correct. This is more easily done if enough sculpting material is added to begin the delineation of the eyelids.

The remaining sculpting is completed by repeatedly trying the pattern on the patient and comparing to the opposite side. It may be that as this activity proceeds some minor modification of the position of the orbital prosthesis may be necessary. Repeated viewing of the sculpting from various angles is necessary to achieve a more realistic effect. The final step in

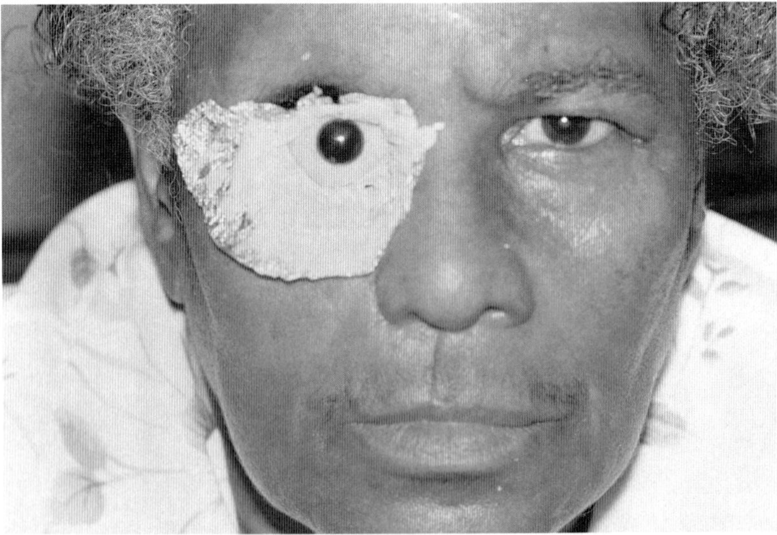

Figure 3. Remaining eye and prosthetic restoration should appear to be "looking" at the same point in space anterior to the face.

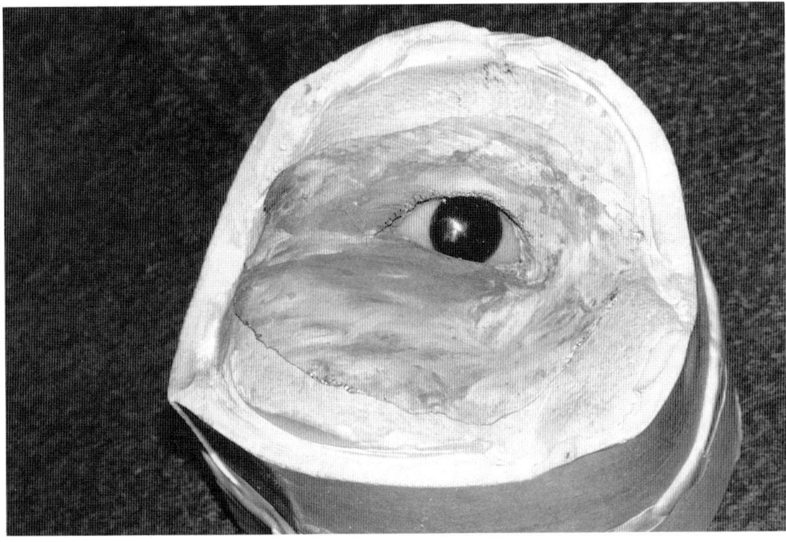

Figure 4. Sculpting of orbital prostheses.

the sculpting process is achieved by creating a skinlike texture on the surface of the wax or clay. This can be accomplished by striking the surface with the bristles of a brush, the pressing of gauze onto the surface and by the use of various sculpting tools (Fig. 4).

An orbital prosthesis, unlike other facial prostheses, involves complicated laboratory pro-

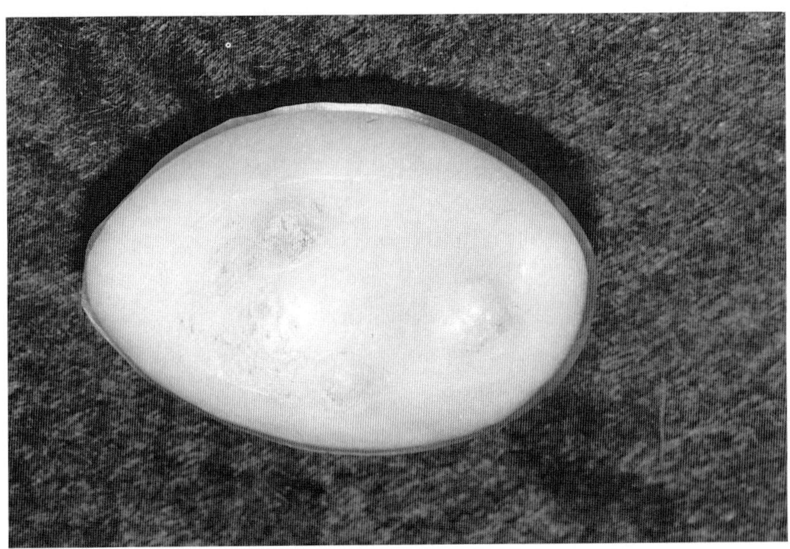

Figure 5. Indices on the undersurface of the resin eye.

cedures in fabricating the mold [9,10]. This is caused by the necessity of maintaining the ocular portion of the prosthesis in the same position throughout the procedure.

Guerra and Canada [11] have described the use of metal molds for the fabrication process. However, because the use of dental stone molds appears more popular, their use will be described. After the sculpting is completed and the margins seated to the master cast, a hole is drilled from the undersurface of the cast to the clay or wax sculpting pattern between the ocular prosthesis and the cast. This hole should be large enough to allow for removal of the sculpting medium to expose the undersurface of the acrylic resin ocular prosthesis. The previously placed depressions on the undersurface and the margins of the acrylic resin eye are exposed (Fig. 5). Dental stone is then poured into the hole avoiding any trapped air. When the stone has set the entire master cast is trimmed to fit within the confines of a denture (processing) flask. Most casts will fit a conventional flask, although jumbo denture flasks are available for larger prosthesis fabrication. For extremely large cases, custom flasks can be fabricated using PVC pipe material as the flask.

Dental stone is placed in one half of the flask and the model with the sculpting in place is seated into the flask. The dental stone is smoothed between the model and the walls of the flask. When the stone has set a separating medium such as petroleum jelly is applied over the dental stone. Care must be exercised so as not to place the petroleum jelly on the sculpting surface as this will distort the final prosthesis. The second half of the flask is then placed into position and dental stone is used to complete the second half of the flask. The dental stone should be allowed to set for approximately 1 to 2 hrs.

The flask is then separated and the sculpting is removed. The acrylic resin eye is replaced on the stone pedestal to which it is keyed on the first half of the flask (Figs. 6 and 7). A small drop of cynoacrylate glue can be used to maintain the eye on the pedestal. A separating medium is then applied to the dental stone to both sides of the flask. A clear noncolored separating medium is preferred so as not to affect the color of the final prosthesis. The separating medium is allowed to dry completely prior to placing the silicone mixture into the flask.

A room temperature vulcanizing material such as Dow Corning, type A adhesive is used as the base material. Dow Corning MDX 2400 is added in varying amounts as a plasticizer. This addition should never exceed 40% by volume of the mixture. As more of the MDX 2400 is added, the physical characteristics in relationship to the softness, tear strength, and edge strength are adversely affected. Flocking of various colors can be added on the surface of the prosthesis by first applying diluted type A adhesive and dusting the flocking to place.

Rare earth pigments which have been diluted in the MDX 2400–Type A adhesive mixture are used to color the material. The total amount of material to be used can be estimated by observing the volume of the sculpting pattern.

FABRICATION

The material used for fabrication of the molds required for the processing of the prosthesis depends on the prosthesis material. Latex, rigid and flexible acrylic resins, urethane, polyvinylchloride, and heat vulcanized and room temperature vulcanized polysiloxanes have all been used to fabricate facial prostheses. Presently, the room temperature vulcanized polysiloxanes offer a more versatile medium. Hutcheson and others [12,13] have described its use.

The MDX 2400 is a clear material and requires a catalyst for setting. (The catalyst is not added into the mixture.) The MDX is used as a plasticizer, and will require an opaquer. Kaoline can be used for this purpose. The MDX mixture is colored by using the diluted rare earth

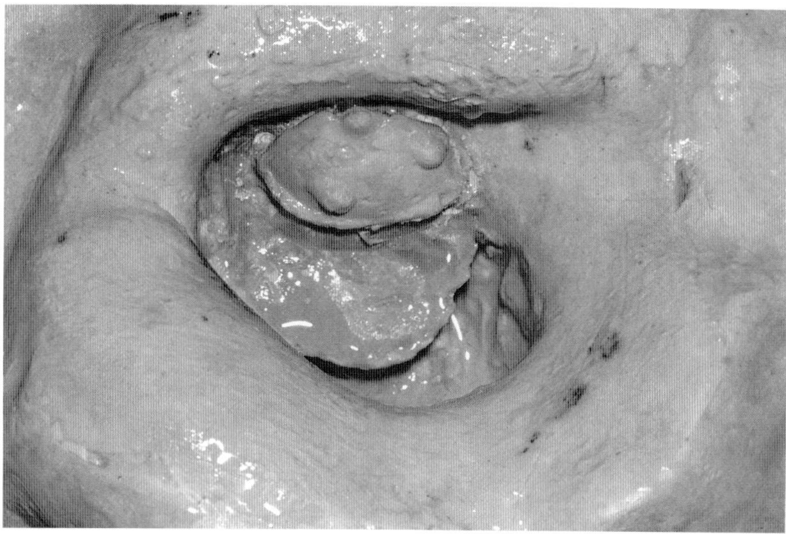

Figure 6. Stone pedestal keyed to receive undersurface of eye.

pigments. This coloring is best done with the patient present, because the goal of this procedure is to reproduce the lightest base shade compatible with the patient. Flocking of various colors can be used to heighten the effect. This is mixed smoothly until the desired color is achieved. Because this represents only 40% by volume of the mixture, it is important that the color be slightly more intense than desired. The type A adhesive is then added and the entire

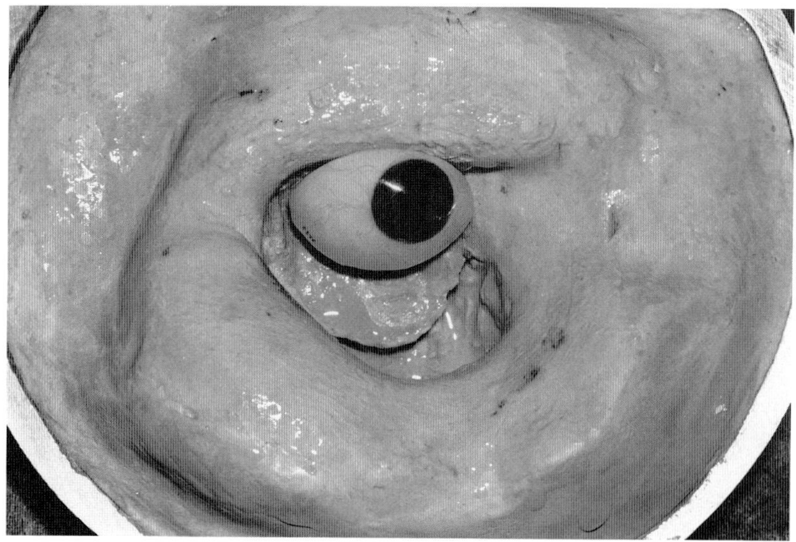

Figure 7. Resin prosthetic eye keyed into position during processing.

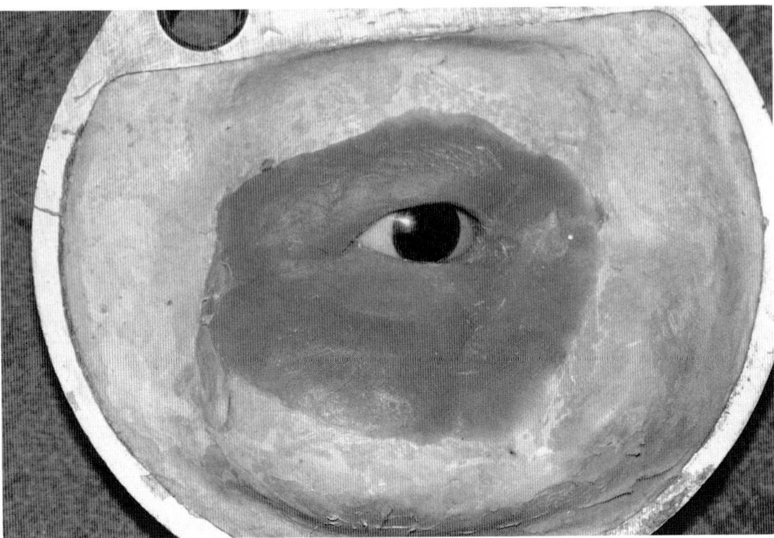

Figure 8. Bottom portion of metal flask with waxed prosthesis in position.

mixture spatulated very smoothly so as not to incorporate air into the mixture. The material is then carefully placed in the mold to ensure that no air is trapped. The opposite side of the flask is then closed. The material requires moisture for setting; thus the flask is set into water overnight. When the flask is separated, the prosthesis is removed gently, preventing tears

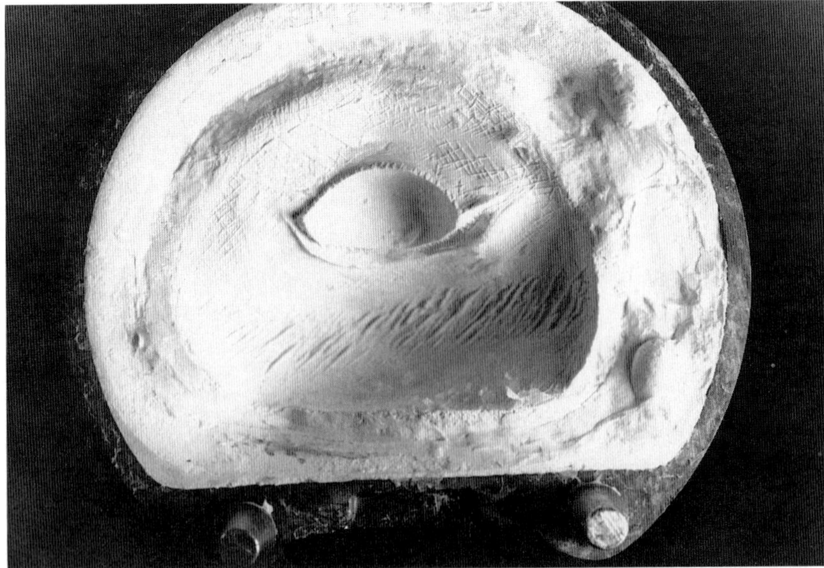

Figure 9. Top half of metal flask with stone capturing anatomical topography of waxed prosthesis.

around the edges possibly trapped in an undercut (Figs. 8 and 9). The prosthesis is then tried on the patient and trimmed to its proper size. Coloring of the prosthesis to a more exact replication of the patient's skin is now accomplished. This is done by diluting the rare earth pigments in type A adhesive which is diluted with either xylene or with cyclohexane.

Eyebrows can be added by using hair. The final tinting is allowed to dry completely.

Several prostheses are given to the patient. The patient is then given instructions on placement of the prosthesis. It is helpful if the spouse or a friend is present so they can also learn the procedure.

The polysiloxane materials are very inert and hence not all surgical adhesives will adhere to them. Various adhesives are available; however, the Hollister adhesive is the one most often used. This adhesive is available in an aerosol can. The patient is instructed not to spray the prosthesis but rather to dispense the adhesive into a cup and pick up the fluid with a cotton ball and apply to the margins of the tissue side of the prosthesis. This avoids having the adhesive on all of the tissue side surface, thus minimizing soiling of the surface. The adhesive adheres on contact and there is no compromise on seating the prosthesis. The patient must learn to use a mirror and anatomic landmarks to aid in correctly seating the prosthesis (Fig. 10). Special emphasis is placed on assuring complete seating around the margins of the prosthesis.

CARE AND MAINTENANCE

To provide longevity of the prosthesis it must be cleaned and the adhesive removed on a regular basis. The prosthesis should be removed at night prior to retiring and washed in a mild soap. The patient is instructed to use a bar of Ivory soap, work up a lather and wash the prosthesis. No harsh or abrasive materials are to be used. The adhesive must be carefully rolled off the prosthesis. The use of the Hollister adhesive remover should be limited as it tends to soften the margins of the prosthesis. Makeup can be applied to the prosthesis but care must

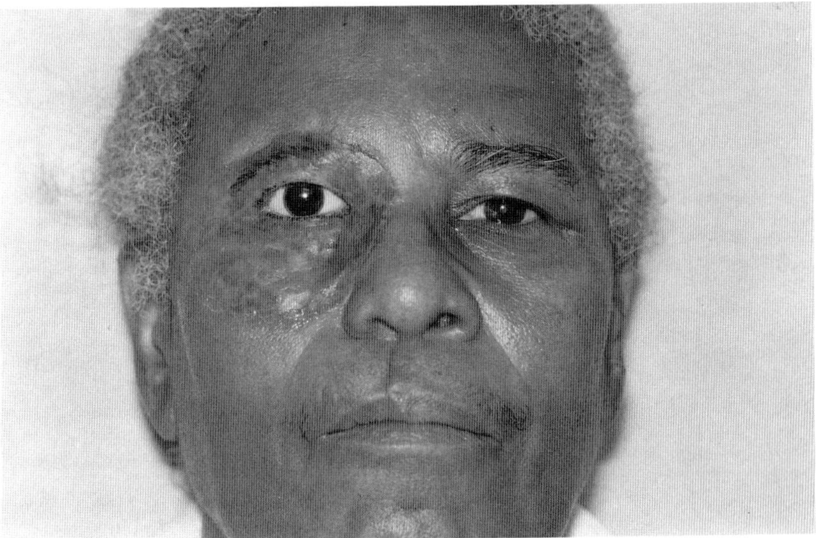

Figure 10. Correctly sealed orbital prosthesis.

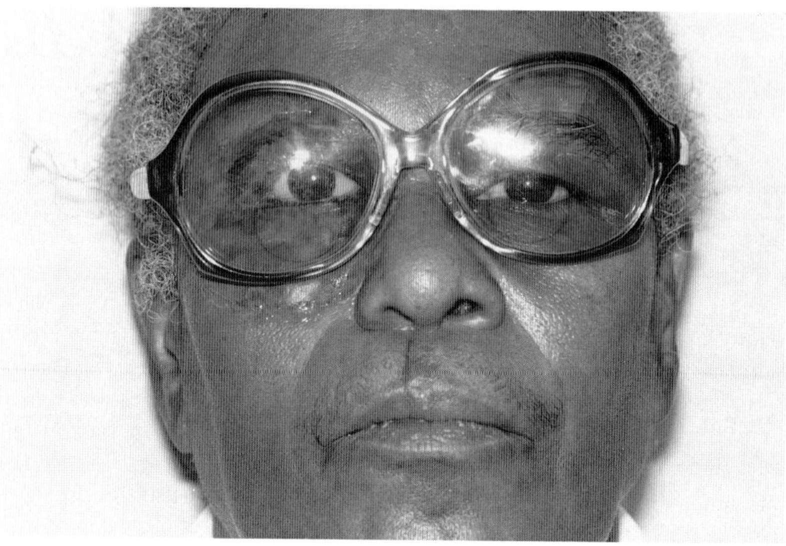

Figure 11. Wide glass frame to assist in covering margins of the prostheses.

be used in the selection of the cosmetics used. Water based cosmetics tend to bead on the silicone material and some oil base materials are difficult to remove and may permanently stain the prosthesis. With good maintenance the prosthesis should be adequate for six to eight months or more. The patient should be given several prostheses so that future scheduling can be done on a yearly basis. Although reactions to the adhesives used are rare, the patient is cautioned that this may occur and should report any untoward reaction immediately. To achieve a more satisfying result the patient is also instructed to turn toward those persons engaged in conversations to reduce movement of the eyes. Finally, the patient is encouraged to use eye glasses if they do not do so at the time. The glass frame chosen should be the widest possible to assist in covering the margins of the prosthesis (Fig. 11).

REFERENCES

1. Joneja OP, Madan SK, Mehra MD, Dogra RN: Orbital prostheses. *J Prosth Dent* 1976; 36:306–311.
2. Barron JB, Rubenstein JE, Archibald D, Manor RE: Two piece orbital prostheses. *J Prosth Dent* 1983; 49:386–388.
3. Udagama A, King GE: Mechanically retained facial prostheses: helpful or harmful? *J Prosth Dent* 1983; 49:85–86.
4. Rouse JA, Chalian VA: Fabrication of hollow extraoral prostheses to enhance retention. *J Prosth Dent* 1985; 53:557–64.
5. Brown KE: Fabrication of orbital prosthesis. *J Prosth Dent* 1969; 22:592.
6. Bulbulian AH: *Facial Prosthetics.* Springfield, IL, Charles C Thomas, 1973:353–363.
7. Chalian VA, Drane JB, Standish SM: *Maxillofacial Prosthetics.* Baltimore, MD, The Williams & Wilkens Company, 1971.
8. Oral K, Zini I, Aramany MA: Construction of orbital prostheses using the silicone pattern technique. *J Prosth Dent* 1978; 40:430–433.
9. Wolfaardt JF, Hacqueboard A, Els JM: A mold technique for construction of orbital prostheses. *J Prosth Dent* 1983; 50:224–226.
10. Shifman A, Levin AC, Levy M, Lepley JB: Prosthetic restoration of orbital defects. *J Prosth Dent* 1979; 42:543.
11. Guerra ON, Canada K: Open cast technique for metal molds in constructing facial prostheses. *J Prosth Dent* 1979; 36:421–425.
12. Hutcheson PE, Udagana A: Surgical nasal prostheses. *J Prosth Dent* 1980; 43(1):78–81.
13. Kanter JC: The use of RTV silicones in maxillofacial prosthetics. *J Prosth Dent* 1970; 24:646.

Osseointegrated Implants in Facial Prosthetics

Barry Shipman, D.M.D., Israel M. Finger, D.D.S., and Luis R. Guerra, D.D.S.

Facial disfigurement secondary to cancer surgery or trauma is functionally and psychologically disturbing for the individuals and family involved. Classically, rehabilitation of patients with facial deformities has been the responsibility of the plastic surgeon, the maxillofacial prosthodontist, or the facial prosthetist. To date, the specific requirements for success with facial prostheses are almost unobtainable. To be successful, facial prosthesis should meet five basis criteria. (a) The prosthesis should meet optimal cosmetic requirements. (b) They should be easy to place and remove. (c) Once placed, prostheses should be stable and easily maintain position. (d) Facial prostheses should remain in an appropriate anatomical position during reasonable activities. (e) They should be durable and easily maintained.

In 1980 and 1981, Tjellstrom, Lindstrom, Hallén, Albrektsson and Branemark [1] presented works on bone anchored auricular prosthesis. They reported background information over 20 years of investigation with implant materials in animals. Tjellstrom et al. acknowledged the introduction by Branemark et al., in 1975 [2] of the concept of osseointegration and the use of titanium fixtures in the mandible and maxillae for the reconstruction of oral structures and the improvement of oral function. Branemark et al. defines "osseointegration" as a histological definition meaning "a direct connection between living bone and a load-carrying endosseous implant at the light microscope level. . . ." [3].

Weiss, on the other hand has complicated the implant controversy with the concept of "fibro-osseous integration" [4]. Denissen, Veldhusis, and van den Hoof [5] experimented with a combination titanium-apatite coated implant in animals and humans and displayed an intimate contact between the hydroxylapatite and bone which was shown as the demonstration of an actual chemical bond between bone and implant. Clinical studies using the hydroxylapatite implant system in facial prosthetics are presently being developed.

There are some limitations associated with the use of osseointegrated implants in the orbital and paraorbital regions. The criteria for placing implants for dental rehabilitation is primarily limited by the quantity and quality of the available bone. Implants can vary in width from 3.3 to 4.0 mm and in length from 4.00 to 15.00 mm. Anatomically the orbit appears to be a suitable site for use of a variety of the osseointegrated implant sizes. Critical evaluation is necessary both by standard and imaging radiographic techniques as well as good clinical digital examination. Presurgical planning is indicated to maximize the placement of implants in appropriate bony sites. The superior and infra-orbital areas and the zygomatic process appear to be good sites for implant placement. The ability to recess superstructures within the orbital cavity improves the aesthetic quality of the orbital or facial prosthesis.

This unique approach of the use of osseointegrated implants in facial prosthetic rehabilitation opens and expands the need for further investigation in the use of the implant in facial prosthetics. The ability to attach a silicone, acrylic, or polyvinyl chloride prosthesis to an implant substructure expands the use and extends the life and flexibility to extraoral prosthesis. The osseointegrated implants, whether pure titanium or hydroxylapatite coated, provide auricular, orbital, or large facial prosthesis attachment by means of clips and magnets to the implant structure. Patients are able to work, play, and sleep without concern about dislodgment or loss.

The authors have personal experience in the treatment of six patients with hydroxylapatite-coated titanium implants over 18 months. The clinical success, although limited, appears good. Additional trials on more patients will be necessary before scientific acceptance of this new rehabilitation procedure becomes as commonplace as osseointegrated implants have become in dental reconstruction.

The dental and medical community is excited about the use of the osseointegrated implants in the area of facial reconstruction. It will offer significant benefits to patients who in the past had to suffer with poorly retentive, removable, extraoral prosthesis, and at best had a guarded acceptance and success.

REFERENCES

1. Tjellstrom A, Lindstrom J, Hallén O, Albrektsson T, Branemark PI: Osseointegrated titanium implants in temporal bone. *Am J Otol* 1981: 2:304.
2. Branemark P, Lindstrom J, Hallén O, Breine U, Jeppson PH, Ohman A: Reconstruction of the defective mandible. Scand *J Reconst Surg* 1975; 9:116.
3. Branemark PI, Zarb G, and Albrektsson T: *Tissue Integrated Prosthesis; Osseointegration in Clinical Dentistry.* Chicago, IL, Quintessence Publ. Co., 1985.
4. Weiss, CM: Tissue integration of dental endosseous implants: Description and comparative analysis of the fibro-osseous integration and osseointegration systems. *J Oral Impl* 1986; 12:169–214.
5. Denissen, H. et al., Hydroxylapatite-titanium implants. Proceedings of the International Congress on Tissue Integration in Maxillofacial Reconstruction. Brussels. *Excerpta-Medica*, 29: 389–394.

Prosthetic Rehabilitation of the Anophthalmic Socket Using Osseointegrated Fixtures

Mark Bowden, D.D.S., M.D.

Since 1979 the retention of craniofacial prostheses to the residual skeleton has been accomplished in Sweden with titanium fixtures (implants) (Figs. 1 and 2). One of many potential uses for the elegant work of Branemark et al., this adaptation of osseointegration may revolutionize anaplastology, the study of replacements of missing body parts. Long-term follow-up studies now show excellent results of jawbone-anchored fixtures used since 1965 for the penetration of oral mucosa and the support of dental prostheses.

In 1988, the multicenter study sponsored by the U.S. FDA began to assess the skin-penetrating uses of the Branemark fixtures. The ability to provide prostheses that can be stabilized without bothersome adhesives and attachments to glasses frames or straps would be of immense advantage to many patients, especially those who are physically active (Figs. 3 and 4).

The combination of meticulous surgical technique to maintain the vitality of the living bone and the unique physical characteristics of the titanium fixtures has produced this remarkable dynamic relationship between foreign bodies (implants) and recipient sites [1]. This dynamic relationship appears to produce with loading, after appropriate bone healing (usually 3–4 months), a capacity to bear increasing stresses. Loads imposed by craniofacial prostheses are far less than those carried by the highly successful jaw implants.

Whether absence of globe and adnexa results from trauma, ablative surgical procedures, or congenital deficit, this technique offers hope for better restoration of appearance and resumption of normal activities (Figs. 5 and 6). Even patients requiring radiotherapy can be treated. Usually their first phase of surgical care is delayed for at least 12 months postirradiation, and healing times are doubled. As expected, more fixtures will fail to osseointegrate in irradiated bone; but to date there have been only localized inflammatory responses managed by removal of the failed fixtures without progression to osteoradionecrosis.

Patients with disease processes that might be expected to interfere with bone healing such as diabetes mellitus can also be treated by increasing the healing period.

Prostheses can be fabricated that offer exceptional esthetic results [2] (Fig. 7). Mechanical retention by clips, magnets, or combinations of both afford a capacity to tailor a prosthesis to the unique needs and physical activities of patients.

REFERENCES

1. Branemark PI, Zarb GA, Albrektsson T: Tissue integrated prostheses. In: *Osseointegration in Clinical Dentistry.* Chicago, IL, Quintessence, 1985:333–342.
2. Parel SM, Holt R, Branemark PI, Tjellstrom A: Osseointegration and facial prosthetics. *Int J Oral Maxillofac Impl* 1986:1: 27–29.

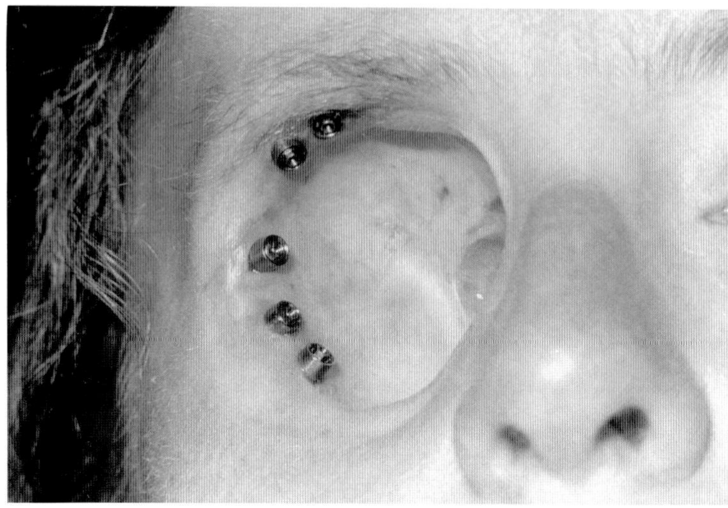

Figure 1. Exenteration socket with osseointegrated fixtures in place.

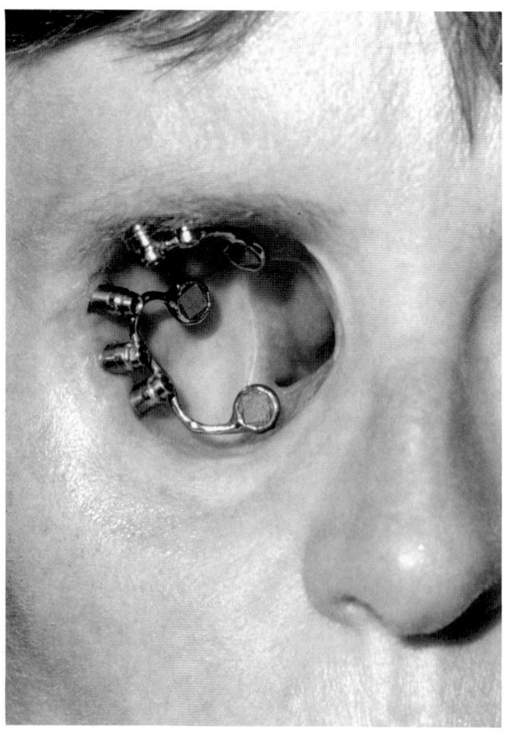

Figure 2. Exenteration socket with fixtures and magnets in place.

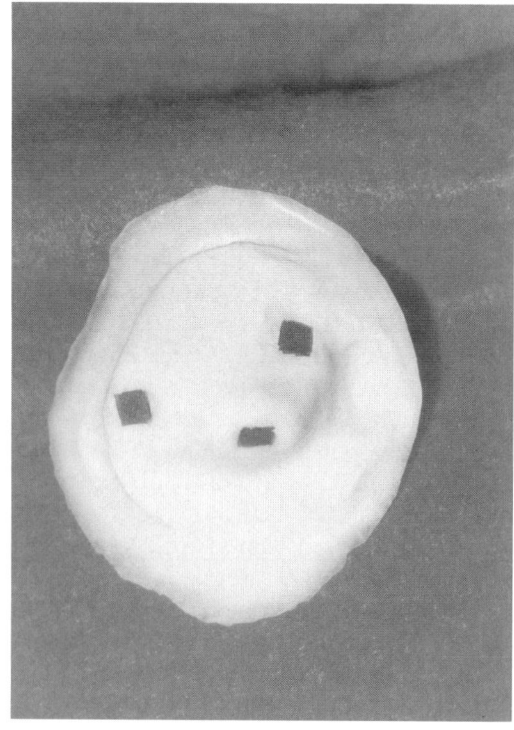

Figure 3. Magnets implanted in posterior surface of prosthesis.

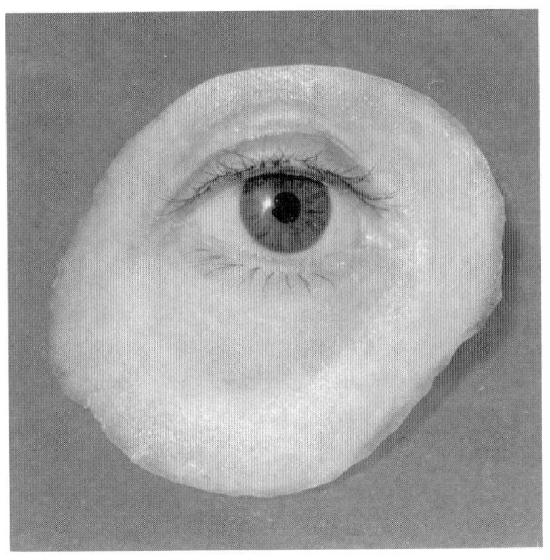

Figure 4. Exenteration prosthesis.

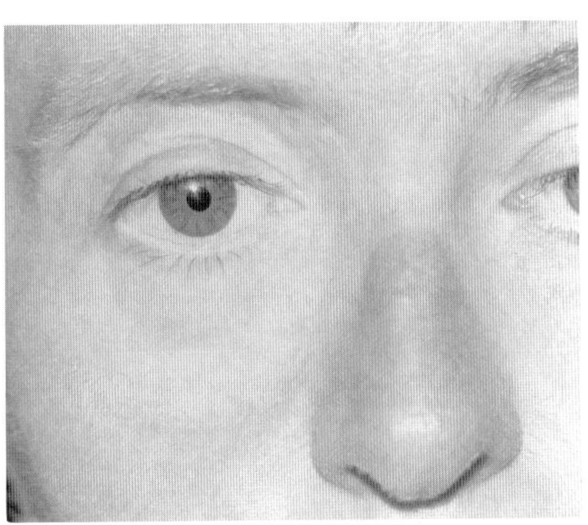

Figure 5. Prosthesis in place.

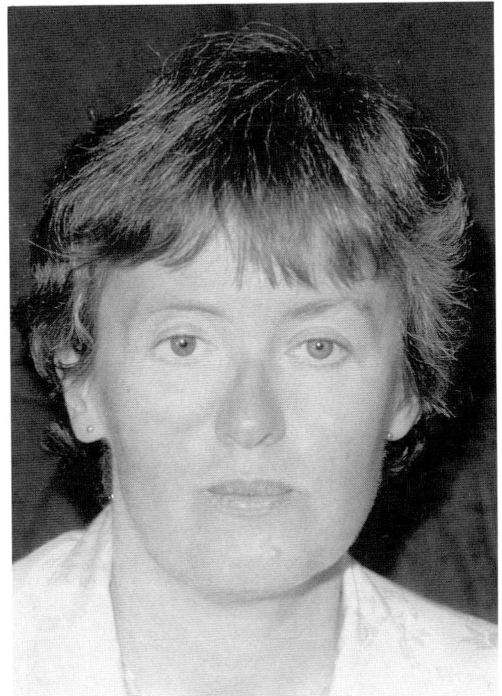

Figure 6. Patient wearing prosthesis without spectacles.

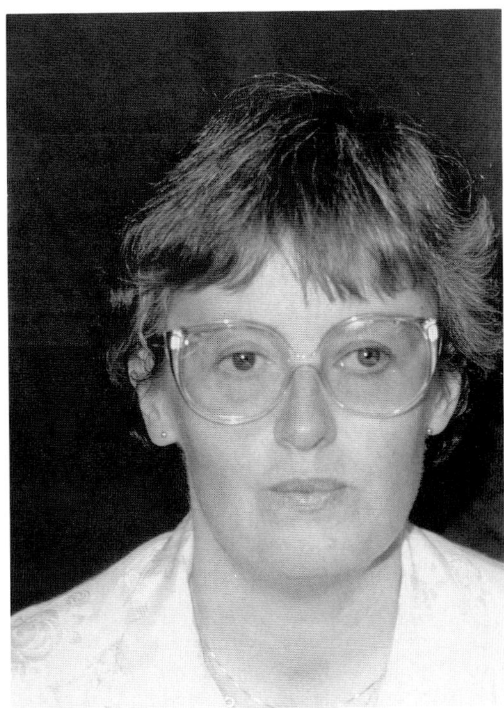

Figure 7. Patient with exenteration prosthesis and spectacles.

Figures courtesy of S. Parel, D.D.S., University of Texas, San Antonio.

INDEX

10 + 13 + 13

NGC - 600

5/5/4 — 13.
(0,5)(5,2)

NGC - 600